War Surgery in Afghanistan and Iraq

A SERIES OF CASES, 2003–2007

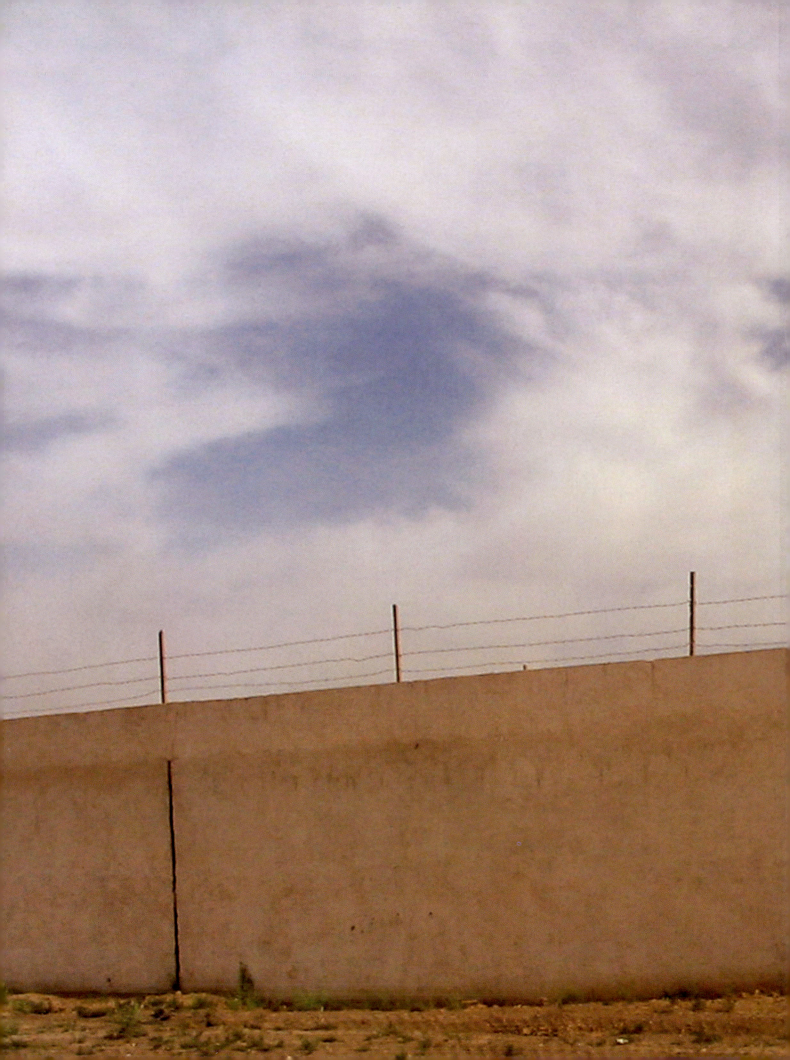

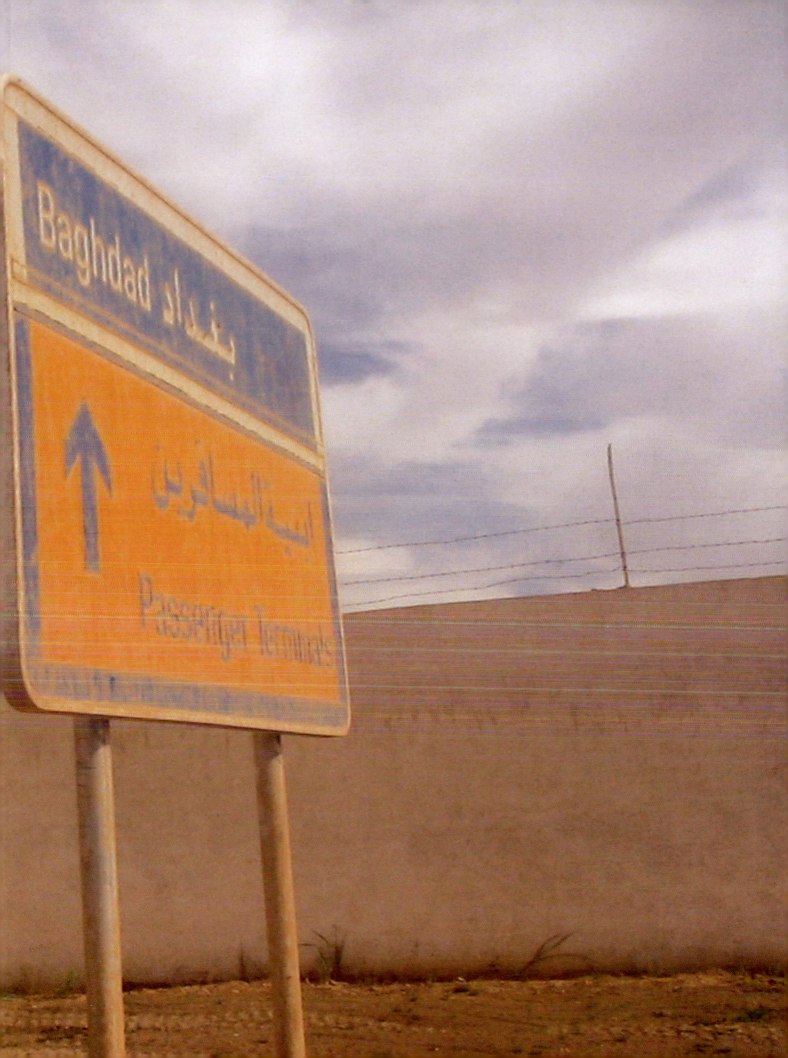

It is impossible to convey to you

the picture of human misery continually before my eye. . . .

While I amputate one man's thigh, there lay at one time thirteen,

all beseeching to be taken next. . . .

It was a strange thing to feel my clothes stiff with blood,

and my arms powerless with the exertion of using the knife! . . .

The view of the field, the gallant sorties, the charges,

the individual instances of enterprise and valour

recalled to me the sense the world has of victory and Waterloo.

But this is transient. A gloomy uncomfortable view of

human nature is the inevitable consequence of

looking upon the whole as I did—as I was forced to do.

—SIR CHARLES BELL (1774–1842)

War Surgery in Afghanistan and Iraq

A SERIES OF CASES, 2003–2007

Edited by

SHAWN CHRISTIAN NESSEN, DO, FACS
LTC, MC, US Army

DAVE EDMOND LOUNSBURY, MD, FACP
COL, MC, US Army (Retired)

STEPHEN P. HETZ, MD, FACS
COL, MC, US Army (Retired)

OFFICE OF THE SURGEON GENERAL
United States Army, Falls Church, Virginia

BORDEN INSTITUTE
Walter Reed Army Medical Center, Washington, DC

A Specialty Volume of the
TEXTBOOKS OF MILITARY MEDICINE

Published by the
OFFICE OF THE SURGEON GENERAL
Department of the Army, United States of America

US ARMY MEDICAL DEPARTMENT CENTER AND SCHOOL
Fort Sam Houston, Texas

TELEMEDICINE AND ADVANCED TECHNOLOGY RESEARCH CENTER
US Army Medical Research and Materiel Command, Fort Detrick, Maryland

Editor in Chief
MARTHA K. LENHART, MD, PhD, FAAOS
Colonel, MC, US Army
Director, Borden Institute
Assistant Professor of Surgery
F. Edward Hébert School of Medicine
Uniformed Services University of the Health Sciences

Developmental & Consulting Editor
DAVE EDMOND LOUNSBURY, MD, FACP
Colonel, MC, US Army (Retired)
Borden Institute
Assistant Professor of Medicine
F. Edward Hébert School of Medicine
Uniformed Services University of the Health Sciences

The Nation today needs men who think in terms of service to their country and not in terms of their country's debt to them.

—GENERAL OMAR N. BRADLEY, 1948

And so, my fellow Americans: ask not what your country can do for you—ask what you can do for your country.

—JOHN F. KENNEDY, 1961

★　★　★　★

TO SERVICE

To the Soldiers, Marines, Airmen, and Sailors

who have sacrificed so much

for their country

EDITORIAL STAFF

Developmental Editor	Dave Edmond Lounsbury, MD, FACP (COL, MC, US Army, Retired)
Creative Director/Production Manager	Christine Gamboa-Onrubia, MBA, Fineline Graphics LLC
Senior Volume Editor	Vivian Mason
Illustrator	Aletta Frazier, MD

Published by the Office of The Surgeon General
Borden Institute, Walter Reed Army Medical Center, Washington, DC 20307-5001

Library of Congress Cataloging-in-Publication Data
War surgery in Afghanistan and Iraq : a series of cases, 2003–2007 /
edited by Shawn Christian Nessen, Dave Edmond Lounsbury, Stephen P. Hetz.
     p. ; cm.
Includes bibliographical references and index.
ISBN 978-0-981822-80-8
1. Surgery, Military—Afghanistan. 2. Surgery, Military—Iraq. 3. Afghan war, 2001—Medical care. 4. Iraq war, 2003—Medical care. I. Nessen, Shawn Christian. II. Lounsbury, Dave Edmond. III. Hetz, Stephen P. IV. United States. Dept. of the Army. Office of the Surgeon General. V. Borden Institute (U.S.) VI. Walter Reed Army Medical Center. [DNLM: 1. Military Medicine—Afghanistan. 2. Military Medicine—Iraq. 3. Military Medicine—United States. 4. Wounds and Injuries—surgery—Afghanistan. 5. Wounds and Injuries—surgery—Iraq. 6. Wounds and Injuries—surgery—United States. 7. Emergency Medical Services—Afghanistan. 8. Emergency Medical Services—Iraq. 9. Emergency Medical Services—United States. 10. Iraq War, 2003—Afghanistan. 11. Iraq War, 2003—Iraq. 12. Iraq War, 2003—United States. 13. Wars—Afghanistan. 14. Wars—Iraq. 15. Wars—United States. WO 800 W253 2008]

RD476.A3W37 2008
617.9'9—dc22

2008011884

Printed in the United States of America

15 14 13   10 9 8 7 6 5 4 3

CONTENTS

CONTRIBUTORS

ORIGINAL CASE CONTRIBUTORS

Todd S. Albright, DO, MPH, LTC, MC, US Army

Kenneth Azarow, MD, COL, MC, US Army

Scott D. Barnes, MD, LTC, MC, US Army

Douglas M. Bowley, FRCS(Eng), FRCS(Gen Surg),
    Lt Col, RAMC

Matthew L. Brengman, MD, MAJ, MC, US Army

William A. Brock, CRNA, LTC, AN, US Army

Chester Buckenmaier, MD, LTC, MC, US Army

Jeffrey S. Bui, MD, Maj, MC, US Air Force

Brennan Carmody, MD, LTC, MC, US Army

Paul R. Cordts, MD, COL, MC, US Army

Steven J. Cyr, MD, Maj, MC, FS, US Air Force

Louis A. Dainty, MD, LTC, MC, US Army

David Danielson, MD, MAJ, MC, US Army

Dennis P. Eastman, MD, COL, MC, US Army

James M. Ecklund, MD, COL, MC, US Army

Mark T. Edney, MD, MAJ, MC, US Army

Jonathan Eliason, MD, Maj, MC, US Air Force

Richard Ellison, MD, COL, MC, US Army

Dion L. Franga, MD, MAJ, MC, US Army

Kirby Gross, MD, LTC, MC, US Army

Marty Harnisch, MD, MAJ, MC, US Army

Stephen P. Hetz, MD, COL, MC, US Army (Retired)

Linda C. Hird, MD, CPT, MC, US Army

Patrick J. Houde, MD, Capt, MC, US Air Force

Ronald A. Hyde, DO, MAJ, MC, US Army

James R. Jezior, MD, COL, MC, US Army

Karen M. Keith, DDS, MD, COL, DC, US Army

Kevin L. Kirk, MD, MAJ, MC, US Army

Kevin J. Kulwicki, MD, MAJ, MC, US Army

Geoffrey S. Ling, MD, PhD, COL, MC, US Army

Juan M. Lopez-Gonzalez, MD, LTC, MC, US Army

Dave Edmond Lounsbury, MD, COL, MC, US Army (Retired)

John D. Lowry, MD, LTC, MC, US Army

Kevin J. Mork, MD, COL, MC, US Army

Shawn Christian Nessen, DO, LTC, MC, US Army

Peter E. Nielsen, MD, COL, MC, US Army

Joel B. Nilsson, MD, Lt Col, MC, US Air Force

John S. Oh, MD, MAJ, MC, US Army

Mary F. Parker, MD, LTC, MC, US Army

George E. Peoples, MD, COL, MC, US Army

Kimberley L. Perkins, DDS, LTC, DC, US Army

Donald W. Robinson, DO, LTC, MC, US Army

Nelson Rosen, MD, MAJ, MC, US Army

Paul J. Schenarts, MD, MAJ, MC, US Army

Brian S. Schultz, DO, MAJ, MC, US Army

Jody Schultz, MD, MAJ, MC, US Army

Niten N. Singh, MD, MAJ, MC, US Army

Richard J. Teff, MD, LTC, MC, US Army

Andrew Wargo, DDS, LTC, DC, US Army

Harry Warren, MD, COL, MC, US Army

Glenn W. Wortmann, MD, COL, MC, US Army

Mark Ziemba, MD, COL, MC, US Army

Joseph J. Zubak, MD, LTC, MC, US Army

OTHER CONTRIBUTORS

Rocco A. Armonda, MD, LTC, MC, US Army

Ronald F. Bellamy, MD, COL, MC, US Army (Retired)

Francis M. Chiricosta, MD, LTC, MC, US Army

James R. Ficke, MD, COL, MC, US Army

Katherine M. Helmick, MS, CNRN, CRNP

John B. Holcomb, MD, COL, MC, US Army

Donald H. Jenkins, MD, Col, MC, US Air Force

John F. Kragh, MD, COL, MC, US Army

Charles R. Mulligan, MD, MAJ, MC, US Army

Clinton K. Murray, MD, MAJ, MC, US Army

Jeremy G. Perkins, MD, MAJ, MC, US Army

Benjamin Potter, MD, CPT, MC, US Army

Evan M. Renz, MD, LTC, MC, US Army

Stephen L. Rouse, DDS, LTC, DC, US Army (Retired)

Deborah L. Warden, MD

ACKNOWLEDGMENTS

PHOTO CREDITS: *Digital cameras are ubiquitous today in both theaters of combat operations. Electronic sharing of snapshots, both clinical and recreational, is widespread. As a consequence, however, it becomes difficult, if not impossible, to accurately attribute each photo. For this and other reasons, we have not attempted to provide photo-by-photo attribution. With few exceptions, clinical photographs were taken and provided by the surgical team attending the case with which they are attached. We are particularly indebted for the large files of nonclinical material provided by the Editors and the following individuals: COL Martha Lenhart, LTC Kenneth L. Ferster, LTC Tommy Brown, and MAJ Adam Hamawy—all MC, US Army. We also thank Dr (PhD) Sanders Marble, Mr Dimitri Doganis, Mr Stefan Radtke, Keith S. Albertson, MD (COL, MC, US Army, Retired), SGT Heather Denman, and Polaris Images Corporation for permission to use Sungsu Cho's photograph that appears on page 403. Where they appear, unblocked facial images are used with permission. All photographs are retained on file at the Borden Institute.*

An edited work such as this is only as good as the efforts of its contributors and production staff. The Editors are deeply grateful to all those who participated in and supported this project.

This textbook would not have been possible without the unflagging support of the Borden Institute under the Directorship of Colonel Martha K. Lenhart.

Ms. Vivian Mason worked tirelessly—often in real time—to interpret and translate innumerable twists and turns in the development of this book.

Ms. Chris Onrubia grasped early the intent of this project and captured that purpose in the design and layout of the final product.

Dr. Aletta Frazier not only provided expert medical illustration, but also her generous time and effort to assist with graphics. We appreciate this more than she knows.

Mr. David Leeson of *The Dallas Morning News* has generously provided stunning nonclinical photographs. Today soldiers unknowingly circulate many of his OIF-1 (2003) photographs, unattributed, and wrongly assumed to be amateur snapshots unprotected by copyright.

The Editors are grateful to all case contributors. We wish to especially acknowledge, however, the generosity of MAJ Kevin J. Kulwicki, LTC Richard J. Teff, LTC Mary F. Parker, LTC Kimberley L. Perkins, MAJ Mark T. Edney, and MAJ Jeffrey S. Bui. Special tribute is extended to SFC John C. Thomas, SGT (Retired) Brian Wilhelm, SFC (Retired) Joseph M. Mosner, SSG (Retired) Brian E. Wells (all US Army), and Sr A (Retired) Brian G. Kolfage for their permissions to reveal personal images.

Others whose efforts, advice, and contributions warrant mention include the following: Dr Paul J. Dougherty (formerly LTC, MC, US Army); Dr James E. Cox (COL, MC, USAF, Retired); Mr Douglas Wise; Mr Bruce Maston; COL Leo Tucker, MC, US Army; and COL Peter Nielsen, MC, US Army.

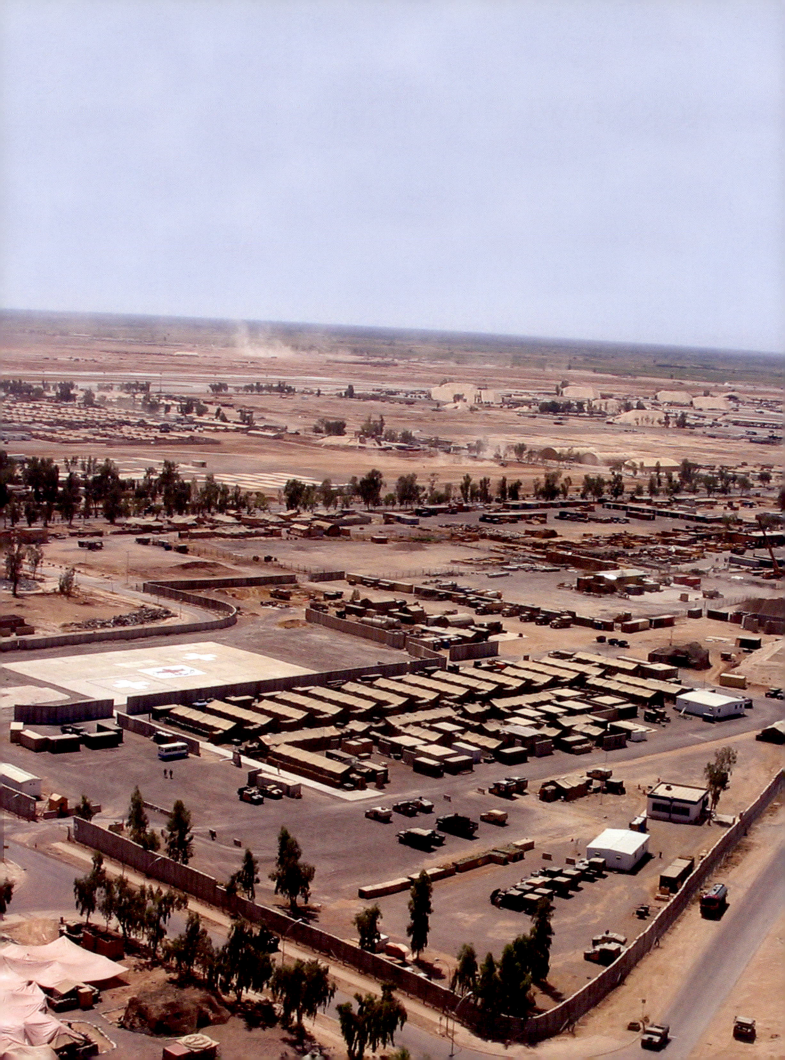

FOREWORD

On January 29, 2006, I was riding on top of an Iraqi APC (armored personal carrier), heading down a road in Taji, Iraq, that was supposed to represent a success story of the war: a collaboration between US and Iraqi forces against the insurgents. As the newly named co-anchor of ABC World News Tonight, I was in Iraq to cover President Bush's State of the Union address and to report on the positive stories of the war—the hard work of the military to train and empower local forces on the ground.

In an instant, an improvised explosive device (IED) exploded about 20 yards from the vehicle, and my life was changed forever, as well as that of my cameraman, Doug Vogt. The force of the blast, a 155-mm shell, shattered my skull over the left temporal lobe. Hundreds of rocks, packed around the IED, were blasted into the side of my face. One rock, the size of a child's marble, sheared my helmet chinstrap in half and traveled through the left side of my neck, coming to rest on the carotid artery on the other side of my head.

For the next 36 days, I would remain in a medically induced coma; but the quick actions and amazing skills of the medics, military doctors, nurses, and assistants would not only save my life, but also save my brain function following this life-threatening injury. Their experiences with such large numbers of those wounded by IEDs, most of whom would not have survived in previous wars, gave them the confidence to make split-second decisions. In the medical barracks of Balad, the doctors did not hesitate, giving me the chance for the best possible outcome.

One of the most amazing stories I heard later, which speaks to me of the dedication of our men and women in uniform, is a story about the MEDEVAC pilots. After the IED exploded, a gunfight ensued and the helicopter pilots were instructed not to land. Unaware of who was on the ground and only knowing that someone needed help, these pilots turned down the radio, ignored the order, and landed. I was then taken to Baghdad, assessed, and then sent to Balad, where—within the hour—my skull flap was removed and my brain began swelling. From Balad, I was sent to Landstuhl Regional Medical Center in Germany, a major way station for wounded soldiers en route to the United States. Just 60 hours after my family arrived there, I was ready to be transported again to neurosurgical care at the National Naval Medical Center (also known as Bethesda Naval Hospital) outside of Washington, DC.

It was there that I received top-notch medical care from an expert team of dedicated military specialists. It was their skill, perseverance, team approach, and kindness that created a platform from which to heal. In writing this foreword, I want to applaud the efforts, bravery, and dedication of the American military. It is well known that much of cutting edge medicine in civilian life comes from the valiant efforts, ingenuity, and pure guts of the battlefield physicians in an effort to save lives under extreme conditions. I am not a hero. I leave that to the men and women serving their country in uniform who put their lives on the line every day for our freedoms. After their wounds, their lives (like mine) are changed forever. What do we owe these men and women? How do we measure our debt to them and their families? What will be our legacy of how we treat those with long-term injuries— such as traumatic brain injury, posttraumatic stress disorder, depression, and other mental illnesses—that can require years of appropriate therapy as the brain heals and the body regenerates?

George Washington, our nation's first Commander in Chief, said, "The willingness with which our young people are likely to serve in any war, no matter how justified, shall be directly proportional to how they perceive the Veterans of earlier wars were treated and appreciated by their nation." Today, in the face of so many injured returning from the wars in Iraq and Afghanistan, we are faced with a wave of wounded, many of them young, all of them returning to a life vastly different than what they left, and families who must learn to deal with a new reality. Are we adequately meeting that charge from our founding father?

Once I passed through the acute stage of my injury, the real work began with my long journey to heal during rehabilitation. Time, energy, commitment, and dedicated professionals supplied the framework to help my brain heal. The love and encouragement of family and friends provided my personal motivation to "get my brain back."

I hope that this book instructs deployed physicians in aspects of the care of initial injuries. But may it also serve as a stepping-off point to focus on continuing that quality of care in the long road to rehabilitation following the injury. My family and I are so appreciative and forever grateful for the medical care that I received from the military. It is our dream that the attention to the wounded remains as focused in the long journey to heal as it is in those white-hot moments in the surgical theater when nothing is spared to save a life.

BOB WOODRUFF
July 2007

PREFACE

It is not uncommon for editors of multiauthored textbooks, and for reviewers of these books, to comment apologetically—or critically—on the inherent bumpiness of such works. We make no such apology here. Indeed, we maintain that the individual nuance and variation among this series of cases are a testament to the collective dedication of the many surgeons, deployed in Southwest Asia, who volunteered their experiences to the effort that produced this textbook.

The photographs were taken mostly in the field by handheld digital cameras. The surgical accounts were typed into e-mails dispatched to the Borden Institute from overseas Forward Surgical Teams (FSTs), combat support hospitals (CSHs), and their equivalent sister Service deployable surgical facilities, or collected from surgeons on their return from these deployments. End-of-chapter peer review commentary has been provided, but the editors have been careful to maintain the individual character of each case as it was presented, as it evolved, as it was managed, and as it was concluded . . . not in every case successfully.

The result of this extraordinary frankness, included in such a broad spectrum of acute trauma surgical presentations, is a textbook unlike any other in the surgical literature. Paired, as it is intended to be, with the 2004 edition of *Emergency War Surgery, Third United States Revision*, this text provides the deploying surgeon, as well as surgical housestaff, with the fundamental principles and priorities critical in managing the trauma of modern warfare; and all medical professionals with insights into the extraordinary technical, clinical, and ethical challenges of their colleagues.

The US Army Medical Department applauds the diligent work of the editors in collecting these cases and providing the necessary instruction and discussion in order to provide optimal forward surgical care—care that is the duty of a great nation to those who serve.

ERIC B. SCHOOMAKER, MD, PhD, FACP
Lieutenant General, Medical Corps, US Army
The Surgeon General

Washington, DC, December 2007

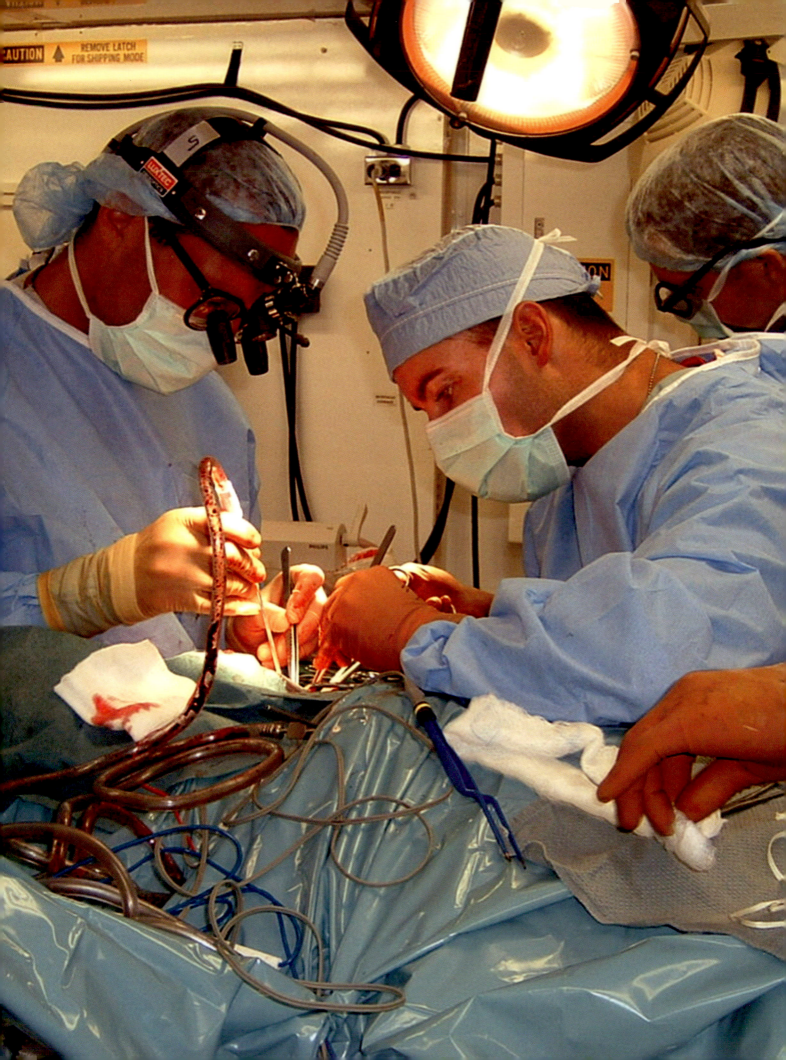

INTRODUCTION

. . . he who would become a surgeon,
therefore, should join the army and follow it.
—HIPPOCRATES

Following terrorist attacks of September 11, 2001 on the United States, US military forces were mobilized and deployed to Afghanistan (Operation Enduring Freedom [OEF]) in 2001 and to Iraq (Operation Iraqi Freedom [OIF]) in 2003. Deployed forces were accompanied by Army field medical assets (eg, the Mobile Army Surgical Hospital [MASH], the Combat Support Hospital [CSH], and the Forward Surgical Team [FST]), as well as their Air Force and Navy equivalents. Almost immediately, these medical units were presented with the casualties, both military and civilian, of insurgent guerilla warfare.

When *Emergency War Surgery, Third United States Revision* (EWS) was published in 2004, it was the intention of the Borden Institute to present this handbook in an electronic version, as well as in a printed format. Although EWS is widely available today, including on the World Wide Web (http://bordeninstitute.army. mil) and as a CD-ROM, plans to incorporate instructional video links proved technically infeasible. Nonetheless, the Borden Institute continued to solicit case reports related to the resuscitation and management of acute trauma in the field. These requests were extended in an ad hoc fashion predominantly to US Army medical units as they rotated in and out of operations in Iraq and Afghanistan.

Today, it is common for deployed physicians to have ready access to personal digital cameras, and to use these to capture presentations and operative stages of their surgical cases. We are grateful for the generous response to our requests. In 2005, with almost 50 cases on file, we decided to collect these into a single series for publication and distribution to surgeons deploying to overseas theaters of war. Our goal was to select cases such that, when paired with the pertinent section of EWS, they would provide important insight and guidance on one or more aspects of the management of acute combat trauma. We believe we have succeeded in this endeavor. Over 80 cases are now captured and presented in identical format with "Teaching Points" describing key aspects that the attending surgeon took away from his or her case. "Clinical Implications" follow. Largely developed by the editors, these points are intended to address the broader issues of all cases similar to the one presented. Due to multiple considerations, the editors decided not to identify contributors at the case level, a reluctant decision not intended to diminish the debt due these dedicated individuals. A single photo without legend at the opening of each case is a deployment scene from Iraq or Afghanistan and is usually <u>un</u>related to the case. Nearly all subsequent clinical photos, however, were taken by staff attending the case presented.

It is important to clarify what this book is not. It is not a comprehensive textbook of surgery. Nor does it substitute for a preparation grounded in the principles of surgery, patient management, or the experience that comes with years at the bedside. We do believe, however, that we have captured the comprehensive spectrum of trauma that characterizes war today, as well as the military medical interventions that have evolved to deliver the wounded from the ferocious destruction of modern warfare. As the history of mankind has been regrettably punctuated in its largest part by the history of war, so have numerous leaps in the advancement of medicine been attributed to lessons learned in war. The present conflicts in Iraq and Afghanistan have proved no exception.

Indeed, the pace of clinical adjustment and improvement in this war is startling and unprecedented. Due to the present availability of high-speed communication, practiced command and control, rapid air evacuation, routine teleconferencing between in-theater level III medical assets and level IV and V facilities (in Germany and the United States, respectively), and (increasingly) computer-based patient tracking, refinement of medical-surgical practice is ongoing rather than gleaned decades after the conflict ends, as was the case in previous wars. A change in the technique for field decompression of suspected pneumothorax and revised thresholds for suspicion of extremity compartment syndromes are two examples of midcourse theater medical corrections.

"... refinement of medical-surgical practice is ongoing rather than gleaned decades after the conflict ends, ..."

Broader changes in treatment are also evident. These often began when anecdotal notice was extended to wider practice if not controlled trials. To be sure, emergency surgical resuscitation in combat does not readily lend itself to placebo-controlled or blinded trials. However, an improving computerized database does permit intratheater outcomes comparisons, as well as theater comparisons to civilian and/or historical norms. As a result, hemorrhage control—the most preventable cause of death on the battlefield—has significantly improved in OIF and OEF, given the introduction of field-applied topical hemostatics (QuikClot and the HemCon Bandage), improved use of prefashioned tourniquets, low-volume and hypertonic resuscitation, newer ratios of packed red cell-to-plasma transfusions, recent (limited) theater availability of apheresis platelets, early resort to fresh whole blood, and perhaps the timely use of human recombinant Factor VIIa.

As important as these interventions, however, has been a wider understanding of the need to recognize early, treat prophylactically, and thereby avoid what has been familiarly called a "triad," but which is, in fact, a relentless vortex of hypothermia, metabolic acidosis, and (hypo)coagulopathy in the severely injured. This approach, known as damage control resuscitation, is transforming the priorities and mechanics of forward acute trauma management fraught with wide practitioner variation to an applied science based on sound physiological principles and with measurable goals and outcomes.

The major precepts of damage control resuscitation are to stop bleeding, minimize contamination, and restore blood flow in order to establish near-normal physiology prior to embarking on definitive repair of injuries. Damage control surgery does not connote haste. Careful attention to a full examination; frequent checks of the patient's evolving physical and mental status; and constant scrutiny for missed sources of bleeding, infection, and compartment syndrome require time and tedium. But explicit in battlefield care is the requirement for resuscitation to be undertaken in the context of timely evacuation to higher echelons of capability.

These then are some of the recurring themes in this book:
- Frequent reference to EWS.
- Setting priorities; emphasis on early consideration of damage control resuscitation.
- Appropriate incorporation of damage control principles into a moving scheme of aeromedical evacuation.
- Defining state-of-the-art combat trauma surgery as practiced in the conflicts in Iraq and Afghanistan.

Another recurring theme is evident in these cases. Battlefield casualties immediately include noncombatant civilians, including women and children, along with host national allies and enemy combatants. All of these individuals are entitled to medical and surgical care. Although all combat casualties are initially resuscitated and stabilized in the immediately available deployed medical facilities, if further definitive care is necessary, US military casualties are evacuated out of theater and rapidly moved along a chain of ever-escalating levels of medical capability. In contrast, host nationals and enemy combatants remain in the combat theater for all of their care, eventually returning to the host country's indigenous medical system (except for enemy combatants who remain in designated US military medical facilities). Since CSHs are designed to provide resuscitation, stabilization, and rapid evacuation for injuries requiring more definitive care, the initially deployed CSHs were neither equipped nor staffed to provide the protracted, resource intensive care necessary for long-term definitive care or rehabilitation. Ad hoc accommodations had to be made for complex orthopaedic, oral-maxillofacial, neurosurgical, and burn care, among many other difficult-to-manage combat wounds. US military physicians would often embark on heroic salvage efforts for severely injured extremities. They understood that in the depleted, underresourced, and overstretched host nation hospitals, amputation of the involved limb was, by far, the most likely outcome. Military general surgeons, in particular, have had to broaden their expertise in order to attend patients whose injuries in a stateside setting would often place them under the care of subspecialty trained colleagues.

These shortcomings of deployed military medical facilities were especially poignant for pediatric casualties. Both experience and equipment were wanting in the care of these injured children. As deployed medical assets have matured in theater, many shortfalls have been corrected. Nonetheless, the dichotomy of different pathways of care for American versus host nation casualties remains an ongoing challenge.

"Battlefield casualties immediately include noncombatant civilians, including women and children, along with host national allies and enemy combatants."

"... attention to the wounded remains as focused in the long journey to heal as it is in those white-hot moments ... when nothing is spared to save a life."

This textbook is not intended to represent an historical account of the US Army Medical Department in the ongoing conflicts in Afghanistan and Iraq. That history waits to be written by others. Nonetheless, we recognize that what is presented here as a clinical-technical work of applied medicine, with time, necessarily becomes an historical reflection of the state-of-the-art and capability of military medicine at the opening of the 21st century.

The editors profoundly share the hope, expressed herein by Mr. Woodruff, that "attention to the wounded remains as focused in the long journey to heal as it is in those white-hot moments . . . when nothing is spared to save a life."

The focus of this book is immediate trauma care. But the wounds attended, as well as the experiences that accompany them, are too often lifelong. Recovery is incomplete. Management becomes rehabilitation. Life is interrupted—forever demarcated in terms of "before" and "after" a split second in war.

SHAWN CHRISTIAN NESSEN, DO, FACS, LTC, MC, US Army
DAVE EDMOND LOUNSBURY, MD, FACP, COL, MC, US Army (Retired)
STEPHEN P. HETZ, MD, FACS, COL, MC, US Army (Retired)

Washington, DC
October 2007

PROLOGUE
Trauma System Development and Medical Evacuation in the Combat Theater

Introduction

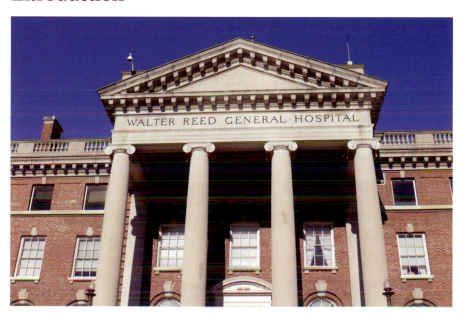

Throughout history, care of the wounded soldier has been the essence of military medicine. The first trauma centers were, by their very nature, military facilities. Many medical advancements have been made during warfare—from the use of a makeshift "ambulance" by Baron Dominique Jean Larré to move casualties off Napoleon's battlefields quickly and back to surgical units in the rear to the advent of blood transfusions during World War I. Lessons learned by military physicians during times of conflict eventually made their way into peacetime practice. In Korea and Vietnam, Mobile Army Surgical Hospitals (MASHs) were deployed to decrease the transit time from the site of injury to definitive surgical treatment. One of the great advances that made the transition from the Vietnam battlefield to the present urban landscape has been the development of similar urban trauma centers and systems.

The helicopter, the advanced training of field medics, and the concentration of surgical resources in a single center all expedited the development of centers for trauma care. The late 1960s to the late 1970s saw the evolution of our modern civilian emergency medical system (EMS) and trauma center capabilities. Few young people learning to be paramedics today could imagine a time when the local undertaker's hearse also doubled as the community ambulance. Over the past few decades, the American College of Surgeons/Committee on Trauma (ACS/COT) has established guidelines to facilitate the development of civilian trauma centers and systems. The US military deployed its medical assets in Iraq and Afghanistan to support its troop dispositions. With these assets in place, the US Army Medical Department then spearheaded joint efforts to connect and operate these separate facilities as much as possible in accord with ACS/COT standards. This latter effort included establishing subspecialty care centers (eg, neurosurgery), on-site wounding and outcomes data collection, and theaterwide Clinical Practice Guidelines (CPGs). The result has been the development and deployment of the world's largest and most complex trauma system.

Trauma System

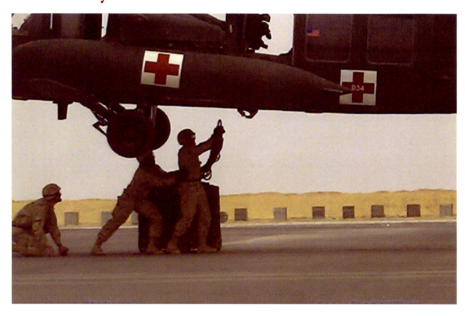

"A trauma system is an arrangement of available resources coordinated for the effective delivery of emergency healthcare services in a geographical region."

ACS/COT emphasizes "optimal care given available resources." This reflects the important and abiding principle that the needs of all injured patients are addressed in as timely a fashion as possible and at the highest standard of care reasonably available. A trauma system is an arrangement of available resources coordinated for the effective delivery of emergency healthcare services in a geographical region. The goal is to "Get the Right Patient to the Right Hospital in the Right Amount of Time"—the motto of the US Central Command Joint Theater Trauma System (JTTS) team.

Military Health System Echelons of Care

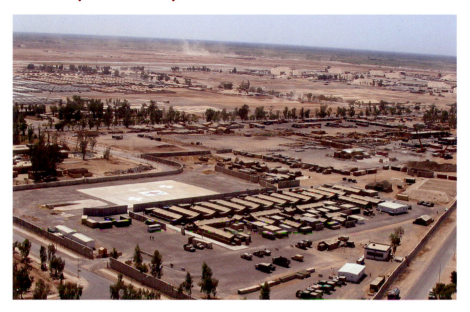

Current routes of patient evacuation, from site of injury to definitive care, include four echelons of care for US forces (Fig. 1):

1. **Level I Echelon of Care**—This unit level, the Battalion Aid Station/Combat Medic, is initiated at the Self-Aid/Buddy Care level, and consists of immediate first aid and transport. It includes care by combat lifesavers, nonmedical soldiers who receive additional training in wound care. Both the medic and the casualty patient may still be under fire, and there is limited medical equipment available. The combat medic has increasingly assumed the responsibility—and capability—of recognizing and treating potentially preventable causes of death: exsanguinating hemorrhage (early tourniquet application, topical hemostatics), pneumothorax (needle angiocatheter), and airway control (oral intubation, cricothyroidotomy). Triage outcome at level I is either return to duty with minimal treatment or evacuate from the battle zone. Casualty evacuation is ideally less than 1 hour to the level II echelon of care.

2. **Level II Echelon of Care**—This level often includes a Forward Surgical Team (FST). Each service provides this level, staffed with from 5 to 20 personnel. The Army FST is typically composed of a 20-person team, with 1 orthopaedic surgeon, 3 general surgeons, 2 nurse anesthetists, 1 critical care nurse, and technicians. The team is able to perform lifesaving resuscitative surgery. This team, when used in its doctrinal configuration, is capable of at least 10 operating room (OR) cases per day and a total of 30 operations within 72 hours. In present operations in Iraq and Afghanistan, it is not uncommon for an FST to be split into two geographically separate facilities. When split, however, its capabilities are degraded. Evacuation to level III care typically occurs as soon as possible after treatment.

> "The combat medic has increasingly assumed the responsibility . . . of recognizing and treating potentially preventable causes of death. . . ."

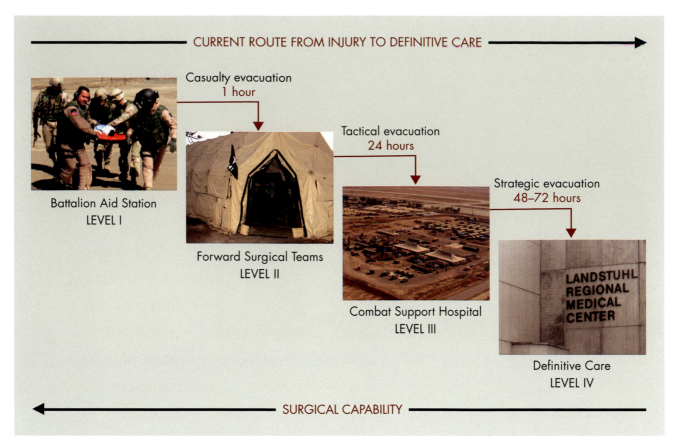

CURRENT ROUTE FROM INJURY TO DEFINITIVE CARE

Battalion Aid Station
LEVEL I

Casualty evacuation
1 hour

Forward Surgical Teams
LEVEL II

Tactical evacuation
24 hours

Combat Support Hospital
LEVEL III

Strategic evacuation
48–72 hours

Definitive Care
LEVEL IV

SURGICAL CAPABILITY

FIGURE 1. *Military system echelons of care.*

3. **Level III Echelon of Care**—Army combat support hospitals (CSHs), but also Navy ships and Air Force theater hospitals, are all capable of further definitive care, and are often located within the combat zone. Level III provides triage, resuscitation, transfusion, initial surgery, definitive and reconstructive surgery, postoperative care, intensive care, and patient holding capacity. Patients are either returned to duty in theater or stabilized for further evacuation. Such facilities are modular and allow for a 44-bed to a full 248-bed configuration as required. In full complement (248 beds), the CSH has six OR tables, allowing 96 operating hours per day. Professional capability routinely includes general, orthopaedic, thoracic, and oral and maxillofacial surgeons; anesthesia providers (as anesthesiologists and certified registered nurse anesthetists [CRNAs]); and internists, emergency medicine physicians, a radiologist, and a psychiatrist. Within 48 to 72 hours, a strategic evacuation can be underway to the next level of care and (in Operation Iraqi Freedom/Operation Enduring Freedom [OIF/OEF]) out of the combat theater. In the shortest timeframes today in Iraq, this can begin less than 12 hours from the time of wounding. Patients who are host nationals, however, are not evacuated out of area and may require definitive surgeries and prolonged hospitalization at a sustained level of care not originally envisioned for the CSH (see Introduction).

TABLE 1. *Echelons of Military Medical Care*

MILITARY DESIGNATION	DESCRIPTION OF US CIVILIAN COUNTERPART	US CIVILIAN DESIGNATION
I. Battalion Aid Station	EMS/corpsman/medic ambulance team	—
IIA. Area medical support facility	Outpatient clinic	—
IIB. FSTs	Community hospital with limited emergency surgery capability	IV
III. Theater hospital in Iraq—eg, Army CSH and (formerly) MASHs	Regional trauma center, limited capability, 30-day ICU holding capability	III
IV. LRMC	Major trauma center	II
V. For example, WRAMC, BAMC, NNMC, WHMC	Major trauma center with teaching and research	I

BAMC: Brooke Army Medical Center (Fort Sam Houston, Texas); CSHs: Combat Support Hospitals; EMS: emergency medical system; FSTs: Forward Surgical Teams; ICU: intensive care unit; LRMC: Landstuhl Regional Medical Center (Landstuhl, Germany); MASHs: Mobile Army Surgical Hospitals; NNMC: National Naval Medical Center (Bethesda, Maryland); WHMC: Wilford Hall Medical Center (Lackland Air Force Base, Texas); WRAMC: Walter Reed Army Medical Center (Washington, DC).

4. **Level IV Echelon of Care**—This definitive care stop is the general hospital that is en route back to the continental United States (CONUS). During the current conflicts in Southwest Asia, this is Landstuhl Regional Medical Center (LRMC) in Germany. (Some would describe LRMC as a level V facility given its location outside of the theater of war. By this criterion, level IV is a definitive surgical capability within the actual theater of war, but outside of the combat zone.) This level IV echelon of care reevaluates and treats all en route patients. The LRMC is staffed and equipped for general and specialized medical and surgical care. Patients not expected to return to duty are stabilized and evacuated to CONUS. Reconditioning and rehabilitating services are provided for those patients who will be returned to duty within theater. LRMC finds itself in a unique position because it is the common pathway node between theater operations in Southwest Asia (OIF/OEF) and CONUS medical facilities. Virtually 100% of US troops evacuated from those two theaters of operations pass through LRMC for additional care. LRMC provides multidisciplinary trauma surgical management to those who have sustained catastrophic injury and is where the first step in the process of rehabilitating the wounded begins. The average length of stay is less than 4 days. Then, the patient is transferred to the **Level V Echelon of Care** in CONUS military medical centers. These levels of care should not be confused with the civilian ACS/COT levels of trauma center designation, which uses these ordinals in reverse order (Table 1).

Aeromedical Evacuation

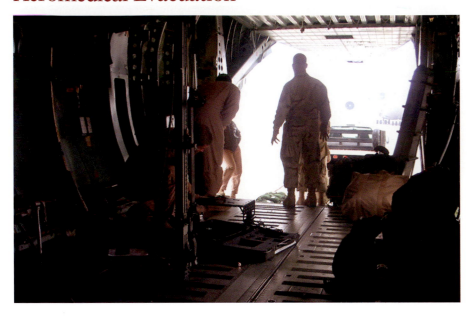

The aeromedical evacuation system is capable of moving more than 1,000 casualties per month from theater operations in Southwest Asia. Critical Care Air Transport Teams (CCATTs) are flying intensive care units with a staff of three (typically, a physician trained in critical care, a critical care nurse, and a respiratory therapist) capable of not only transporting a ventilated critically ill casualty, but also able to continue resuscitation and advance the care of the casualty patient en route to the next echelon of care. From September 2001 through September 2007, there have been more than 44,000 air evacuation/ CCATT patients transported by the US Air Force aeromedical evacuation system from OIF/OEF. This capability, which did not exist more than 10 years ago, undergoes continual scrutiny and refinement.

Movement of severely injured patients is always a critical event that requires appropriate timing and careful attention to minute details. Determining the optimal time of transfer in the continuum of military medical care requires balancing the benefit of resources available at the next echelon against the risks inherent in moving a critical patient with all the necessary tubes, lines, monitors, and equipment in a ground and/or air ambulance. Many patients are initially too unstable to be placed in a system in which the present air evacuation component (from Southwest Asia) often exceeds 10 hours of flight time. The system, however, is evolving. Traditional air evacuation moved *stable* patients who required little intervention outside preflight orders. CCATT enables the safe transport of *stabilized* patients—stability that depends on ongoing intervention, such as ventilator management, sedation, pressors, etc.

Ideally, each of these parameters should be met prior to transfer of any patient:
- Heart rate < 120.
- Systolic blood pressure > 90.

- Hematocrit > 27%.
- Platelet count > 50,000.
- INR < 2.0.
- pH > 7.30.
- Base deficit < 5.
- Temperature > 35°C.

When any one or more of these criteria is not met, the responsible physician should hold the patient and continue treatment or document the limitations at the current facility that compel urgent, high-risk transfer.

Combat Trauma System Implementation

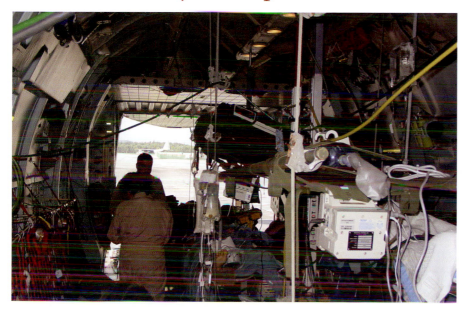

Organizing and appointing working groups to implement an ACS/COT-like trauma system within the US Army Medical Department doctrine were pivotal to the successful development and implementation of a modern combat trauma system. In addition to providing a rapidly deployable, mobile, modular, and sustainable infrastructure, such a system would need to constantly improve coordination of care, provide data to address and answer operational questions, predict manpower needs, and provide medical situational awareness (ie, injury patterns and evaluate protection/prevention maneuvers). Such data could be collected to evaluate outcomes, assess training, improve continuity of care, and facilitate system-wide, data-driven, and real-time improvements.

The goal was to develop and implement a trauma system modeled after recent successes of stateside civilian systems (which, in turn, were modeled on experiences from the Vietnam War), but leavened by the realities of combat. A trauma system director and a team of trauma nurse coordinators have been utilized for just this purpose. One tenet used to guide trauma care algorithms and the location and

> "A modern combat trauma system provides a rapidly deployable, mobile, modular, and sustainable infrastructure that coordinates care, provides data to address and answer operational questions, predicts manpower needs, and provides medical situational awareness."

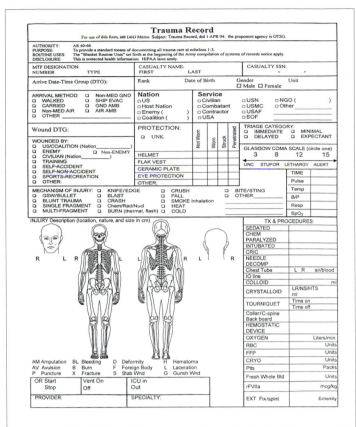

Figure 2.
(Front) *Theater
trauma registry.*

capability of resources equates to the following: elapsed time from injury to lifesaving surgery is to be as short as possible; but, in every case, less than 2 hours (ie, "deliver the right casualty to the right care at the right place and in the right time").

Care for injured soldiers in current theater operations has been the focus of the JTTS. Additionally, the JTTS continues to work on performance improvement issues. Some of the responsibilities of the trauma system director include the following:

- Recommending optimal placement of surgical assets within theater.
- Developing triage criteria for casualty evacuation to the appropriate level of care.
- Ensuring adequate communication at/between military treatment facilities at every level of care.
- Standardizing approaches to common battle injury patterns across theater.

JTTS also has the responsibility to review and maintain a Joint Theater Trauma Registry (Fig. 2), conduct and collate morbidity and mortality reporting and operative case reporting, and develop a Performance Improvement Program and initiatives for the entire trauma system. This includes evaluating the Casualty Evacuation/Air Evacuation System (evacuation times and casualty outcomes) and assisting with development of the clinical information management scheme for theater.

Trauma Record
DISCHARGE SUMMARY

MEDICATIONS:	LABS:	X-RAYS:	PMH: Allergies:

REGION	DIAGNOSIS, PROCEDURES, and COMPLICATIONS
Face	
Head & Neck (incl C-spine)	
Chest (incl T-spine)	
Abdomen (incl L-spine)	
Pelvis UPPER /LOWER Extremities	
Skin	

DISPOSITION DTG:	□ EVAC to ____________ □ RTD □ DECEASED (see below)	Evacuation Priority □ ROUTINE □ PRIORITY □ URGENT

Damage Control Procedures? Y / N Hypothermic (< 34°C)? Y / N Coagulopathy? Y / N

Cause of Death at ____________

ANATOMIC:
□ Airway □ Head □ Neck □ Chest □ Abdomen □ Pelvis □ Extremity (Upper/Lower)
□ Other

PHYSIOLOGIC:
□ Breathing □ CNS □ Hemorrhage □ Total Body Disruption □ Sepsis □ Multi-organ failure

COMMENTS: SURGEON: (Printed Name)

FIGURE 2. (Back) *Theater trauma registry.*

Areas for system improvement have been identified in the need for smoother transmission of healthcare information along the multiple and physically distant echelons of care and a smoother transition between healthcare teams when units rotate into and out of theater (ie, retention of operational memory). The requirement is to educate all healthcare providers in the importance of information flow, standardize documentation of health forms, and have a central electronic patient data repository. This patient data repository is intended to have all available medical records scanned at the level III echelon of care and then placed on a secure Web site, thus giving providers access to critical healthcare information at all echelons of care.

"Areas for system improvement have been identified in the need for smoother transmission of healthcare information along the multiple and physically distant echelons of care and a smoother transition between healthcare teams when units rotate into and out of theater. . . ."

Stateside, where civilian casualties typically present one at a time, we are challenged with documenting patient encounters adequately. It is difficult to imagine how daunting a task it is for a field medic—under fire, with multiple injured comrades, as well as numerous enemy casualties—to document even the simplest of clinical findings or events on the battlefield. Recordkeeping is much more difficult at aid stations or FST locations, where military healthcare is conducted under the most austere conditions. Documentation there is often, necessarily, an afterthought.

Trauma Registry

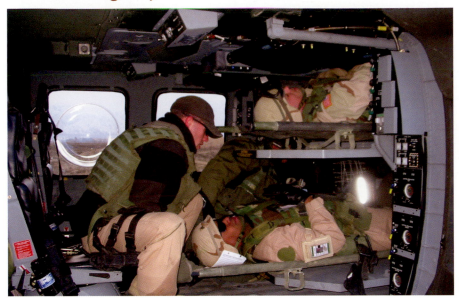

"To . . . capture documentation and evaluate injury patterns, as well as the care provided, the US Army Institute of Surgical Research has developed the Joint Theater Trauma Registry."

To optimally capture documentation and evaluate injury patterns, as well as the care provided, the US Army Institute of Surgical Research has developed the Joint Theater Trauma Registry. This repository is collected on forms developed exclusively for use by the deployed military while, at the same time, designed to facilitate completion of nurse and physician examinations and treatment records. (See Fig. 2 for an early version of this form.)

This field clinical information—collated, tabulated, dissected, analyzed, and thoughtfully reviewed—will become the database of battlefield casualty management in Iraq and Afghanistan.

SUGGESTED READING

Appendix 3: Theater Joint Trauma Record. In: *Emergency War Surgery, Third United States Revision*. Washington, DC: Department of the Army, Office of The Surgeon General, Borden Institute; 2004.

Chapter 2: Levels of medical care. In: *Emergency War Surgery, Third United States Revision*. Washington, DC: Department of the Army, Office of The Surgeon General, Borden Institute; 2004.

Chapter 4: Aeromedical evacuation. In: *Emergency War Surgery, Third United States Revision*. Washington, DC: Department of the Army, Office of The Surgeon General, Borden Institute; 2004.

Hetz SP. Introduction to military medicine: a brief overview. *Surg Clin North Am.* 2006;86:675–688.

ARE WE DOING BETTER?
Assessing Combat Casualty Data

Combat casualty data are readily available during the present war in Afghanistan and Iraq, with some newspapers even publishing summaries of the numbers of Americans killed and wounded on a daily basis. It is common to read analyses of these data in which they are interpreted to show remarkable improvement in the outcome of the management of combat injury compared with historical norms. However, caution is needed when coming to such a conclusion because deaths in combat are determined by a multitude of factors, of which the effectiveness of the deployed medical system is only one. Certainly, the total number of combat casualties has little to do with medical care, but has everything to do with the number of warriors at risk and the casualty-generating potential of the battlefield (ie, the weapons used and the war-fighting tactics). One might think that the ratio of the killed in action (KIA) to wounded is closer to telling us the effect of medical care, but this proportional mortality more likely reflects the lethality of the weapons. The unprecedented use and effectiveness of today's protective equipment (all other factors being equal) should make for a less lethal battlefield because armor decreases the lethality of weapons. When a blunt index of injury severity is used (the number of wounded divided into those who returned to duty quickly and those who did not), we are closer to assessing the effect of medical care. Because combat casualty care is unlikely to affect casualties with only minor injuries, the ratio of KIA to those surviving with wounds of severity preventing rapid return to duty is likely to be more affected by the excellence of combat casualty care.

The unprecedented use and effectiveness of today's protective equipment (all other factors being equal) should make for a less lethal battlefield because armor decreases the lethality of weapons.

Combat casualty care can and does prevent deaths. However, the lethality of the weapon and the anatomical location of wounds remain dominant. Most of those who are killed in combat die quickly and before lifesaving surgery is possible. Perhaps the index most sensitive to the quality of combat casualty care is the fraction of those with potentially fatal wounds who are evacuated from the battlefield alive, but who then die in the hospital (ie, died of wounds [DOW]). But even this measure will be affected by the lethality of weapons and the speed of the evacuation from the battlefield. Indeed, fast evacuation of the very severely injured—those likely to die despite aggressive care—may even increase the number of casualties who are ultimately categorized as DOW.

With these factors in mind, it is interesting to calculate some indicators of mortality outcome in the present conflict in Iraq. Data on DOW in Iraq (US Army and Marines) from March 2003 through the end of June 2007 are as follows:
- total DOW for all services—663; and
- total wounded not returned to duty within 3 days—11,831.[1,2]

DOW mortality is calculated to be 5.3%. Data for the conflict in Vietnam are as follows:
- total DOW for all services—5,289; and
- total wounded not returned to duty within 1 day—153,303.[3]

DOW mortality is calculated to be 3.3%. It appears that medical treatment facility mortality outcome was better in the Vietnam War; however, this conclusion seems implausible. It may be that, in the present war, better treatment of the gravely wounded is vitiated by more lethal injuries and more rapid evacuation of the mortally wounded. Or, it may be that the difference is a statistical artifact because the same time periods are not used for data collection (ie, return to duty in 1 day for Vietnam, 3 days for the present war).

The second index mentioned previously (ratio of KIA to casualties with wounds of such severity that rapid return to duty is prohibited) also needs to be considered, even though it is less likely to reflect the influence of medical treatment. Data of American KIA as of June 2007 are as follows:
- total KIA for all services—2,265; and
- total wounded not returned to duty within 3 days—11,831.[1,2]

KIA mortality is calculated to be 16.1%. Data for the conflict in Vietnam are as follows:
- total KIA for all services—40,934; and
- total wounded not returned to duty within 1 day—153,303.[3]

> *The military has made enormous efforts to improve*
> *battlefield first-aid training and equipment.*
> *It is likely that at least some of the decrease in the*
> *number of KIA reflects this effort.*

KIA mortality is calculated to be 21.1%. Clearly, casualties in the present war are less likely to die before reaching a medical treatment facility than in the Vietnam War. Why? It cannot be due to better medical care in a medical treatment facility, but it could and probably is at least partially due to better battlefield first aid at the site of wounding. The military has made enormous efforts to improve battlefield first-aid training and equipment. It is likely that at least some of the decrease in the number of KIA reflects this effort. A second explanation involves battlefield lethality. The explosive devices used by terrorists have a fearsome reputation, and therein lays a paradox. If the weapons are more lethal, the proportion of those injured who are KIA should increase. The fact that the proportion is actually less clearly points to the excellent protection afforded by the military's wide use of individual body armor. Historical data indicate that penetrating missile wounds of the trunk were responsible for about one third of combat deaths.[4] Defeating even one half of such threats might well be expected to decrease mortality and therefore accord with the observed percent KIA.

However, until more data are made available,
it will remain difficult to separate conclusively the effect of
medical care on mortality from battlefield factors,
such as weapons lethality.

The widespread belief that mortality has been reduced in the present war—compared with historical norms—appears, then, to be well founded. However, until more data are made available, it will remain difficult to separate conclusively the effect of medical care on mortality from battlefield factors, such as weapons lethality and armor. It is certainly possible that evacuation in the present war is so fast that many more casualties with potentially fatal wounds reach hospital-level care and are saved by modern surgery than in past wars. But only data on evacuation time and, ideally, quantitative injury severity assessment will allow this question to be addressed.

—RONALD F. BELLAMY, MD, FACS, COL, MC, US Army (Ret.)

REFERENCES

1. Global War on Terrorism—Operation Iraqi Freedom: By Casualty Category Within Service, March 19, 2003 Through June 30 2007. Available at: http://siadapp.dmdc.osd.mil/personnel/CASUALTY/OIF-Total.pdf. Accessed December 2007.

2. Operation Iraqi Freedom (OIF) U.S. Casualty Status—Fatalities as of: June 29, 2007, 10 a.m. EST.* Available at: http://www.defenselink.mil/news/casualty.pdf. Accessed December 2007. [*The KIA category given by the DefenseLink Web site appears to include DOW, as well as KIA.]

3. Military Casualty Information. U.S. Military Casualties in Southeast Asia—Vietnam Conflict. Vietnam Conflict—Casualty Summary, as of June 15, 2004. Available at: http://siadapp.dmdc.osd.mil/personnel/CASUALTY/OIF-Total.pdf. Accessed December 2007.

4. Bellamy RF. Combat trauma overview. In: Zaitchuk R, Grande CM, eds. *Anesthesia and Perioperative Care of the Combat Casualty. Textbook of Military Medicine.* Washington, DC: Department of the Army, Office of The Surgeon General, Borden Institute; 1995: 1–42.

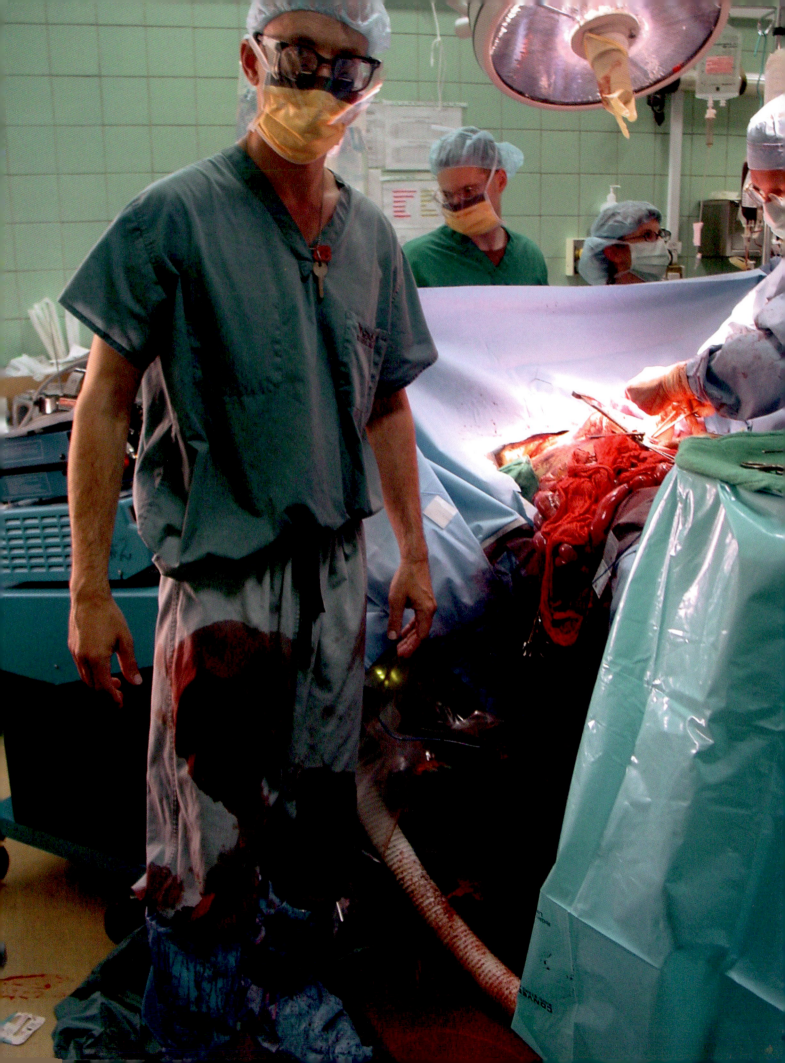

War Surgery in Afghanistan and Iraq

A SERIES OF CASES, 2003–2007

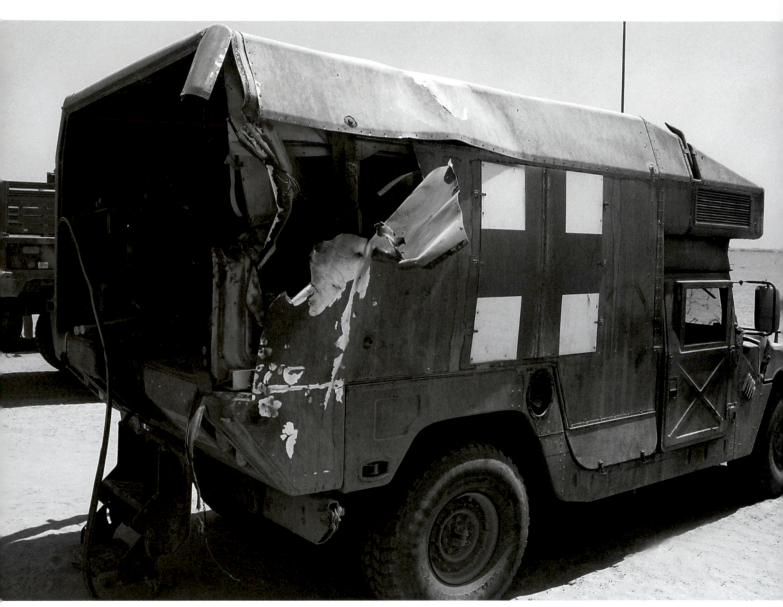

This four-litter ambulance was struck by an RPG en route to the 28th CSH in Iraq. The medic on board placed himself across his casualty and was killed in the attack.

Chapter I
ACUTE RESUSCITATION AND CRITICAL CARE

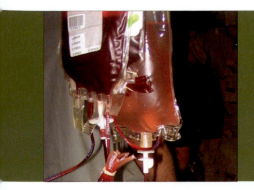

I.1
Forward Resuscitative Surgery: An Introduction to Polytrauma

CASE PRESENTATION

Two soldiers were standing guard when they sustained multiple gunshot wounds by unknown assailants. Both individuals were treated in the field by a medic and transported to a Forward Surgical Team (FST) facility in nonmedical vehicles. The two soldiers were brought in by their units. Emotions ran high. Their unit had been notified, and several members met these soldiers on arrival at the FST. The first soldier suffered a single, high-velocity wound to the head. On quick inspection, he had agonal breathing and had not been intubated. He was intubated, and the dressing that had been placed around his head was removed. Half of his left cranium was missing, with protrusion of macerated brain matter (an obviously mortal injury). The second soldier sustained multiple wounds, including a partial traumatic amputation of his left hand. High-velocity wounds (see sidebar on page 23) were present with entries and exits to both thighs and scrotum. Rapid assessment of this second soldier revealed that he was awake, alert, and answering questions appropriately. He maintained his own airway and moved air freely. He had no apparent chest or abdominal wounds. Tourniquets were placed just above his left hand and high on the upper portions of both thighs. Intravenous (IV) access was rapidly established, with large-bore IVs in both upper extremities. Initial vital signs revealed mild tachycardia and a systolic blood pressure of around 100 mm Hg. This soldier did have some oozing through dressings that had been placed over his bilateral thigh wounds. Fluid resuscitation was initiated while a secondary survey was completed. No additional upper body injuries were identified. His pelvis appeared stable. His right upper extremity was without injury; he had a partial traumatic amputation just above his left wrist. Lower extremities examination revealed entrance and exit wounds to both upper thigh areas, with apparent bilateral femur fractures. He also had an open scrotum with exposed testicles. His phallus appeared intact. In his lower extremities, the patient had no sign of injury below the thighs. However, he had poor perfusion of both lower extremities. Chest X-ray (CXR) revealed no pneumothoraces. The FAST (Focused Abdominal Sonography for Trauma) exam was negative for free fluid in the abdomen. The pelvis film revealed no pelvic fractures or foreign bodies. Although the patient remained hemodynamically stable, he became progressively combative. The surgeons judged that the patient was on the verge of hemodynamic collapse. Consequently, while receiving fluid and blood resuscitation,

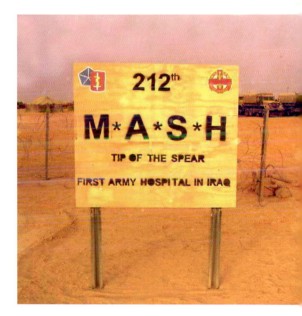

TO OPERATE OR TO TRANSPORT?

This soldier was severely wounded when a vehicle-borne improvised explosive device (IED) exploded near a vehicle where he was standing. The left lower extremity was nearly amputated by the explosion. The right lower extremity was severely injured with multiple fragments, fractures, and a popliteal artery injury. The soldier was treated with a tourniquet above the knee, splinted, and immediately transported to a nearby FST, arriving within 10 minutes of the injury. At the FST, the wounds were assessed. Significant blood loss and hypotension required immediate transfusion of PRBCs and saline. The patient was stabilized. A 45-minute helicopter transport to a CSH was immediately available. The senior surgeon elected to operate on the patient at the FST. Vascular repair was attempted, and an extensive external fixator was placed. The operation lasted approximately 4 hours, and the blood available to the FST was exhausted during the procedure. The patient was

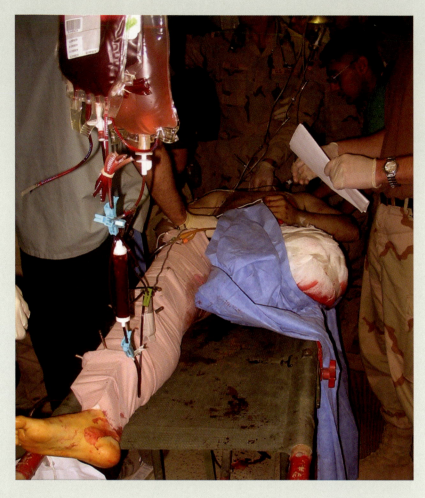

then transported via MEDEVAC helicopter to the CSH. En route (approximately 20 minutes into the flight), the patient had a cardiac arrest. Despite attempts at resuscitation, he died.

TEACHING POINTS

1. It is likely that this patient succumbed from the lethal triad of hypothermia, acidosis, and coagulopathy.

2. The surgical mission of an FST is extremely difficult, and difficult to delimit. Although the capability and equipment necessary to perform a wide variety of resuscitative and definitive surgical procedures are available at the FST, the fundamental principle of military surgery makes it imperative that patients who can tolerate transport to the next level of care are stabilized and moved expeditiously to more robust surgical facilities.

3. The judgment of the senior surgeon can be severely tested. Patients should only undergo extensive surgical procedures at the FST if, in the judgment of the senior surgeon, the patient will not survive transport to the next level of care. Even when such dire circumstances prevail, the goal is stabilization such that the patient can tolerate transport to the next level of care.

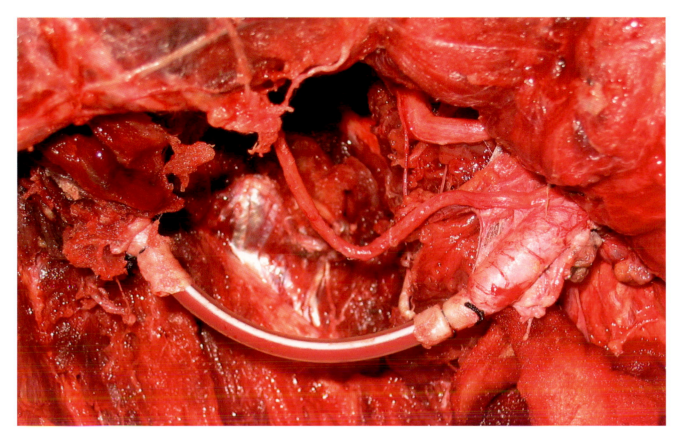

FIGURE 1. *Extensive loss of tissue associated with a high-velocity wound. A shunt is in place in the SFA.*

he was taken urgently to the operating room (OR) for further evaluation and exploration of his multiple extremity wounds. The "walking blood bank" was mobilized because of the anticipated need for whole blood. In the OR, a pneumatic tourniquet was placed above the dressing and completion amputation of the left hand was rapidly performed. The pneumatic tourniquet was released with no evidence of ongoing bleeding from the extremity. The left thigh had diffuse oozing below the field tourniquet, and a pneumatic tourniquet could not be placed proximally. Therefore, the wound was explored with the field tourniquet in place. The tourniquet was gradually released, and the major sources of bleeding were identified. The superficial femoral vein (SFV) had been transected, and was ligated both distally and proximally. The superficial femoral artery (SFA) was initially in spasm, but began to bleed profusely once the tourniquet was released. The transected ends were identified, and an Argyle shunt was rapidly placed (Fig. 1). Doppler signals were obtained in the dorsalis pedis and posterior tibial arteries. Attention was then directed to the right lower extremity. The SFA appeared

intact, but the SFV was transected. The vessel was ligated and bleeding controlled. Exploration of both lower extremity wounds took approximately 1 hour to complete, during which time the patient received 6 units of packed red blood cells (PRBCs) and 4 units of whole blood. Preparation for transport was initiated. External fixators were placed on both lower extremities and fasciotomies performed (Fig. 2). The vascular shunt was reassessed to ensure it had not become dislodged during the previously described procedures. While awaiting transport, the patient's testicles were protected by placing them inside the injured scrotum and loosely approximating the scrotal edges. A repeat FAST exam was performed, which was negative. Because of the severity of the patient's injuries and the need for ongoing resuscitation, one of the FST surgeons accompanied the patient in-flight to the combat support hospital (CSH). The second surgeon called the receiving surgeon and relayed information about the nature of the injuries, status of the patient, and operative procedures performed. Treated expectantly, the first casualty succumbed to his wounds.

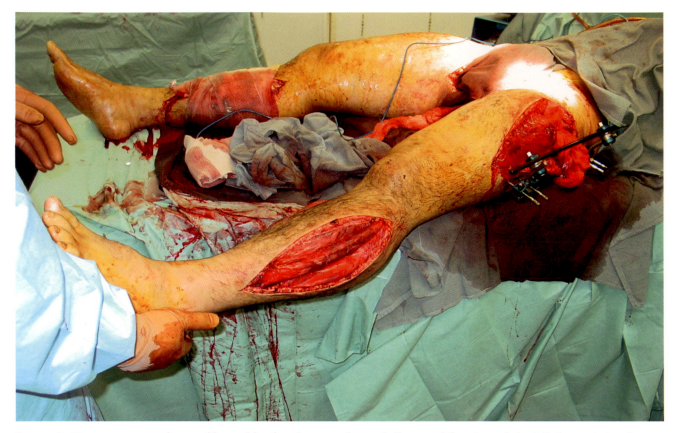

FIGURE 2. *Compartment release of lateral leg has been performed. External fixation of the left femur is in place.*

TEACHING POINTS

1. This introductory case provides insight into the dynamics of the rapid, reasoned, sequential approach required in the acute management of complex battlefield trauma. Faced with a crowded emergency area and the emotional chaos of the moment, the surgeon nonetheless walks us through a process of: rapid initial assessment, triage, reassessment with attention to the ABCs, exposure, IV placement, early call for a walking blood bank, secondary survey, plain films of the chest and lower extremities, the FAST exam, the move to the OR, distal upper extremity amputation, attention to the lower extremities, control of venous and arterial bleeding to include placement of an arterial shunt, confirmation of distal flow, transfusion, external fixator placement, prophylactic lower extremity fasciotomies, reassessment and repeat FAST exams, transport, and communication.

2. Specifically: Clear the emergency area of all non-medical personnel, including commanders. Do not allow nonmedical personnel—including those who are injured, their buddies, or their commanders—to become involved with medical triage.

3. The FST has its own blood stock, but it consists of only PRBCs. Neither the FST nor CSH normally has access to fresh frozen plasma or platelets. Whenever it is determined that someone may become coagulopathic, whole blood is drawn.

4. The FST is not traditionally equipped with X-ray capability. In FSTs without X-rays, external fixators are placed based on known landmarks. This procedure requires skill and experience. General surgeons should be capable of performing this procedure.

5. In a combat situation, all possible avenues of communicating pertinent and essential information must be attempted when transporting patients to the next level of care. This may include writing on the patient and/or the bandages (see Fig. 5, page 175), informing accompanying transport and personnel, radiocommunication, e-mail, written records, or even accompanying the patient when exceptional circumstances permit.

6. Combativeness may be an impending sign of hypovolemic shock and hemodynamic decompensation. It is often misinterpreted as sequelae of a closed-head injury, which seldom, if ever, is the case.

7. General surgeons have responsibility for the overall management of polytrauma patients at the FST. Airway management and resuscitation are critical priorities in conjunction with control of hemorrhage.

8. Once bleeding is controlled, external fixation of fractures may be appropriate. Fracture alignment stabilized with external fixators may improve distal perfusion. Definitive vascular repair may be delayed by placing a temporary vascular shunt. If transport times to the next level of care are short (1 hour or less) and the patient can be stabilized, temporizing with the use of tourniquets and splints and rapid transport to the next level of care should be strongly considered (see sidebar on page 20).

CLINICAL IMPLICATIONS

Often, combat wounds will present to the surgeon in a highly chaotic and emotionally charged environment. As demonstrated in this case, adherence to sound principles of military surgery—including triage, resuscitation, damage control surgery, and evacuation with concise communication to the next level of care—is critical to achieving a successful outcome.

DAMAGE CONTROL

This case is representative of the type of damage control surgery performed by an FST. In this case, after appropriate triage, resuscitation was started, hemorrhage was controlled, and evacuation accomplished. Placement of external fixators and lower extremity fasciotomies fall well within the scope of the FST. Definitive vascular repair was performed later at the CSH.

SUMMARY

This case demonstrates well how quickly a small surgical team can become engaged in a life-and-death struggle to save wounded soldiers. In this case, the FST was successful because they understood the signs of impending cardiovascular collapse, studied previous lessons learned from austere environments, and implemented protocols unique to war trauma. This case captures the confusion and chaos small teams must overcome in combat.

SUGGESTED READING

Chapter 3: Triage. In: *Emergency War Surgery, Third United States Revision*. Washington, DC: Department of the Army, Office of The Surgeon General, Borden Institute; 2004.

Chapter 12: Damage control surgery. In: *Emergency War Surgery, Third United States Revision*. Washington, DC: Department of the Army, Office of The Surgeon General, Borden Institute; 2004.

DR JANICE MENDELSON AND THE BALLISTICS OF WOUNDING

In this book and elsewhere, trauma surgeons frequently use the phrase "high-velocity wound." Indeed, modern munitions attain extraordinary velocities. But to better understand the mechanics of wounding, the reader should think in terms of "high-energy transfer." It is not the velocity, but the kinetic energy of the projectile, transferred to the tissue, that produces tissue disruption. High-velocity rifle bullets that traverse tissue undeformed and in a stable trajectory may transfer only a small fraction (< 20%) of their kinetic energy, whereas bullets that break up while traversing tissue (and blast fragments) transfer considerably more of their kinetic energy (> 40%), thus resulting in a larger wound. Energy transfer usually is not uniformly distributed along the wound tract. This is because the projectile may yaw, ricochet, fragment, and/or deform in transit. In addition, the casualty presents nonhomogeneous tissue (garments, skin, fat, muscle, organs of varying densities, and bone) with different viscoelastic properties. It is quite possible to produce a massive wound with a (relatively) slow heavy missile that has an unstable trajectory.

This understanding of energy transfer rather than velocity per se as the determinant of the extent of wounds was largely described by scientists at the US Army's Ballistics Research Laboratory at Edgewood Arsenal in Aberdeen, Maryland. One of the investigators responsible for this work was Colonel Janice A. Mendelson. She served as Chief of the Trauma Investigation Branch (Biophysics Division) at Edgewood from 1958 to 1966. Dr Mendelson was one of the first female surgeons in the Army Medical Corps. She was lead investigator for a number of studies concerning the clinical course of military injuries—studies to which our greater understanding today can be attributed. During the Vietnam War, she deployed as a staff surgeon (1970–1971) and worked in a Vietnamese burn unit where she demonstrated the remarkable efficacy of topical mafenide hydrochloride (Sulfamylon).

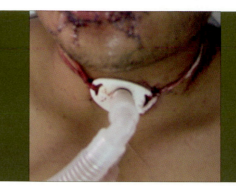

I.2
Emergency Surgical Airway Management

CASE PRESENTATION

This host nation male was injured by an improvised explosive device (IED) and brought to the combat support hospital (CSH). He sustained extensive facial injuries (Figs. 1 and 2), including a maxillary fracture, a comminuted mandibular fracture, and tongue and soft-tissue injuries. There were also fragment wounds in his abdomen and flank. The patient could only breathe sitting up and was able to maintain his oxygen saturation above 90%. He resisted efforts to place him in the supine position. Consequently, the anesthesiologist could not orally intubate the patient. The decision was made to perform a cricothyroidotomy. While in a sitting position, the patient's neck was prepared with betadine solution. He was given propofol, placed in the supine position, and an immediate cricothyroidotomy performed. The procedure took less than 1 minute. During this time, the patient's oxygen saturation dropped to 45%, but quickly returned to normal once his trachea was intubated (Figs. 3 and 4). With the airway secure, the patient underwent exploratory laparotomy that revealed no intraabdominal injuries. A gastrostomy tube was placed, and facial reconstruction was performed. Within 48 hours, the cricothyroidotomy was converted to a tracheostomy, and the patient recovered well postoperatively without complication.

TEACHING POINTS

1. This case provides an example of a patient who required an emergency surgical airway. The patient was able to maintain adequate oxygen saturation until arrival at a level III (see Prologue) medical treatment facility that had an experienced surgical staff. If this patient had been unconscious, it is likely that a surgical airway might have been needed at the site of injury.

2. Cricothyroidotomy is a simple procedure that is typically performed in a stressful environment. The procedure is taught to nonsurgeons working at a level I or level II medical treatment facility (see sidebar on page 25).

3. Tracheostomy should be avoided in this scenario because it is a multistep procedure that includes dividing strap muscles and dividing or elevating the thyroid isthmus. The patient, who cannot be preoxygenated, might not survive the additional time needed to perform a tracheostomy.

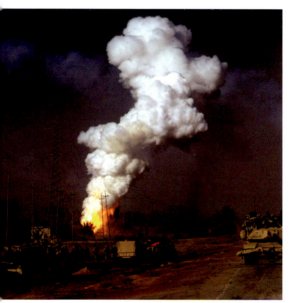

Courtesy David Leeson, *The Dallas Morning News*

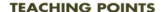

STEPS OF SURGICAL CRICOTHYROIDOTOMY

1. Identify cricothryroid membrane between cricoid cartilage (or cricoid ring) and thyroid cartilage (A).
2. Prep skin widely.
3. Grasp and hold trachea, stabilizing the airway.
4. Make a vertical skin incision down to the cricothyroid membrane (use a no. 10 or no. 11 blade).
5. Bluntly dissect the tissues to expose the membrane.
6. Make a horizontal membrane incision (B).
7. Open the membrane with forceps or the scalpel handle.
8. Insert a small, cuffed endotracheal tube (6.0–7.0 inner diameter) to just above the balloon (C).
9. Confirm tracheal intubation.
10. Suture the endotracheal tube in place and secure it with ties that pass around the neck.

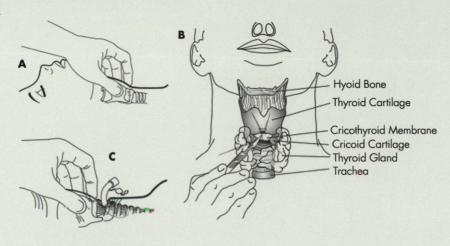

4. Ten to fifteen percent of battle casualties present with maxillofacial trauma. Although establishing an emergency surgical airway is well within the capabilities of a general surgeon, complex maxillofacial reconstruction is not. This case demonstrates the need for an oral and maxillofacial surgeon or equivalent at the level III medical treatment facility.
5. This case also shows the not infrequent need for definitive reconstructive surgical procedures to be performed at the CSH.

CLINICAL IMPLICATIONS

Cricothyroidotomy is the procedure of choice for emergent surgical airway management. Indications for cricothyroidotomy include the following:

1. Maxillofacial trauma that precludes intubation.
2. Inability to secure the airway for any reason in hypoxic patients.

A nasopharyngeal airway (NPA) may be an alternative to surgery in the emergent management of oral and maxillofacial injuries.

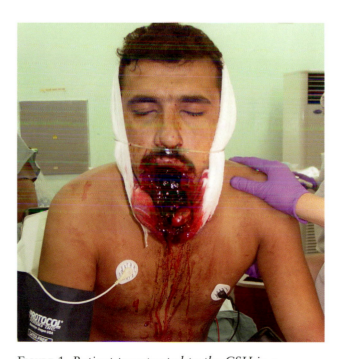

FIGURE 1. *Patient transported to the CSH in a sitting position. This position allowed the patient to maintain his own airway until experienced trauma personnel could secure his airway.*

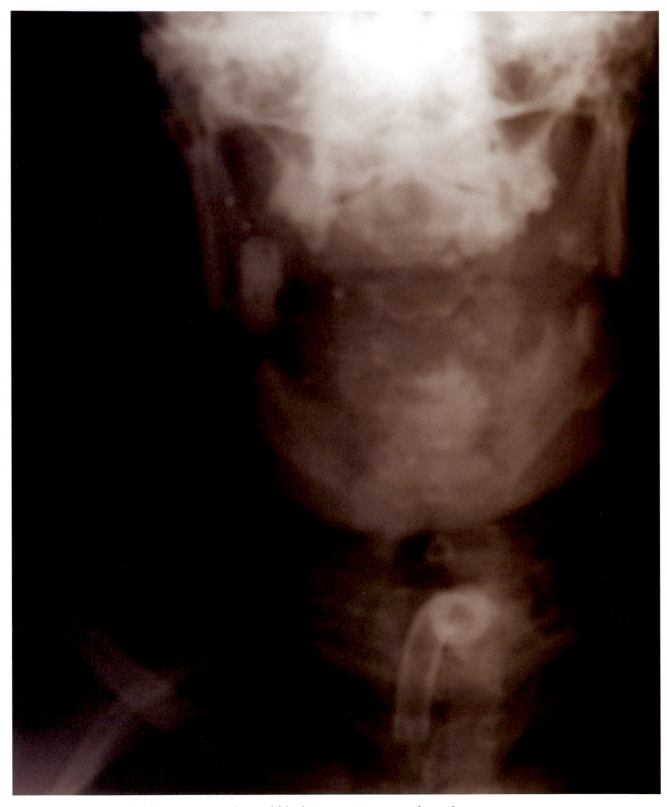

FIGURE 2. *Radiograph of a comminuted mandible fracture. Note cricothyroidotomy.*

> ***Contraindications*** *to an NPA:*
> Coagulopathy, midface trauma, basilar
> skull fracture, and suspected elevated
> intracranial pressure.

DAMAGE CONTROL

Cricothyroidotomy is an essential damage control technique used to secure an airway that cannot be orally intubated. An endotracheal tube (6.0–7.0 inner diameter) or a tracheostomy tube (no. 4 or no. 6 Shiley tracheostomy tube) can be used.

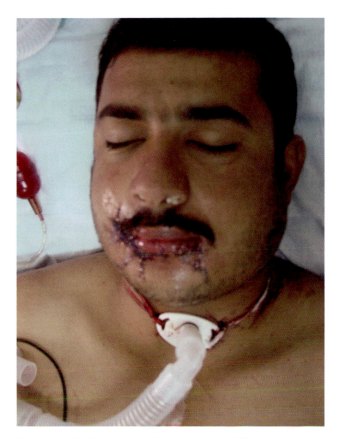

FIGURE 4. *Patient immediately post-op. The cricothyroidotomy was converted to a tracheostomy within 48 hours.*

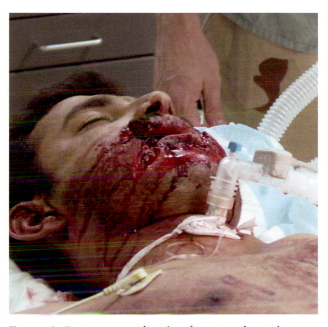

FIGURE 3. *Patient immediately after cricothyroidotomy.*

SUMMARY

This patient required an emergent surgical airway. Medical personnel deployed to combat environments must be trained to perform surgical airways at the site of injury. Cricothyroidotomy is the surgical procedure of choice.

SUGGESTED READING

Chapter 5: Airway/breathing. In: *Emergency War Surgery, Third United States Revision.* Washington, DC: Department of the Army, Office of The Surgeon General, Borden Institute; 2004.

Chapter 13: Face and neck injuries. In: *Emergency War Surgery, Third United States Revision.* Washington, DC: Department of the Army, Office of The Surgeon General, Borden Institute; 2004.

Chapter 22: Soft-tissue injuries. In: *Emergency War Surgery, Third United States Revision.* Washington, DC: Department of the Army, Office of The Surgeon General, Borden Institute; 2004.

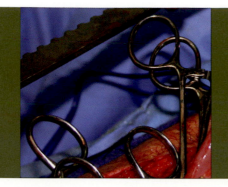

I.3
Devastating Burn, Blast, and Penetrating Injury

CASE PRESENTATION

On admission, this male patient presented with burns covering approximately 60% of his total body surface (Fig. 1). The mechanism of injury was unclear. He received initial care (including intubation because of face and neck burns) and was evacuated to a level III medical treatment facility (combat support hospital [CSH]) that had been established in an austere environment. His oxygenation status remained poor despite intubation and supplemental oxygen. The patient was also tachycardic and hypotensive. Chest wall escharotomies were performed because of decreased chest wall compliance. Aggressive fluid resuscitation was initiated. No gross extremity deformity was noted. However, closer inspection of his left posterolateral chest revealed a fragment wound. Despite fluid and blood infusion, the patient became more hypotensive until all pulses were lost. In the presence of penetrating chest injury and witnessed loss of vital signs, resuscitative thoracotomy was indicated and performed. Open cardiac massage was performed, and resuscitation was successful. Thoracotomy revealed that the left diaphragm had been traversed by the fragment. Consequently, the patient underwent laparotomy in which splenic, gastric, and hepatic injuries were found. Expeditious splenectomy and closure of stomach wounds were performed. The patient required 14 units of blood. He had lost much of his body heat due to the combined effects of burns, fluid resuscitation, thoracotomy, and laparotomy. Despite active rewarming and other aggressive, lifesaving efforts, the patient died.

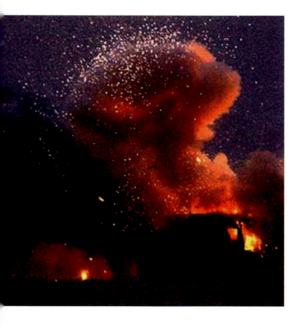

TEACHING POINTS

1. Combat trauma patients may sustain any combination of penetrating, blunt, and thermal injuries as a result of blasts from explosive munitions. Injuries depend on the proximity of the individual to the detonation.

2. Explosive munitions have three mechanisms of injury (Fig. 2); all mechanisms were present in this patient because he was in close proximity to the epicenter of the explosion:

   a. A burn covering approximately 60% of his total body surface.
   b. Evidence of a primary blast injury to the lungs (as observed during resuscitative thoracotomy).
   c. A thoracoabdominal fragment injury (evidence of a ballistic injury).

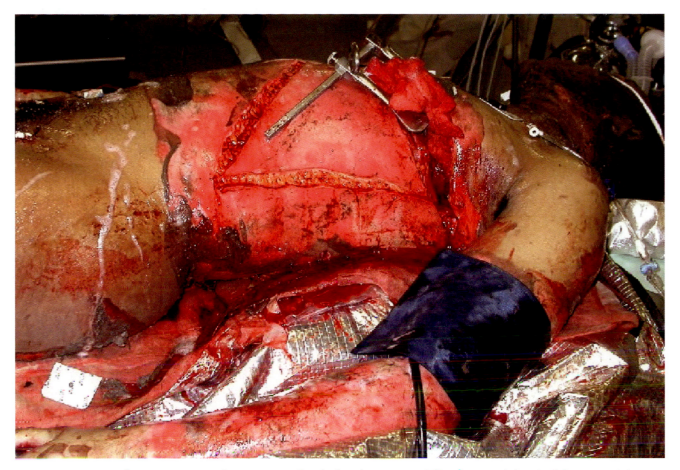

FIGURE 1. *Patient after resuscitative thoracotomy (but before laparotomy) for thoracoabdominal fragment injury.*

CLINICAL IMPLICATIONS

Identifying all weapon effects is not easy. Consider the following points:

1. Thermal injury is usually easily identified, but blast injury is not obvious on superficial examination.
2. The ears, lungs, and gastrointestinal tract are at greatest risk for blast effects.
3. A major thermal injury can obscure a penetrating wound.
4. Thorough secondary survey is mandatory to avoid missing life-threatening injuries resulting from explosive munitions.
5. Trauma patients with burn injuries, who do not respond to fluid resuscitation, must be reassessed for missed injuries.

DAMAGE CONTROL

The use of resuscitative thoracotomy in the combat zone should be limited to patients in extremis with penetrating thoracic injuries and then only under the most favorable circumstances (eg, small penetrating injury, minimal associated injuries, abundant resources, no other urgent patients). Even in these circumstances, patient salvage is rare. In this case, in which a laparotomy was required for control of ongoing bleeding, the absolute minimal intervention (packing, bowel stapling, ligation of bleeding vessels) is essential.

SUMMARY

This case demonstrates a common difference between combat trauma and civilian trauma. Civilian trauma is typically characterized as penetrating or blunt injury. Combat-injured patients often present with combinations of penetrating, blunt, and thermal injuries. As in civilian trauma, combat-injured patients require thorough secondary surveys to ensure that all life-threatening injuries are identified early in the resuscitation phase. Decisions to forego or undertake basic, aggressive resuscitative efforts, as in this case, are always difficult and include considerations of

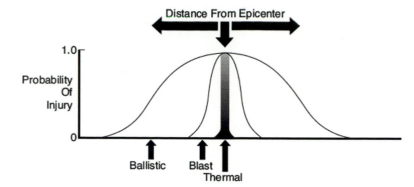

FIGURE 2. *Combat blast injuries often depend on the proximity of the individual to the detonation. In the case examined here, the patient was in close proximity to the epicenter of the explosion.*

INDICATIONS FOR EMERGENCY THORACOTOMY

- Penetrating thoracic trauma.
  - Traumatic arrest with previously witnessed cardiac activity (pre-hospital or in-hospital).
  - Unresponsive hypotension (blood pressure < 70 mm Hg).
- Blunt thoracic injury.
  - Unresponsive hypotension (blood pressure < 70 mm Hg).
  - Rapid exsanguination from chest tube (> 1,500 mL).
- Suspected systemic air embolism.

CONTRAINDICATIONS FOR EMERGENCY THORACOTOMY

- Blunt thoracic injuries with no witnessed cardiac activity.
- Multiple blunt trauma.
- Severe head injury.
- Severe multisystem trauma.

triage, resource availability, nature of the injuries, and individual expertise.

SUGGESTED READING

Chapter 3: Triage. In: *Emergency War Surgery, Third United States Revision.* Washington, DC: Department of the Army, Office of The Surgeon General, Borden Institute; 2004.

Chapter 16: Thoracic injuries. In: *Emergency War Surgery, Third United States Revision.* Washington, DC: Department of the Army, Office of The Surgeon General, Borden Institute; 2004.

Chapter 28: Burns. In: *Emergency War Surgery, Third United States Revision.* Washington, DC: Department of the Army, Office of The Surgeon General, Borden Institute; 2004.

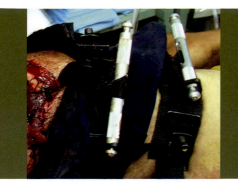

I.4
To Shunt, Repair, or Amputate . . . ?

CASE PRESENTATION

A 23-year-old male sustained multiple blast injuries while riding in a bus when an improvised explosive device (IED) was detonated. The patient arrived at the Emergency Medical Treatment (EMT) section of a combat support hospital (CSH) unit approximately 65 minutes after the attack. He was incoherent and hypotensive on arrival, with a temperature of 97.2°C and a heart rate of 120 beats per minute. His injuries included an open right mandibular fracture, an open right first metacarpal fracture, an open left foot wound, and a large through-and-through medial left thigh wound with a large soft-tissue defect and arterial bleeding. No tourniquet was present, and an attendant was holding direct pressure on the wound. No evidence of left femur fracture was present, and minimal bleeding was noted from the hand, foot, and facial wounds.

PREOPERATIVE ISSUES

1. Obvious arterial injury (likely superficial femoral artery [SFA]).
2. Hypotension/hypovolemia.
3. Associated extremity injuries.

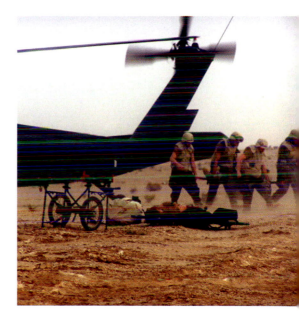

After initial resuscitation via large-bore IVs, the patient was taken to the operating room (OR). A right internal jugular cordis was inserted. Both extremities were prepped while pressure was maintained on the left thigh point of hemorrhage. His initial hematocrit was 24%. Exploration of the wound revealed near transection of the SFA and transection of the femoral vein. Atraumatic clamps were applied to gain proximal and distal control of the SFA, and the vein was ligated. Bleeding was effectively stopped following these measures.

DECISION POINT

*Repair vascular injury vs shunt vascular injury
vs primary amputation*

Given the patient's hemodynamic stability with ongoing resuscitation and the cessation of significant bleeding, arterial repair with an interposition of reversed femoral vein was performed. The anesthesia team administered 4 units of packed red blood cells during the repair, and the laboratory prepared

4 units of fresh frozen plasma (FFP). Palpable pulses were not present, but an intraoperative arteriogram revealed flow to the foot. After release of the clamps, the patient demonstrated clinical evidence of coagulopathy by diffuse bleeding, and his blood pressure dropped. This condition was treated with additional warmed crystalloid and 2 units of whole blood; a shortage of FFP and difficulties thawing the available plasma precluded transfusion of concentrated factors. The patient's coagulopathy and acidosis worsened, and efforts to staunch nonsurgical bleeding from transected muscle and wound edges were unsuccessful. His body temperature fell to 34°C, and acidosis and hypotension did not respond to resuscitation. A damage control approach was taken: efforts to halt bleeding were aborted, all wounds were packed, a dopamine drip was initiated, and the patient was taken to the intensive care unit (ICU). Because no standard active warming devices were available, an improvised heater resembling a Bair Hugger was constructed using biohazard bags and a space heater. The patient received additional warmed whole blood and FFP; and sodium bicarbonate was also administered. Hypotension worsened and an epinephrine drip was started. His blood pressure could not be maintained despite additional pressors, and he became asystolic soon afterward. Further advanced cardiac life support measures were unsuccessful; and, despite aggressive resuscitative efforts, the patient died.

LEARNING POINTS

1. Before undertaking vascular reconstruction, all aspects of the patient's status (hemodynamic, coagulation parameters, urine output, and core body temperature) should be evaluated to determine if repair can/should proceed at that time. Not all of these data were or will be simultaneously available. Once a vascular repair has begun, it becomes difficult to break the operative flow and consider additional information (current core temperature, trend in coagulation parameters, response to ongoing resuscitation). It also becomes psychologically difficult to stop a repair once it has been initiated. Therefore, it is critical to communicate effectively with the anesthesia staff and to accurately assess the patient's condition before making the decision to repair, shunt, or amputate.

2. Hypothermia can be insidious but deadly, and can contribute to coagulopathy and acidosis. In this case, the OR heater was inoperable long after the case had started. Improvised active heaters, fluid warmers, and other adjuncts (IV bags warmed in a microwave and placed alongside the body, etc) should be used when standard equipment is unavailable.

3. The release of clamps after a vascular repair can severely impact a patient who was previously stable. Communication with the anesthesia staff to warn them of the impending return of flow (with potassium, metabolic acids, and inflammatory mediators) can help them prepare for the hemodynamic sequelae of clamp release. Do not assume that the anesthesia personnel are aware of the surgeon's actions or intentions.

SUMMARY/DAMAGE CONTROL

In retrospect, this patient's chances of survival would have been significantly improved if the SFA had been shunted or ligated and damage control had been implemented by packing the soft-tissue wounds and moving the patient to the ICU for resuscitation and warming.

SUGGESTED READING

Chapter 13: Face and neck injuries. In: *Emergency War Surgery, Third United States Revision*. Washington, DC: Department of the Army, Office of The Surgeon General, Borden Institute; 2004.

Chapter 22: Soft-tissue injuries. In: *Emergency War Surgery, Third United States Revision*. Washington, DC: Department of the Army, Office of The Surgeon General, Borden Institute; 2004.

Chapter 23: Extremity fractures. In: *Emergency War Surgery, Third United States Revision*. Washington, DC: Department of the Army, Office of The Surgeon General, Borden Institute; 2004.

Chapter 26: Injuries to the hands and feet. In: *Emergency War Surgery, Third United States Revision*. Washington, DC: Department of the Army, Office of The Surgeon General, Borden Institute; 2004.

Chapter 27: Vascular injuries. In: *Emergency War Surgery, Third United States Revision*. Washington, DC: Department of the Army, Office of The Surgeon General, Borden Institute; 2004.

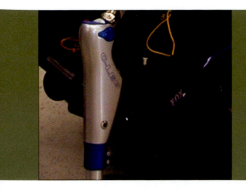

1.5
Extremity Trauma With Profound Shock

CASE PRESENTATION

A US serviceman on a secure compound was within 10 feet of the impact point of a large mortar round and suffered severe injuries. He remained conscious and had an adequate airway despite severe bleeding that could not be completely controlled at the scene with direct pressure. He was transported immediately to a combat support hospital (CSH) that was less than a mile away. In the resuscitation area, pressure that was applied at the wounding scene was maintained by medical personnel despite minimal bleeding. He had sustained severe extremity and soft-tissue wounds, including a traumatic amputation of the right hand, a left arm radial artery injury with soft-tissue injury to the hand, a near amputation of the left leg, and severe injuries to the right leg (Fig. 1). The patient underwent rapid resuscitation by the assembled trauma team, which included emergency room and critical care physicians, nurses, medics, surgeons, and anesthesia providers. He was intubated, a right subclavian central line was inserted, and 4 units of packed red blood cells (PRBCs) were rapidly transfused. The walking blood bank was activated immediately so that fresh whole blood would be available within 45 minutes. The patient was transported immediately to the operating room (OR), where his resuscitation continued (Fig. 2).

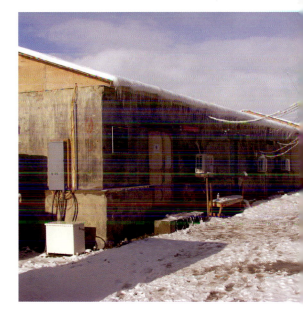

An end femoral artery arterial line was placed because no other sites were immediately available. His initial arterial line pressure was 80/40 mm Hg. The near amputation of the left leg was completed, requiring a hip disarticulation. Because of the extensive soft tissue, bone, nerve, and vascular damage to the right leg—as well as the patient's critical condition—a transfemoral amputation was performed quickly. A rapid laparotomy was done and a loop colostomy fashioned. The right arm stump was debrided, as was the soft-tissue injury to the left thenar eminence. The left radial artery, which now began to bleed profusely, was ligated after it was clear that the hand was adequately perfused by the ulnar circulation. Wounds were dressed by sponges held in place by stapling expandable mesh dressing to the skin (Fig. 3). The patient's intraoperative hematocrit (after the initial 4 units of PRBCs) was 15, and he was transfused with additional units of fresh whole blood that were available. He was taken to the intensive care unit (ICU) where warming and further resuscitation were continued. Once stable, the patient was evacuated by a standby Critical Care Air Transport Team to the level IV medical treatment facility in Landstuhl, Germany. After

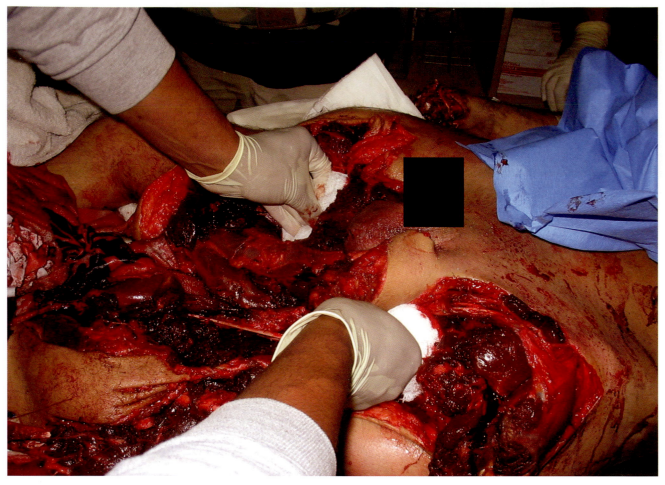

FIGURE 1. *Patient at arrival to the Emergency Medical Treatment (EMT) area. Note direct pressure applied to the transected ends of both femoral arteries.*

a brief stopover, he was evacuated to a level V medical facility in the United States, where he arrived just 36 hours after leaving the CSH (Fig. 4). After multiple surgical procedures and extensive rehabilitation (Figs. 5 and 6), he was medically retired and is currently fully employed (Fig. 7).

CLINICAL IMPLICATIONS

1. Because of the relative youth of most combat casualties, the initial vital signs (heart rate, blood pressure) and ongoing bleeding may not alert the resuscitation team to the degree of hypovolemic shock at initial presentation. Immediate recognition of profound shock in severe combat injuries, particularly those created by large explosions (improvised explosive devices [IEDs] and mortar/artillery munitions), is critical to patient survival.

2. Patients who arrive with massive injuries (traumatic amputations; open abdominal or chest injuries;

large, soft-tissue wounds of multiple extremities) are in profound shock virtually at the moment of wounding and require aggressive, immediate resuscitation (see end-of-chapter Commentary).

TEACHING POINTS

1. Severely wounded patients with multiple areas of injury benefit from a team approach to trauma care. From the initial scene of wounding through resuscitation, surgery, stabilization, and critical care in the ICU, through continuation of critical care during evacuation and definitive care and rehabilitation, an experienced team of healthcare providers offers the greatest chance of survival and functional outcome for those who suffer from war wounds. Teams at each level of care, as well as the entire team of the military healthcare system extending from the battlefield to stateside medical centers, are critical to patient survival and outcome.

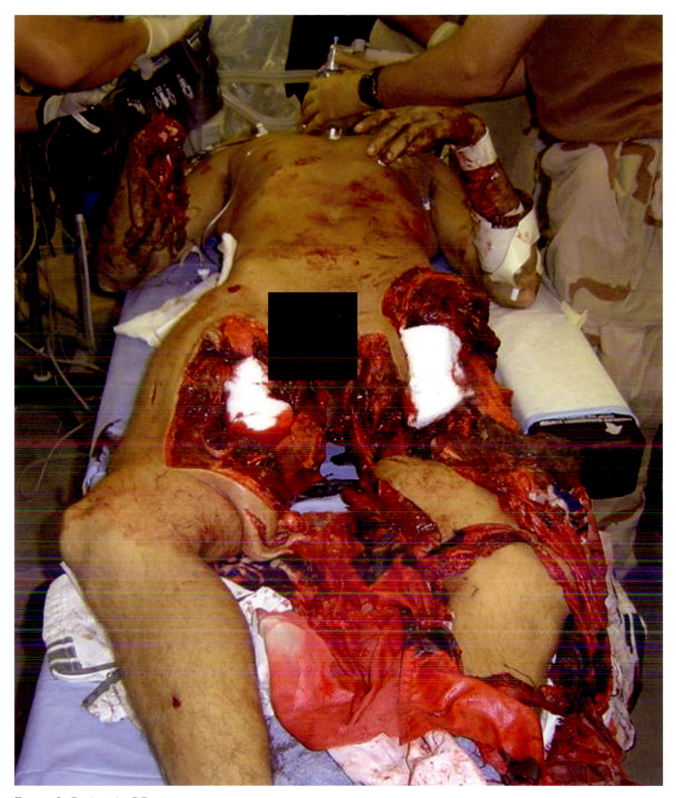

FIGURE 2. *Patient in OR.*

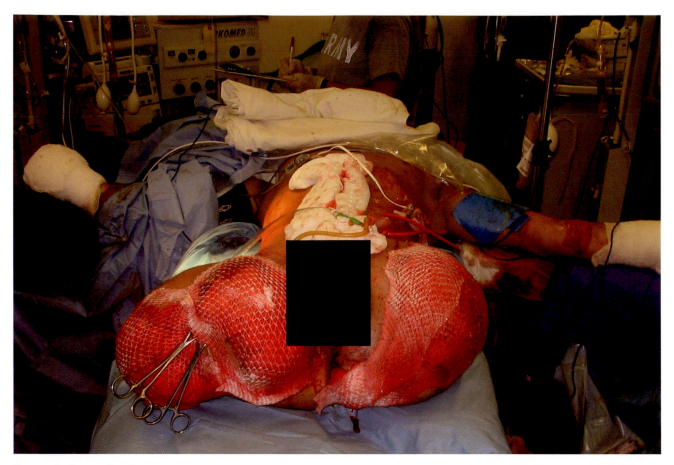

FIGURE 3. *Immediately post-op.*

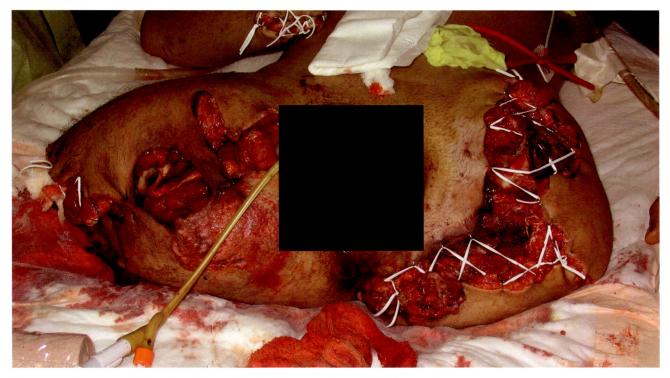

FIGURE 4. *Patient at Walter Reed Army Medical Center during initial examination.*

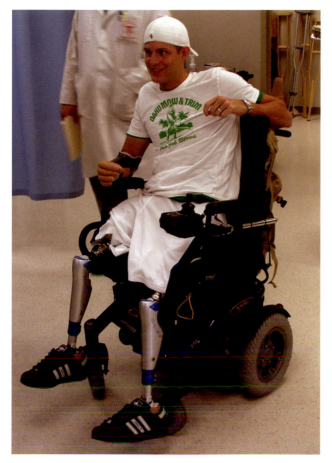

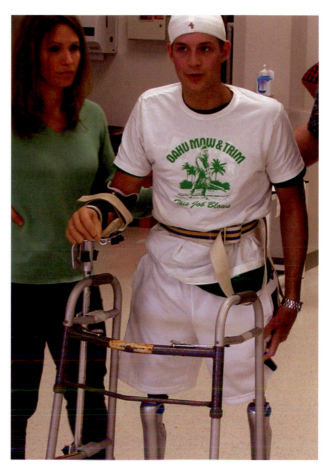

FIGURE 5. *Several months after wounding during rehabilitation.*

FIGURE 6. *Further rehabilitation.*

2. In the deployed setting, the OR is often the best location to resuscitate a patient with severe wounds, allowing excellent 360-degree patient access to multiple providers, superior airway control (anesthesia personnel), monitoring, temperature control, and pain control. Even if a surgical procedure is not needed, or deferred because of damage control considerations, the patient can be assessed quickly and resuscitation initiated in this location.

DAMAGE CONTROL

1. In the face of severe hemorrhage and extensive tissue injury, hypothermia, coagulopathy, and acidosis are ever-present threats to patient survival. An early decision for damage control—using abbreviated surgery with the goal of controlling hemorrhage, stopping contamination, and removing nonviable tissue—often proves to be critical to a favorable outcome.

2. Once the patient achieves physiological stability in the ICU, a return to the OR for further definitive surgery can be considered. In addition, patients may be transported to a higher level of care once stabilized, as in this case.

SUMMARY

Extensive combat wounds often result in profound shock, requiring immediate assessment, recognition, and resuscitation. Having an experienced trauma team assembled and prepared is critical to patient survival. Resuscitation in the OR offers many advantages for a critically injured patient over that available in a crowded resuscitation area. An early decision to use damage control techniques, based on the patient's physiological condition, is often the most important link to avoiding the deadly triad of hypothermia, coagulopathy, and acidosis. The "chain of custody" for the wounded patient—from the point of wounding

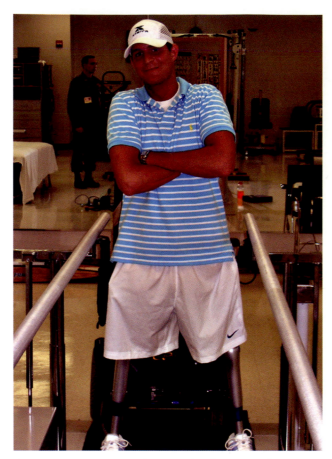

FIGURE 7. *Approximately 2 years after wounding.*

COAGULOPATHY

Clinical evidence of coagulopathy may be seen as "microvascular bleeding," a diffuse bleeding from surgically cut or traumatically damaged tissue surfaces, and bleeding from mucosal surfaces and around intravascular catheters. Laboratory evidence of coagulopathy is often said to be elevated prothrombin time (PT) or partial thromboplastin time (PTT), without specifying how much elevation. Published guidelines suggest using a cutoff of 1.5 times normal (midrange of PT reference or upper end of PTT). The suggested dose of fresh frozen plasma to correct coagulopathy is 10 to 15 mL/kg of patient body weight, usually 4 to 6 units of fresh frozen plasma for the average adult.

The use of the international normalized ratio (INR) is not advocated. The INR was developed and validated with respect to anticoagulation with coumadin. In any event, the PT value is arbitrary. It should be recognized that the PT value is a crude evaluation of a complex hemostatic system.

on the battlefield, through resuscitation, initial surgery, further resuscitation, critical care transport to definitive care, and final rehabilitation—requires a global team effort provided by the US military.

SUGGESTED READING

Chapter 7: Shock and resuscitation. In: *Emergency War Surgery, Third United States Revision*. Washington, DC: Department of the Army, Office of The Surgeon General, Borden Institute; 2004.

Chapter 11: Critical care. In: *Emergency War Surgery, Third United States Revision*. Washington, DC: Department of the Army, Office of The Surgeon General, Borden Institute; 2004.

Chapter 17: Abdominal injuries. In: *Emergency War Surgery, Third United States Revision*. Washington, DC: Department of the Army, Office of The Surgeon General, Borden Institute; 2004.

Chapter 22: Soft-tissue injuries. In: *Emergency War Surgery, Third United States Revision*. Washington, DC: Department of the Army, Office of The Surgeon General, Borden Institute; 2004.

Chapter 24: Open joint injuries. In: *Emergency War Surgery, Third United States Revision*. Washington, DC: Department of the Army, Office of The Surgeon General, Borden Institute; 2004.

Chapter 27: Vascular injuries. In: *Emergency War Surgery, Third United States Revision*. Washington, DC: Department of the Army, Office of The Surgeon General, Borden Institute; 2004.

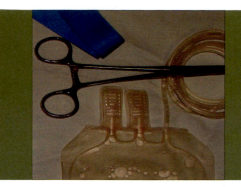

I.6
Massive Blood Transfusion in a Patient With Hemoperitoneum

CASE PRESENTATION

A Forward Surgical Team (FST) in remote Afghanistan was notified approximately 30 minutes prior to the arrival of a 24-year-old US soldier with multiple AK-47 gunshot wounds. The patient was reported to be tachycardic, hypotensive, and in severe distress. A whole blood drive was initiated immediately, and 4 units of fresh frozen plasma (FFP) were thawed in preparation for an anticipated requirement for massive transfusion. On arrival, the patient was noted to have been shot through the right chest, and the right and left lower extremities. He arrived tachycardic with a heart rate of 150 beats per minute and a blood pressure of 90 systolic with an obviously distended abdomen. He had a 14-gauge needle thoracostomy in the second intercostal space of the right chest. Resuscitation with packed red blood cells (PRBCs) and FFP was initiated immediately, and a chest tube was placed in the right chest with little return of blood. A right subclavian cordis was placed, and the patient was taken to the operating room (OR) for exploratory laparotomy. Prior to induction with general anesthesia, a Foley catheter was placed, and he was prepped with betadine solution from the neck to the ankles. The surgeons and assistants were gowned, and the patient was draped in anticipation of a profound drop in blood pressure after induction. The patient's blood pressure dropped to 70 systolic at induction. The abdomen was rapidly opened through a midline incision, and massive hemoperitoneum was encountered. All four quadrants were immediately packed. The hemoperitoneum was the result of severe injuries of the liver, duodenum, stomach, colon, and segmental mesenteric arteries. Pulsatile bleeding from the mesenteric arteries was rapidly controlled by ligation. The packs were then removed from the liver. A large, grade 4, stellate laceration could not be controlled by packing. Therefore, a Pringle maneuver was performed, and the large, segmental hepatic veins were identified and eventually controlled with ligation using suture and surgical clips. During this portion of the operation, blood loss was significant. The patient ultimately received 12 units of fresh whole blood (FWB), 12 units of PRBCs, 13 units of FFP, 5 units of cryoprecipitate, and 7.2 mg of recombinant Factor VIIa. With the liver bleeding controlled, the liver was packed and the patient's heart rate almost immediately decreased. His blood pressure normalized. Laboratory values at the time of the patient's most profound shock were significant for a base deficit of 14. The stomach and duodenal injuries

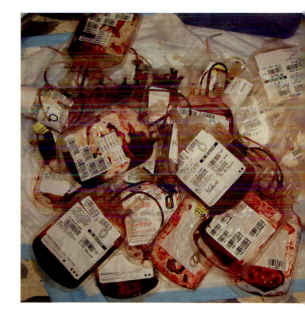

PLASMA

Plasma for transfusion is obtained from volunteer human donors by collection into bags with an anticoagulant preservative mixture. The plasma, or noncellular portion of the blood, is usually separated by centrifugation of a whole blood unit, but can be separated by filter or centrifugation using an automated device. The procedure, known as apheresis, can collect as many as 3 times the volume of plasma as that obtained from a single unit of whole blood, while simultaneously returning the cellular component to the donor.

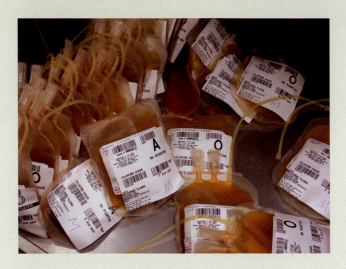

Plasma has been used to treat the combat-injured since World War II. Historically, the initial intent was to use it as a colloid for volume replacement. However, its usefulness to replace coagulation factors in bleeding patients with factor deficiency has been advocated in routine civilian practice for trauma and nontrauma conditions. There is little scientific evidence supporting the practice or to suggest the best practice. However, it seems rational that, in a patient with laboratory or clinical evidence of coagulopathy associated with bleeding, replacement with plasma may correct the factor deficiency and reduce bleeding.

Plasma is separated from the cellular portion of blood and frozen (fresh frozen plasma) within 8 hours of collection. Because of the sometimes long distances between organized blood drives and the fixed facilities with equipment for separation and freezing, the 8-hour requirement cannot always be met. In this case, separation of the plasma still occurs within 8 hours, but freezing may occur up to 24 hours after collection. Either variety, once thawed before transfusion, has essentially the same concentrations of key plasma proteins. These two varieties are similar to liquid plasma never frozen. There is a very small decrement in Factor V concentration and a larger decrement in Factor VIII when stored as a liquid over time. Refrigeration slows the degradation of plasma proteins, and coagulation factors remain little changed for as long as 5 days. Therefore, any of these types of plasma, kept liquid and refrigerated up to 5 days, can be used for the same indications. (The exception is use of the stored plasma for Factor V replacement. This use is not relevant for treating the coagulopathy of a trauma patient.)

The details of collection, processing, and storage may differ, but the different variations produce little significant clinical variation overall. Each unit of plasma has much the same concentration of plasma proteins as normal plasma, and the variation from unit to unit is that of normal human variation. Keeping in mind unit-to-unit variation, plasma as a single unit of fresh frozen plasma has the following qualities:

- Overall volume: 190–220 mL (includes about 25 mL of anticoagulant preservative).
- Coagulation factors, including anticoagulants and fibrinolytic activity in normal concentrations.
- Plasma proteins, including antibodies, notably the red cell major group (ABO) isohemaglutinins, an antibody that is usually and predictably present based on the donor's blood type:

Type A donor plasma:	anti-B.
Type B donor plasma:	anti-A.
Type AB donor plasma:	no anti-ABO.
Type O donor plasma:	anti-A, anti-B, anti-AB.

Consideration of ABO Type

Plasma from AB donors has no anti-A or anti-B, and should cause no direct incompatibility with the red cells of any blood type. Type O donor plasma has both anti-A and anti-B, and thus is incompatible with the majority of patients of the other types (A, B, and AB). Therefore, when the need for emergency plasma transfusion is infrequent, the choice of plasma for prethawing and emergency transfusion should be AB. However, when plasma is frequently transfused to patients without known ABO type, the use of AB plasma will quickly deplete the inventory, and AB recipients who need more plasma will not have any available.

When large numbers of plasma units are transfused, the best choice of type that balances resources with risk to recipient is **plasma of type A donors**. For those situations, type A plasma should be chosen for the prethawed emergent transfusion. Type A plasma is compatible with O and A recipients. Incompatible recipients (B and AB) make up a minority of the general population. Because the B antigen has weaker antibody affinity and is present in lower numbers on red cells than A, the anti-B in A plasma is less likely to cause problems in an incompatible recipient. Further mitigating immediate incompatibility due to transfused anti-B, plasma also contains the B (or A) antigen of a person's blood type. The B antigen in a recipient's plasma provides a neutralizing substance that reduces antibody availability to bind red cells.

The volume of incompatible plasma should be limited, because continued transfusion of incompatible plasma will eventually coat red cells and can cause hemolysis. Type-specific plasma should be given as soon as possible, and only the initial 2 units or so should be given as type A, prethawed.

Recent retrospective study of transfusion patterns and clinical outcomes in the Operation Iraqi Freedom and Operation Enduring Freedom (Afghanistan) conflicts suggests an approach, or a guide, to dosing fresh frozen plasma in bleeding patients with coagulopathy. In a retrospective comparison of red cell and plasma transfusion patterns and mortality, a packed red cell to plasma unit ratio of 1–2:1 was associated with the lowest mortality. (See sidebar on pages 44–45.)

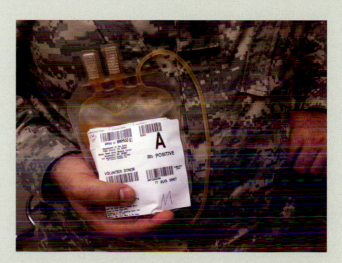

Based on this observation and existing guidelines, the following recommendation is reasonable: For a patient with laboratory and clinical evidence of coagulopathy, the early use of plasma to treat bleeding may use a ratio of packed red cells to plasma of 1–2:1. However, the use of this ratio should <u>not</u> be applied for all patients, or any bleeding patient without coagulopathy. Such an unrestrained practice would contribute to a depletion of resources without expected benefit—a use of resources that should be reserved for the coagulopathic patient with uncontrolled hemorrhage.

—Francis M. Chiricosta, MD, LTC, MC, US Army

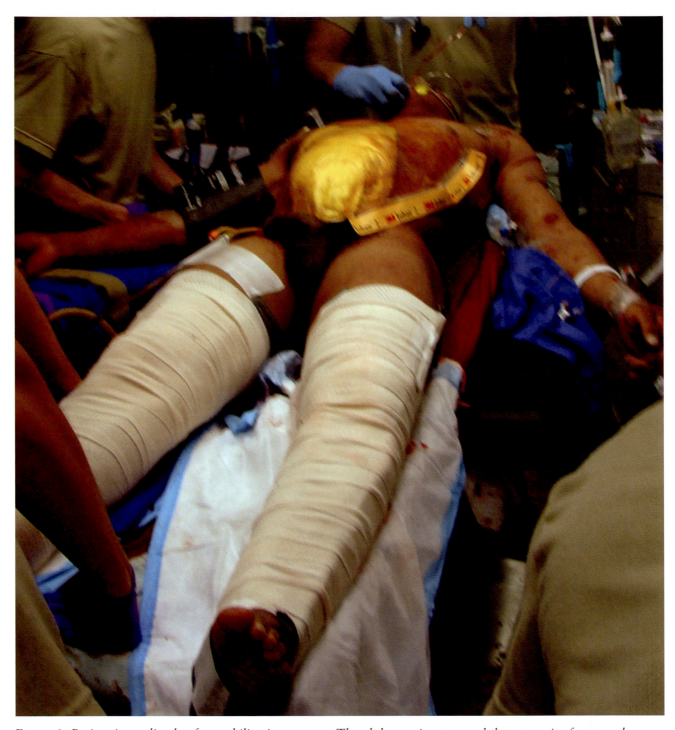

FIGURE 1. *Patient immediately after stabilization surgery. The abdomen is open, and the extremity fractures have been splinted, deferring additional surgery until the patient is stable.*

were controlled with staples, and colon and bowel injuries were resected without creation of anastomoses. The abdomen was closed with a Bogota bag after being washed out with saline. The patient's extremity wounds were then rapidly assessed. Bleeding from the open wounds was controlled with chitosan dressings and packing, and his fractures were splinted (Fig. 1). He was taken to the post-op recovery area. Labs drawn in the immediate post-op period were significant for a base deficit of 3, with a hematocrit of 32%. The patient's heart rate was consistently less than 100, and his systolic blood pressure was consistently above 120 mm Hg. Within 1 hour of surgery, the patient was transferred to a level III military medical treatment facility for ongoing care.

TEACHING POINTS

In patients with massive hemoperitoneum shock, profound hypotension at the time of anesthesia induction and surgical opening must be anticipated. Meticulous attention to detail will allow the surgical team to respond to this predictable event.

1. Prepare (sterilely) and drape the patient prior to induction of anesthesia. The loss of sympathetic tone during induction will result in an acute drop in the patient's blood pressure. Opening the abdomen and releasing the peritoneal tamponade will exacerbate the hypotension. The requirement for blood products will likely increase during this time until the source of hemorrhage is controlled.
2. Establish effective intravenous access. Two large-bore intravenous catheters may be inadequate, and placement of a cordis central catheter should be strongly considered.
3. Begin the transfusion of blood products prior to surgery, if possible. Thaw FFP, and call for FWB or platelets as early as possible. Warm all fluids to 40°C and minimize crystalloid infusion. Use recombinant Factor VIIa with the initial transfusions.
4. Transfer the patient to the OR as soon as possible. This facilitates rapid entry into the chest or abdomen in the event of acute decompensation. Resuscitation of the shock trauma casualty should be considered an urgent OR event and should not be delayed by emergency room evaluation and resuscitative endeavors.

5. Control intraabdominal hemorrhage initially with tight packing of all quadrants. Then, address bleeding sites one quadrant at a time.
6. Place sponges (when packing the liver) in such a way as to approximate the fractured lobes of the liver and compress bleeding sites. This frequently requires posterior packing and may require mobilization of the liver to varying degrees. A Pringle maneuver may be helpful.
7. Note: When bleeding is arrested, rapidly control any source of peritoneal contamination from bowel injury. Do not attempt to create any anastomosis, and stomal creation is unwise. Pack the abdomen and leave the abdominal fascia open. Place a Bogota bag or wound VAC and plan to evacuate or return to the OR when the patient has stabilized.

CLINICAL IMPLICATIONS

Uncontrolled hemorrhage remains the leading cause of potentially preventable death in the present conflicts in Southwest Asia. Massive transfusion is administered to approximately 7% to 8% of combat casualties. Combat surgeons must be familiar with the blood product resources available to them, and they must also be experts in the administration of blood products and know the indications for their use. In austere environments, blood products are available in varying amounts; but, trained blood bank technicians may not be available, thus leaving the physician completely responsible for the safe administration of this lifesaving resource. When combat-wounded patients require transfusion, the following guidelines apply:

1. Begin resuscitation with PRBCs. If four or more units of PRBCs are required, transfuse FFP at a ratio (PRBCs:FFP) of 1:1 or 2:1. Minimize resuscitation with crystalloid, which can cause a dilutional coagulopathy.[1]
2. If massive transfusion (defined as 10 units or more of PRBCs) is anticipated, then platelets should also be administered. If platelets are not available, then FWB should be given.[2]
3. FWB is blood that has been recently drawn. It provides red blood cells, plasma, clotting factors, and platelets. One unit of FWB is the equivalent of 1 unit of PRBCs and 1 unit of FFP. It contains the equivalent of 20,000 to 30,000 plts/cc.[3] FWB is indicated for use in an austere environment where component

PLATELETS vs FRESH WHOLE BLOOD IN MASSIVE TRANSFUSION

In the treatment of coagulopathy and bleeding in trauma patients, the use of plasma alone cannot always be effective. Progressive thrombocytopenia is associated with continued bleeding and transfusion. Platelet transfusion can be helpful.

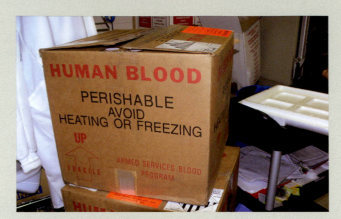

Civilian trauma centers in the United States have available a variety of blood components to treat bleeding. Commonly used among these components are platelets. Conversely, although fresh whole blood (FWB) use is limited in the United States, the military routinely utilizes FWB in the setting of massive transfusion (MT) as both a source of platelets and other factors when large quantities of blood are required.

Surgeons have anecdotally reported rapid correction of microvascular bleeding after infusion of FWB. However, there are drawbacks and dangers to FWB transfusion that can be avoided or lessened by the use of separated platelets.

An emergency whole blood drive ("walking blood bank") requires the commitment of many healthcare workers and donors, taking them away from other duties at the precise time of high demand to treat trauma. Platelets, on the other hand, can be precollected at a scheduled time of the platelet collector's and donor's choosing. Freshly collected whole blood cannot be adequately tested for transfusion-transmitted disease. With platelet collections, donors can be tested ahead of time and once shown to be test-negative, a single donor can donate twice a week, providing many doses for treatment over the course of 2 months. A donor of whole blood can safely donate only 1 unit in that time, and it is not pretested. The ABO type of whole blood must be type-compatible with the recipient. Safe practice (typing of the donor, ensuring the unit is labeled with that type, typing the recipient, and ensuring that the correctly typed unit goes to the correctly typed recipient) is a many-step process with a high likelihood of error in a stressful emergency or mass casualty setting. The type compatibility of a platelet unit can be obtained carefully and double-checked in the quiet between emergencies. ABO-incompatible platelet transfusion is much less likely to cause a fatal hemolytic reaction than an incompatible whole blood transfusion.

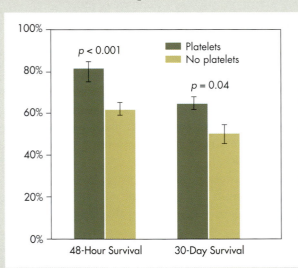

FIGURE 1. *48-hour and 30-day survival by platelet vs no platelet groups. Groups compared using chi-square. Forty-eight-hour survival: platelet group—218/266, 82 ± 2%; no platelet group—90/137, 66 ± 3%; p < 0.001. Thirty-day survival: platelet group—121/196, 62 ± 4%; no platelet group—53/107, 50 ± 5%; p = 0.04.*

In a study of transfusion patterns and outcomes in Operation Iraqi Freedom/Operation Enduring Freedom (performed by MAJ Jeremy Perkins), the use of whole blood or the use of apheresis platelets (aPLTs; collected in theater) in massively transfused patients resulted in lessened mortality than in patients without the use of either. The outcome was similar whether whole blood or platelets were used (in addition to packed red cells and plasma). Because platelet units maintain usefulness and safety only if stored for less than 5 days, and given the long time it takes to transport supplies from the United States to a deployed military medical treatment facility in theater, if platelets were to be transfused in Iraq and Afghanistan by US medical treatment facilities, they would have to be collected in theater.

In November 2004, the combat support hospital (CSH) in Baghdad, Iraq, acquired the capability to collect (by apheresis) and provide platelets (aPLTs) onsite. This offered a unique opportunity to compare not only outcomes of patients managed with and without platelets, but also to compare outcomes for patients who received FWB as compared with those receiving aPLTs. Records for trauma admissions to the CSH in

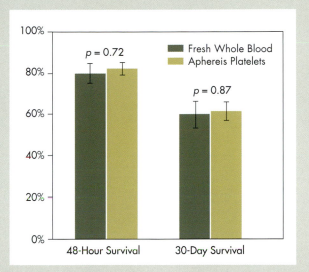

FIGURE 2. *48-hour and 30-day survival by FWB vs aPLT groups. Groups compared using chi-square. Forty-eight-hour survival: FWB—56/70, 80 ± 5%; aPLT group—143/174, 82 ± 3%; p = NS. Thirty-day survival: FWB—36/60, 60 ± 6%; aPLT group—72/117, 62 ± 5%; p = NS. NS: not significant.*

Baghdad between January 2004 and December 2006 who required an MT were reviewed. MT, defined as transfusion of 10 units of packed red blood cells and/or FWB in 24 hours, was administered to 708/8,618 (8.2%) trauma admissions. Of the 708 requiring MT, records were available for 535 patients. Of these, another 101 patients were excluded because they were managed at Forward Surgical Team (FST) facilities or did not receive total transfusion in the first 24 hours. Of the remaining 434 patients, 285 received platelets either as FWB or as aPLTs, and 149 patients received no platelets (neither FWB nor aPLTs). Forty-eight-hour (82% vs 66%, p < 0.001) and 30-day (62% vs 50%, p = 0.04) survival were higher in patients receiving platelets, compared with those who did not receive platelets (Fig. 1). Analysis of FWB and aPLT subgroups showed no differences for 48-hour (80% vs 82%, p = 0.7) or 30-day (60% vs 62%, p = 0.9) survival (Fig. 2). Multivariate logistic regression was performed and showed that both FWB and aPLTs were independently predictive of survival. In this regression, higher fresh frozen plasma/red blood cell ratios were independently predictive of improved survival at 48 hours, consistent with data published by Borgman et al.[1]

Transfusion of platelets either in the form of aPLTs or FWB is associated with improved survival in patients requiring MT. There do not appear to be survival differences between patients managed with FWB, compared with aPLTs (in addition to packed red blood cells and plasma). Because of an easier collection process and its better safety profile, the use of platelets as part of the transfusion treatment of coagulopathy and bleeding should be preferred over the use of whole blood when the former is available.

At facilities where aPLTs or other blood components are unavailable, FWB is an acceptable alternative for the management of coagulopathy in patients requiring MT.

—MAJ JEREMY PERKINS, MD, AND FRANCIS M. CHIRICOSTA, MD

1. Borgman MA, Spinella PC, et al. The ratio of blood products transfused affects mortality in patients receiving massive transfusions at a combat support hospital. *J Trauma*. 2007;63:805–813.

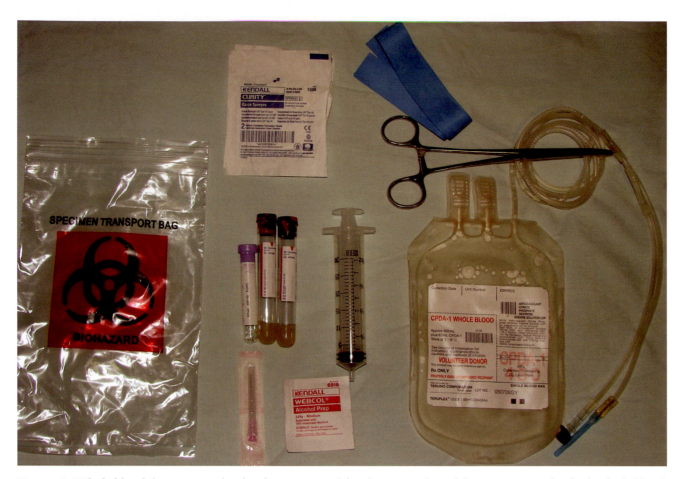

FIGURE 2. *Whole blood donation set that has been prepared for the eventuality of the requirement for fresh whole blood.*

therapy is not available. In the current operating environments in Southwest Asia, it is primarily used by level II FSTs to provide platelets in patients requiring massive blood transfusions. It may also be used in lieu of PRBCs, FFP, and cryoprecipitate when these components are in short supply or exhausted.

4. Prior to the present conflicts in Southwest Asia, FWB transfusion was considered nondoctrinal. Training small units, such as FSTs, the technique of drawing and administering blood was not done despite the frequent use of FWB in previous conflicts. Special equipment is required, such as single donor collection bags and blood tubes (Fig. 2), and a centrifuge is required to prepare blood tubes collected for viral testing prior to shipment.

5. The primary concern with the use of FWB is the risk of infectious disease transmission. US service members are prescreened for human immunodeficiency virus (HIV) and are vaccinated for hepatitis B virus (HBV). However, they are not prescreened for hepatitis C virus

(HCV), human T-cell leukemia, or syphilis. There is also the risk of transmission of local endemic diseases (eg, malaria). The risk of transmitting infectious disease is thought to be less than 1%, whereas the risk of dying from hemorrhagic shock is greater than 30% (unpublished data from the Joint Theater Trauma System Clinical Practice Guidelines for Fresh Whole Blood). Therefore, the use of FWB is indicated when pretested component therapy is not available. In combat patients who require massive transfusion, administration of platelets has been shown to improve survival. There is no significant difference in survival in patients who received apheresis platelets versus those who received platelets from FWB transfusion.[1] Rapid screening tests are available for blood type, HBV, HCV, syphilis, and HIV. These tests are not approved by the US Food and Drug Administration, but are still useful in prescreening donors when time permits and if personnel are trained in their use. Blood should be drawn from all donors for

EMERGENCY FRESH WHOLE BLOOD COLLECTION PROCEDURE

The Walking Blood Bank

1. Develop (when possible) a roster of prescreened donors. In all cases, have the donors complete a DD Form 572—Blood Donation Record. Exclude high-risk donors. Prior blood donors have been screened previously for transmittable disease. Donors with recent laboratory confirmation of blood type are ideal, because identification tags (dog tags) are incorrect 2% to 11% of the time.
2. Clean the donor's arm with povidone-iodine or chlorhexidine solution for 1 minute.
3. Draw the blood from an arm vein into a single donor blood collection bag containing anticoagulant, such as citrate, phosphate, dextrose, adenine (CPDA) solution. Draw about 450 cc of blood until the bag is almost full.
4. Draw tubes of blood for typing and crossmatching (EDTA [ethylenediamine tetraacetic acid] purple top) and for testing of blood-borne infectious disease (two serum separator tubes, red and gray tops). The serum separator tubes should be centrifuged for 20 minutes prior to shipment.
5. Inform the operating team (before transfusing blood) that emergency draw fresh whole blood is about to be transfused and confirm blood type and pertinent patient history.
6. Document clearly who the blood was donated from and to whom it was transfused.
7. Obtain and follow any additional theater guidelines and policies for the transfusion of fresh whole blood.

Equipment Required for Fresh Whole Blood Collection (see Fig. 2)

- Blood recipient set (collection bag), indirect Tx Y-type.
- Stopcock, IV therapy three-way, with Luer.
- Serum separator blood tubes.
- EDTA blood tubes.
- Centrifuge.

posttransfusion testing. A record of donation should be kept for both the recipient and the donor in the event that postscreening testing reveals an infectious disease.

6. Type O PRBCs are the only blood type available to FSTs. Doctrinally, FSTs carry 20 units of PRBCs and have a blood refrigerator as organic equipment. FFP is not doctrinally used by FSTs. However, in the current (2007) operating environment, FFP and cryoprecipitate have been made available. This requires a nonstandard blood freezer and a plasma thawing unit. Type O-negative PRBCs are usually reserved for female patients. There is no absolute blood type match for FWB transfusion. However, because patients at the FST almost always receive several units of type O PRBCs before they receive FWB, usually type O FWB is transfused. Ideally, patients receiving FWB would receive type-specific blood. In local national patients and often in coalition forces, the patient's blood type is unknown and type O blood is used.

7. If ongoing bleeding is anticipated and recombinant Factor VIIa is indicated, then it should be administered early when the patient has a pH above 7.1 and is more likely to have adequate functioning coagulation factors.

8. At level II, there is no specifically trained medical director of the blood bank. The commander or surgeon is entirely responsible for the safe administration of blood products. There are many guidelines that attempt to instruct the surgeon on when the administration of whole blood is appropriate. In fact, the decision to administer FWB is a clinical decision that must be made before the onset of coagulopathy and

exsanguination. Allowing the patient to become coagulopathic prior to administering the appropriate blood products will almost always result in the death of the patient. The surgeon must anticipate a delay of up to 1 hour for the transfusion of FWB.

DAMAGE CONTROL

FWB is the most expeditious source of red cells, platelets, and clotting factors in the acute management of combat trauma. The need for massive blood transfusion must be determined early, sometimes before the patient arrives. If FWB use is likely, call for donors early and begin thawing FFP immediately.

SUMMARY

Hypotension and shock from blood loss remain common problems in battlefield trauma. Replenishment of blood either as components or FWB is fundamental to the successful treatment of these patients. All physicians deploying to a war theater must understand the basic principles of transfusion.

REFERENCES

1. Borgman MA, Spinella PC, et al. The ratio of blood products transfused affects mortality in patients receiving massive transfusions at a combat support hospital. *J Trauma.* 2007;63:805–813.
2. Ketchum L, Hess JR, Hiippala S. Indications for early fresh frozen plasma, cryoprecipitate, and platelet transfusion in trauma. *J Trauma.* 2006;60(suppl 6): S51–S58.
3. Repine TB, Perkins JG, et al. The use of fresh whole blood in massive transfusion. *J Trauma.* 2006;60(suppl 6): S59–S69.

Damage Control Resuscitation

by COL John B. Holcomb, MD

Although the vast majority of bleeding trauma patients who arrive in emergency departments (EDs) are either hypercoagulable, or only slightly injured with normal coagulation parameters, a small number of trauma patients (approximately 10%) are hypocoagulable (international normalized ratio [INR] > 1.5).[1,2] This minority constitutes about 50% of those who receive any blood products and represent the majority of in-hospital trauma deaths. Death increases threefold after receiving more than 4 units of blood. Patients are occasionally hypothermic and have acidosis-induced coagulation factor and platelet dysfunction, combined with coagulation factor consumption, culminating in a profound coagulopathy. Although it has been long recognized that the lethal triad of hypothermia, acidosis, and coagulopathy is associated with a significant increase in mortality,[3] coagulopathy has been viewed as a byproduct of resuscitation, hemodilution, and hypothermia. Based on civilian trauma and military combat casualty data, we now know that coagulopathy is, in fact, present on admission.[4-6]

Current resuscitation practice focuses primarily on rapid reversal of acidosis and prevention of hypothermia, whereas concurrent surgical interventions focus on controlling hemorrhage and contamination with sutures and packs. Early intravascular treatment of coagulopathy has been relatively ignored. Standard resuscitation methods are appropriate for the 90% of trauma patients who are not in shock and are hypercoagulable after injury.[7] However, for the 10% of patients who constitute the most seriously injured, are in shock, and are coagulopathic (hypocoagulable), plasma has been identified as the best resuscitation fluid.[8,9] Unfortunately, clinicians are still being taught never to use plasma as a resuscitation fluid.[10]

Recent studies have shown the following:
- Coagulopathy of trauma is present at a very early stage after injury.[1-6]
- Ringer's lactate solution and normal saline increase reperfusion injury and leukocyte adhesion.[11]
- Increased transfusion is associated with increased risks.[12]
- Massive transfusion in military and civilian casualties is associated with an increased risk of death.[13,14]

Taken together, these observations suggest that the most severely injured patients will likely benefit from a new resuscitation strategy focused on optimal timing and modulation of the metabolic, inflammation, and coagulation pathways.

Over the last 6 years, the US Army has gained considerable experience in resuscitation of combat casualties. Based on previous civilian clinical studies, recommendations of an international consensus conference on early, massive transfusion for trauma,[15] and the cumulative experience of experts in the current war, it is possible to rapidly identify patients at high risk for coagulopathy on admission and promptly treat hypothermia, acidosis, and coagulopathy (see Appendix D). This strategy, known as "damage control resuscitation," addresses the entire lethal triad immediately on admission in concert with aggressive hemostatic interventions.[16] Damage control resuscitation as a structured intervention begins immediately after rapid initial assessment in the ED and progresses through the operating room (OR) into the intensive care unit (ICU). Interventions directed at normalizing the INR, base deficit, and temperature included the following:

- Repeated point-of-care testing.
- Commercial warming devices.

- Use of multiple blood products.
- US Food and Drug Administration-approved drugs readily available in theater (albeit in new ratios and amounts).

Compared with civilian damage control surgery resuscitation strategies, deployed resuscitation efforts are largely completed in the OR, with little resuscitation required in the ICU. Achieving this goal quickly in the OR may ultimately allow a shift from limited damage control surgery to earlier, aggressive surgical interventions, including sophisticated limb salvage techniques and improved outcomes.

Damage control resuscitation consists of two parts and is initiated within minutes of arrival in the ED. First, resuscitation volume is limited to keep systolic blood pressure at approximately 90 mm Hg, preventing renewed bleeding from recently clotted vessels.[17–22] Second, intravascular volume restoration is accomplished by using thawed plasma as a primary resuscitation fluid in at least a 1:1 ratio with packed red blood cells (PRBCs).[8,9,23–25] Recombinant Factor VIIa may be used along with the very first units of red blood cells, thawed plasma, and platelets, if indicated by the clinical situation (see Clinical Practice Guidelines for Damage Control Resuscitation at Levels IIb and III [Appendix D]).[26] For casualties who will require continued resuscitation, the blood bank is notified to activate the massive transfusion protocol. This protocol results in the delivery of 6 units of plasma, 6 units of PRBCs, 6 packs of platelets, and 10 units of cryoprecipitate stored in individual coolers. For the most severely injured with refractory bleeding, fresh warm whole blood from the walking blood bank is resorted to as a primary resuscitative fluid.[27,28] Crystalloid use is significantly limited and serves mainly as a carrier to keep lines open between the units of blood products. The very first data from Iraq describing the initial implementation of this approach revealed a decrease in long-term mortality, from 65% to 19%, by using plasma in a 1:1 ratio with PRBCs.[29]

Damage control resuscitation is summarized then as:
- Early diagnosis of hemorrhage/hypovolemic shock in the ED.
- Early diagnosis and aggressive treatment in the ED of the lethal triad.
- A 1:1:1 ratio (thawed plasma:red blood cells:platelets) throughout resuscitation.
- ED/OR/ICU use of recombinant Factor VIIa, as needed.

- Massive transfusion protocol that delivers fixed ratios of products until stopped by the surgeon.
- Rapid use of fresh whole blood in most critical patients with ongoing hemorrhage.
- THAM (tris-hydroxymethyl aminomethane; also known as tromethamine) and Ca^{2+} in the OR to normalize ionized Ca^{2+} and keep the pH > 7.2.[30]
- Minimize crystalloid.[31,32]
- Allow hypotension until definitive (operative) hemorrhage control.

The recommendations described previously are a snapshot of "best in theater resuscitation practice" in June 2006. It is anticipated that these practices will be improved upon as new data are available. Progress in trauma care requires continuous improvement in everyday patient management, based on good clinical studies. Many of our most basic trauma care principles are founded on tradition rather than on evidenced-based best practice. Current resuscitation practices fall into this category, and only now are data emerging in the civilian trauma literature documenting the deleterious effects of aggressive crystalloid resuscitation.[31,32] As in past wars, observation, discussion, analysis, and recommendations from experienced military medics, nurses, physicians, and scientists—together with our civilian trauma colleagues—will provide the basis for new medical practice, grounded in appropriate and relevant preclinical and human studies.[33,34] Injury, procedure, and outcome data collated in the Joint Theater Trauma Registry will provide hypothesis-generating information for years to come. Further experience, research, development, and prospective randomized studies will generate new information and ongoing modifications.

REFERENCES

1. Schreiber MA, Perkins J, et al. Early predictors of massive transfusion in combat casualties. *J Am Coll Surg*. 2007;205:541–545.
2. Niles SE, McLaughlin DF, et al. Increased mortality associated with the early coagulopathy of trauma in combat casualties. Forthcoming.
3. Moore EE. Thomas G. Orr Memorial Lecture. Staged laparotomy for the hypothermia, acidosis, and coagulopathy syndrome. *Am J Surg*. 1996;172:405–410.
4. Faringer PD, Mullins RJ, et al. Blood component supplementation during massive transfusion of AS-1 red cells in trauma patients. *J Trauma*. 1993;34:481–485.

5. Brohi K, Singh J, et al. Acute traumatic coagulopathy. *J Trauma*. 2003;54:1127–1130.

6. MacLeod JB, Lynn M, et al. Early coagulopathy predicts mortality in trauma. *J Trauma*. 2003;55:39–44.

7. Kiraly LN, Differding JA, et al. Resuscitation with normal saline (NS) vs. lactated Ringer's (LR) modulates hypercoagulability and leads to increased blood loss in an uncontrolled hemorrhagic shock swine model. *J Trauma*. 2006;61:57–64.

8. Hirshberg A, Dugas M, et al. Minimizing dilutional coagulopathy in exsanguinating hemorrhage: A computer simulation. *J Trauma*. 2003;54:454–463.

9. Ho AM, Dion PW, et al. A mathematical model for fresh frozen plasma transfusion strategies during major trauma resuscitation with ongoing hemorrhage. *Can J Surg*. 2005;48:470–478.

10. American Society of Anesthesiologists. Practice guidelines for perioperative blood transfusion and adjuvant therapies: An updated report by the American Society of Anesthesiologists Task Force on Perioperative Blood Transfusion and Adjuvant Therapies. *Anesthesiology*. 2006;105:198–208.

11. Cotton BA, Guy JS, et al. The cellular, metabolic, and systemic consequences of aggressive fluid resuscitation strategies. *Shock*. 2006;26:115–121.

12. Rhee P, Wang D, et al. Human neutrophil activation and increased adhesion by various resuscitation fluids. *Crit Care Med*. 2000;28:74–78.

13. Hebert PC, Wells G, et al. A multicenter, randomized, controlled clinical trial of transfusion requirements in critical care. Transfusion requirements in critical care investigators, Canadian Critical Care Trials Group. *N Engl J Med*. 1999;340:409–417.

14. Como JJ, Dutton RP, et al. Blood transfusion rates in the care of acute trauma. *Transfusion*. 2004;44:809–813.

15. Holcomb JB, Hess JR. Early massive trauma transfusion: Current state of the art. *J Trauma*. 2006;60(suppl 6):S1–S59.

16. Holcomb JB, Jenkins D, et al. Damage control resuscitation: Directly addressing the early coagulopathy of trauma. *J Trauma*. 2007;62:307–310.

17. Cannon WB, Fraser J, Cowell EM. The preventive treatment of wound shock. *JAMA*. 1918;70:618–621.

18. Beecher HK. Preparation of battle casualties for surgery. *Ann Surg*. 1945;21:769–792.

19. Bickell WH, Wall MJ, et al. Immediate versus delayed fluid resuscitation for hypotensive patients with penetrating torso injuries. *N Engl J Med*. 1994;331:1105–1109.

20. Dutton RP, Mackenzie CF, Scalea TM. Hypotensive resuscitation during active hemorrhage: Impact on in-hospital mortality. *J Trauma*. 2002;52:1141–1146.

21. Holcomb JB. Fluid resuscitation in modern combat casualty care: Lessons learned from Somalia. *J Trauma*. 2003;54(suppl 5):S46–S51.

22. Sondeen JL, Coppes VG, Holcomb JB. Blood pressure at which rebleeding occurs after resuscitation in swine with aortic injury. *J Trauma*. 2003;54(suppl 5):S110–S117.

23. Ketchum L, Hess JR, Hiippala S. Indications for early fresh frozen plasma, cryoprecipitate, and platelet transfusion in trauma. *J Trauma*. 2006;60(suppl 6):S51–S58.

24. Malone DL, Hess JR, Fingerhut A. Massive transfusion practices around the globe and a suggestion for a common massive transfusion protocol. *J Trauma*. 2006;60(suppl 6):S91–S96.

25. McMullin NR, Holcomb JB, Sondeen JL. Hemostatic resuscitation. In: Vincent JL, ed. *Yearbook of Intensive Care and Emergency Medicine 2006*. Berlin: Springer-Verlag; 2006: 265–278.

26. Perkins JP, Schreiber MA, et al. Early versus late recombinant factor VIIa in combat trauma patients requiring massive transfusion. *J Trauma*. 2007;62:1095–1099.

27. Kauvar DS, Holcomb JB, et al. Fresh whole blood transfusion: A controversial military practice. *J Trauma*. 2006;61:181–184.

28. Repine TB, Perkins JG, et al. The use of fresh whole blood in massive transfusion. *J Trauma*. 2006;60(suppl 6):S59–S69.

29. Borgman MA, Spinella PC, et al. The ratio of blood products transfused affects mortality in patients receiving massive transfusions at a combat support hospital. *J Trauma*. 2007;63:805–813.

30. Martini WZ, Dubick MA, et al. Evaluation of tris-hydroxymethylaminomethane on reversing coagulation abnormalities caused by acidosis in pigs. *Crit Care Med*. 2007;35:1568–1574.

31. Wiedemann HP, Wheeler AP, et al. Comparison of two fluid-management strategies in acute lung injury. *N Engl J Med*. 2006;354:2564–2575.

32. Balogh Z, McKinley BA, et al. Supranormal trauma resuscitation causes more cases of abdominal compartment syndrome. *Arch Surg*. 2003;138:637–643.

33. DeBakey ME. History, the torch that illuminates: Lessons from military medicine. *Mil Med*. 1996;161:711–716.

34. Pruitt BA. Combat casualty care and surgical progress. *Ann Surg*. 2006;243:715–729.

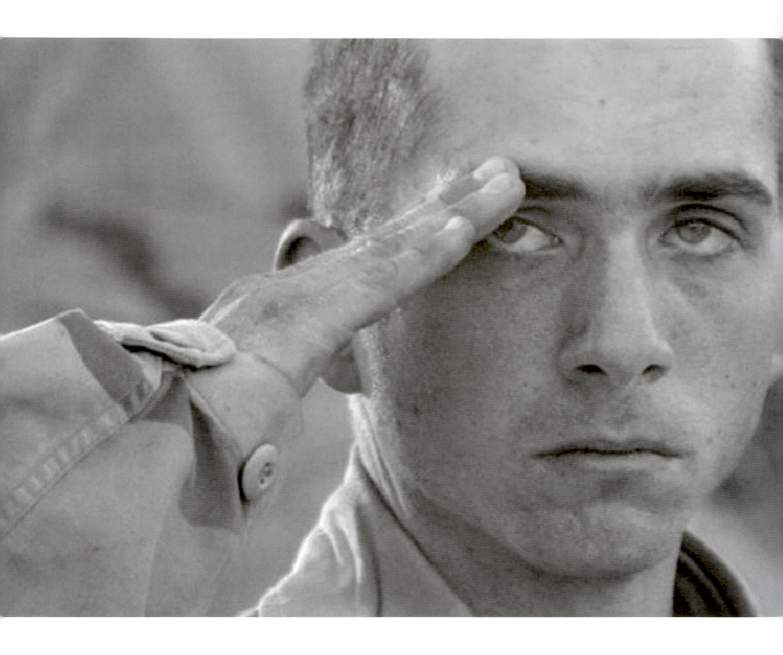

Chapter II
FACE, NECK, AND EYE TRAUMA

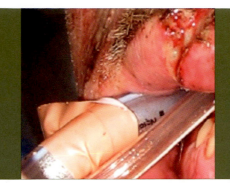

II.1
Complex Facial Wounds

CASE PRESENTATION

A male soldier in his mid-thirties was injured by an improvised explosive device (IED) detonated close to him while he stood near a concrete barrier. He sustained multiple injuries to the face (Figs. 1 and 2), scalp (Fig. 3), and extremities. The patient was orally intubated in the field. A thorough examination that included radiographs revealed macerated facial and scalp wounds impregnated with rocks and dirt, and a partially degloved mandible (Fig. 2). Although exposed, there was no damage to the bony facial skeleton. His vision was intact. During surgery, massive irrigation and debridement of his wounds were performed. Devitalized tissue was debrided, the penetrated tissue was explored, and rocks and dirt were removed with meticulous care. The intraoral mucosa was sutured to cover the exposed mandible and to separate the oral cavity from the face. Moist wet-to-dry sterile dressings were placed on the patient's scalp and face. He was taken to the intensive care unit (ICU) for continued care. The patient was evacuated by air to a level IV medical facility for further treatment.

TEACHING POINTS

1. Note that immediate recognition and appropriate management of airway compromise are critical to survival. A survey for associated eye (proptosis, pupil size), ear (ruptured tympanum), and head trauma is imperative. Patients exposed to blasts may experience iridoplegia (paralysis of the pupil), which does not indicate secondary effect of a central nervous system mass lesion or herniation.

2. Perform wound debridement to thoroughly evaluate the extent of the injury.

3. Perform complete intraoral and extraoral examinations to rule out facial fractures.

4. Cleanse wounds thoroughly with scrub solutions and saline. Use a scrub brush to remove all dirt particles from the dermis. Copious irrigation, forceps (curette and no. 11 blade tip, among other instruments), and strong suction are keys to effective cleansing.

5. Remove foreign bodies with meticulous care in order not to provoke injury to underlying structures. The more time taken initially will improve the cosmetic outcome for the patient.

6. Treat vascular injuries using methods from direct pressure to dissection and ligation of the offending vessel. Blind clamping of bleeding areas should be avoided because critical structures, such as the facial nerve

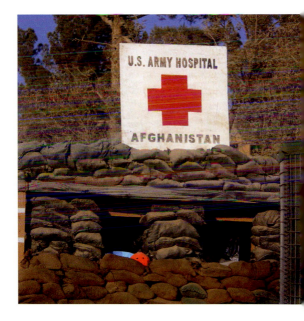

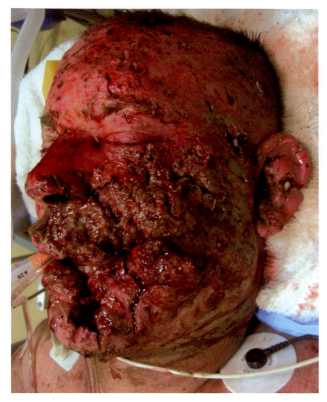

FIGURE 1. *Multiple facial wounds impregnated with sand, rocks, and debris.*

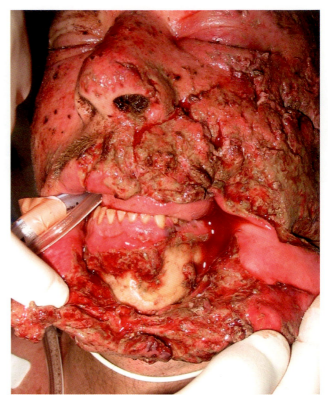

FIGURE 2. *Degloved mandible and extent of wounds.*

and parotid duct, are susceptible to injury. Use sharp debridement of wound edges that are devitalized.

7. Use antibiotics with gram-positive coverage for penetrating injuries to decrease the incidence of infection and to help promote optimal wound healing. Consider tetanus toxoid.

8. In general, in contrast to extremity wounds, primary closure is an important aspect of managing facial lacerations. When primary closure is possible, the wound should be reapproximated in proper layers to optimize an esthetic outcome for the patient (Figs. 4 and 5). In this case, the wounds were so contaminated that primary closure was delayed, and additional irrigation and debridement were required.

CLINICAL IMPLICATIONS

In contrast to similar wounds of other body regions, primary closure of small facial wounds is recommended following thorough cleansing. Closure of deep wounds involving many layers or hasty closure before adequate irrigation and debridement, however, can lead to the following adverse outcomes:

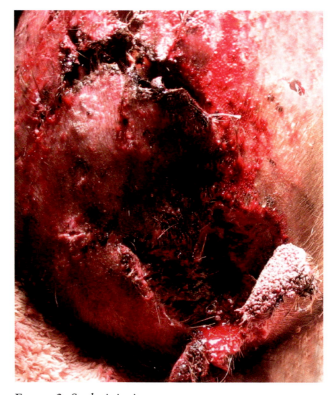

FIGURE 3. *Scalp injuries.*

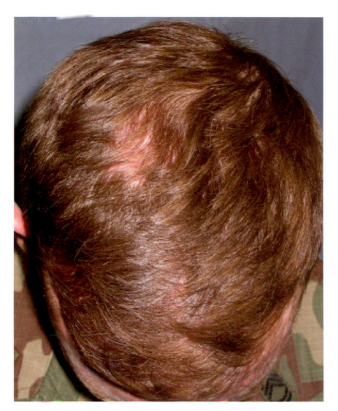

FIGURE 4. *Scalp healing 1-year post-op.*

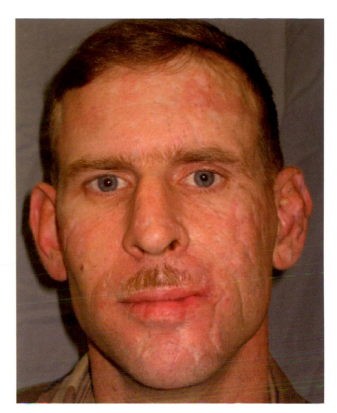

FIGURE 5. *Facial wound healing 1-year post-op.*

1. Infected wounds.
2. Devitalized tissues being inadvertently incorporated into the wounds.
3. Inadequate debridement of wounds with retention of foreign bodies.
4. Tattooing as a result of inadequate dirt removal.

DAMAGE CONTROL

For mild bleeding, use compression. For significant bleeding, perform ligation of the vessel. Direct visual location of the vessel is necessary before vessel ligation to prevent damaging the parotid duct or facial nerve. Meticulous irrigation and debridement of grossly contaminated wounds are vital to prevent infection.

SUMMARY

Attempt to remove all obvious debris from wounds during the first operation to facilitate a more favorable outcome for the patient. If the tissue margin looks dead or macerated beyond repair, it should be removed up to 1 to 2 mm to facilitate a more esthetic wound closure. Because of the highly vascular tissue in the face, small pedicles of tissue can survive. Native tissue will always look better than flaps and grafts. Although the face is very vascular,

it is not recommended that deeply contaminated wounds be primarily closed during initial surgery. In heavily contaminated wounds, multiple rounds of irrigation and debridement are recommended with delayed primary closure, if possible. Rotational flaps and skin grafts may be necessary to obtain optimal results.

SUGGESTED READING

Chapter 13: Face and neck injuries. In: *Emergency War Surgery, Third United States Revision*. Washington, DC: Department of the Army, Office of The Surgeon General, Borden Institute; 2004.

Chapter 22: Soft-tissue injuries. In: *Emergency War Surgery, Third United States Revision*. Washington, DC: Department of the Army, Office of The Surgeon General, Borden Institute; 2004.

Fonseca R, Walker R. *Oral and Maxillofacial Trauma*. 2nd ed. Philadelphia, Pa: W. B. Saunders; 1997.

Rowe N, Williams J. *Maxillofacial Injuries*. 2nd ed. New York, NY: Churchill Livingstone; 1994.

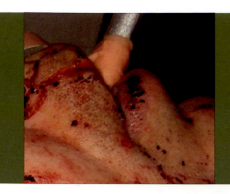

II.2
Facial Lacerations

CASE PRESENTATION

A 35-year-old male soldier sustained facial injuries from debris hurled from a car bomb explosion. Multiple soft-tissue wounds were apparent, with the most significant being a right cheek laceration (Fig. 1). Because of the location of the wounds, evaluations of the parotid duct and facial nerve were indicated. Bleeding was controlled with direct wound compression. The patient was alert and oriented. Physical and neurological examinations revealed no gross evidence of facial nerve weakness. There was no evidence of injury to the bony facial skeleton. During surgery, no evidence of damage to the parotid duct (of Stenson) was found. Manual manipulation of the gland produced an adequate flow of saliva. The duct was cannulated with lacrimal probes and catheter tubing. No disruption of the duct was seen. The patient's wound and vital structures were explored. Foreign bodies were removed, and tissues were closed in layers. He recovered without complications (Fig. 2).

TEACHING POINTS

1. Vascular injuries must be ruled out and repaired before proceeding with the laceration repair.
2. Facial bleeding should be controlled initially with compression. Ligation of the vessels may be necessary. However, direct visual location of the vessel is necessary before performing ligation to prevent damage to the facial nerve or parotid duct.
3. The importance of wound exploration needs to be stressed. There are multiple, underlying vital structures that can be damaged in a facial/cheek laceration. The wound must be carefully examined to identify and evaluate the integrity of the facial artery and nerve and its branches, the buccal fat pad, and the parotid gland and duct.
4. Although not always necessary, if sialography is performed, use a water-soluble contrast media (which is less toxic) instead of methylene blue.
5. Care should also be taken to ensure the sterility of the procedure and to prevent introduction of oral bacteria into the parotid duct.
6. Parotid duct lacerations require stent placement, with suturing of the lacerated ends (see Fig. 4, page 68). Careful monitoring of parotid gland injuries should be performed to rule out the formation of a parotid fistula or sialocele, which can be treated with antisialogogues and pressure dressings.

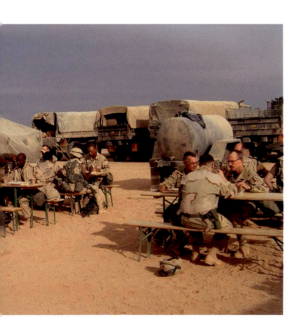

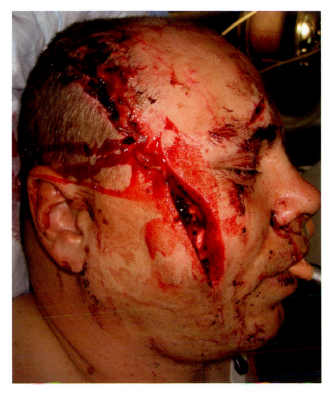

FIGURE 1. *Cheek, scalp, and facial lacerations.*

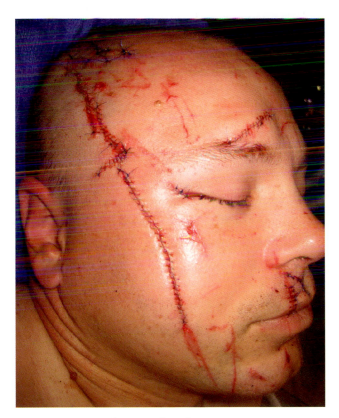

FIGURE 2. *Wounds immediately post-op.*

7. Repair facial nerve lacerations that occur proximal to a perpendicular line drawn from the lateral canthus of the eye.

8. Wound closure is important in managing facial lacerations. Copious irrigation, removal of foreign bodies, and antibiotics with gram-positive coverage are necessary to decrease infection and to help promote optimal wound healing. Try to maintain the buccal fat pad, if possible, to prevent cosmetic defects (eg, hollowing of the cheek). When primary closure is possible, the wound should be reapproximated in proper layers to optimize an esthetic outcome for the patient (Figs. 3 and 4).

CLINICAL IMPLICATIONS

1. Simple cheek lacerations that are superficial in depth should be managed like any other facial laceration in an esthetic zone once a neurological examination has been performed.

2. Large through-and-through lacerations are wounds that may potentially involve injury to any of the structures listed below, and injury to any of these structures may require additional procedures:

   a. Facial nerve injuries.
   b. Damage to the parotid gland and duct.
   c. Damage to the facial artery and its branches.
   d. Damage to the buccal fat pad.

DAMAGE CONTROL

Check vital structures. In a conscious patient, document the neurological examination of the facial nerve before administering local anesthesia. In an unconscious patient, a nerve stimulator can be used to assess facial nerve damage. Control bleeding: use compression for mild bleeding and use ligation of the vessel for significant bleeding. Soft tissue should be closed in multiple layers. Although talking can be uncomfortable, severe pain is not characteristic of maxillofacial injuries. Avoid oversedation.

SUMMARY

Facial lacerations should be thoroughly evaluated to rule out injury to significant underlying structures, specifically the facial nerve and parotid duct. If the clinical situation allows, immediate reconstruction of these structures is recommended. In this case, the patient did well without any significant complications. Although some patients may request scar revision after the appropriate amount of healing time, this patient declined further treatment and proudly wears his scars as a badge of courage.

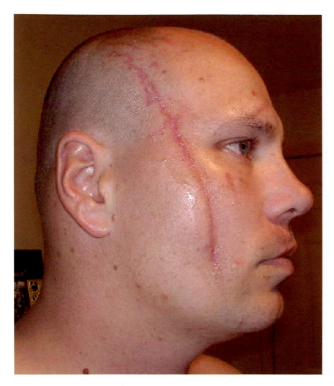

FIGURE 3. *Six months post-op.*

SIALOGRAPHY

Sialography is the radiographic examination of the salivary glands. With the patient in a supine position, it normally involves slowly injecting a nonionic water-soluble contrast medium (350 mg iodine/mL) directly into the salivary duct system. The injection is stopped when the patient feels discomfort or after 1 mL has been injected. (Note: plain films should be taken before injecting the contrast medium to identify any calculi. Also of particular benefit is placing dental film in the buccal sulcus outside the upper molars at the parotid duct orifice.) Using metal probes, the salivary duct opening is explored and dilated. Routine postcontrast X-rays should include oblique lateral and true lateral views, a posterior-anterior view of the parotid gland, or a mandibular occlusal radiograph of the submandibular duct.

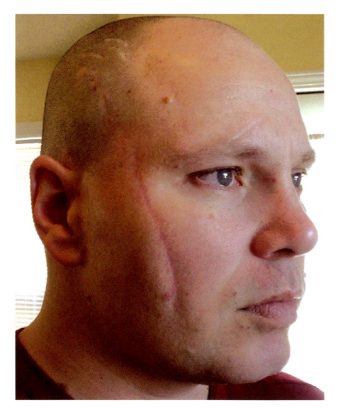

FIGURE 4. *One year post-op.*

SUGGESTED READING

Chapter 13: Face and neck injuries. In: *Emergency War Surgery, Third United States Revision.* Washington, DC: Department of the Army, Office of The Surgeon General, Borden Institute; 2004.

Chapter 22: Soft-tissue injuries. In: *Emergency War Surgery, Third United States Revision.* Washington, DC: Department of the Army, Office of The Surgeon General, Borden Institute; 2004.

Fonseca R, Walker R. *Oral and Maxillofacial Trauma.* 2nd ed. Philadelphia, Pa: W. B. Saunders; 1997.

Rowe N, Williams J. *Maxillofacial Injuries.* 2nd ed. New York, NY: Churchill Livingstone; 1994.

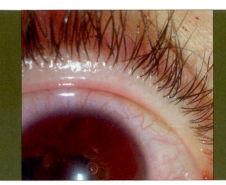

II.3
Corneal Perforation

CASE PRESENTATION

This 19-year-old male soldier sustained a femoral vessel laceration and a penetrating ocular injury from an improvised explosive device (IED). On presentation to the combat support hospital (CSH), examination of the eye revealed a small stellate perforation of his right cornea (Fig. 1). A fragment was present in the vitreous cavity, and a portion of iris and vitreous humor plugged the wound. His lens was partially dislocated, and he had a traumatic cataract. The anterior chamber had blood obscuring much of the iris details (hyphema). After the extremity hemorrhage was controlled, a Weck cell vitrectomy was performed. Because it was less than 6 hours from the time of injury, the small portion of iris was reposited into the globe. Blood was washed out of the anterior chamber. Butyl cyanoacrylate (corneal glue) was unavailable, and suturing the stellate perforation would have left such significant astigmatism that potential visual acuity would have been poor. 2-Octyl cyanoacrylate, given its similar properties to butyl cyanoacrylate, was used to close the wound.

TEACHING POINTS

1. Linear corneal lacerations are fairly straightforward to repair. However, a small stellate (or puncture wound) might pose a more difficult suture repair. Even though the wound might be small, the mechanics of closure may have a more deleterious effect on postoperative visual acuity. This situation occurs because vector forces cause irregular warpage of the cornea (astigmatism) as a result of the tension necessary to close a round or somewhat circular defect in a curved cornea.

2. Butyl cyanoacrylate (Fig. 2) is available in many countries, but it is not approved by the US Food and Drug Administration (FDA), and is unavailable in the United States. However, 2-octyl cyanoacrylate (Fig. 3) is approved by the FDA for skin use. Although they are different compounds, they have similar adhesive properties (eg, flexibility, strength, etc).

3. For glue to adhere to the cornea, the overlying epithelium must be removed. Usually, this procedure is performed easily in an injured cornea because a defect is already present in the epithelium. The process simply involves enlarging the surrounding exposed area.

4. It is important to apply the glue to a dry surface because any liquid tends to solidify the glue. Both corneal glue and skin glue will remain in liquid

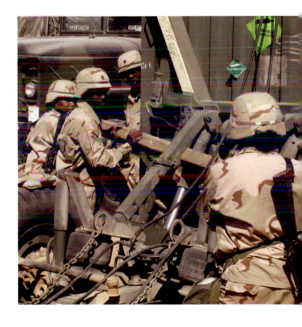

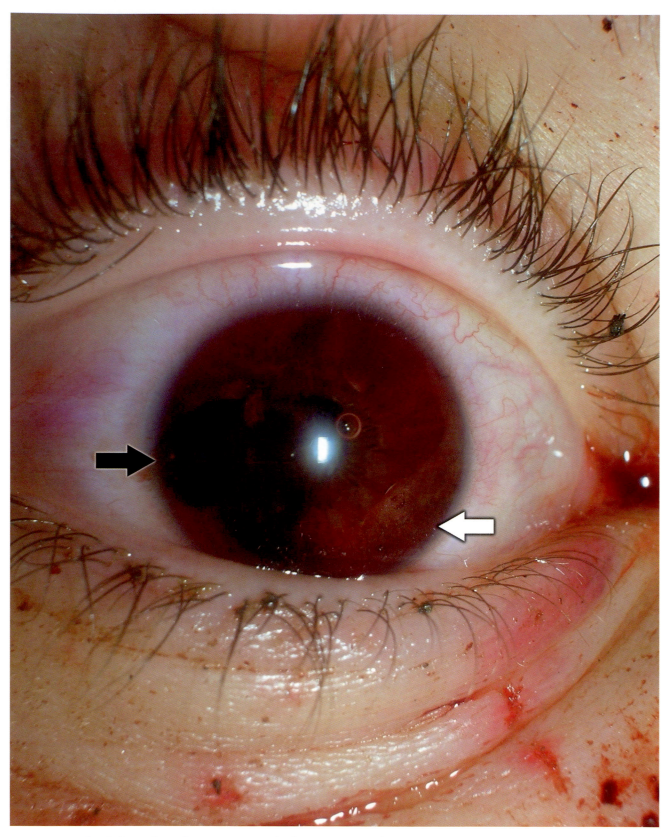

FIGURE 1. *Right globe with perforation at 9 o'clock accompanied by the loss of at least two clock hours of iris* (black arrow). *A portion of the iris and vitreous humor appears as a fine brownish halo at the edge of the cornea protruding from the anterior chamber* (white arrow), *which is filled with blood and an air bubble at 2 o'clock.*

form until contact with fluid or moisture. In this case, the surgeon squeezed the skin glue onto the plastic cover of a specimen cup. He used a 30-gauge needle on a tuberculin syringe to draw up a small amount of it. A Weck cell sponge was used to dry the corneal surface at the perforation. The drop of glue gently touched the surface of the defect, which caused a slight spreading. The aqueous humor quickly began to solidify the glue from the inside. [Note: Add a drop of saline solution to solidify the outer portion of the glue if the tear film does not already do this. The defect may require several drops (as in this case presentation) to cover the defect completely. Be sure that no intraocular contents (eg, iris, vitreous humor, lens material, etc) are protruding through the defect, or it will adhere to the glue.]

5. Dried glue presents a rather hard and irregular surface that is painful to lid movement. Even if the glue dried to a fairly smooth surface, the lid movement can dislodge the glue before sufficient healing has occurred. Therefore, always use a bandage contact lens for protection and comfort (Fig. 4). The best option is use of a specific therapeutic lens that has no refractive power and is larger in diameter (18–24 mm). However, low-power, standard contact lenses can also be used (generally between 13–15 mm) as a bandage. As long as the patient is treated with a broad-spectrum antibiotic (ie, fluoroquinolone or polymyxin/neomycin) 2 to 4 times a day, the contact lens can remain in place.

6. As the defect heals and the epithelium covers the area, the glue will be automatically dislodged. Generally, this process requires 4 to 6 weeks, depending on the

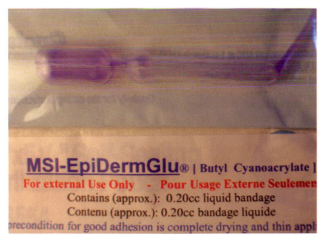

FIGURE 2. *Butyl cyanoacrylate or corneal glue (MSI-EpiDermGlu, Medisav Services, Inc, Markham, Ontario, Canada).*

DERMABOND

This topical skin adhesive is a sterile, liquid wound adhesive designed to repair lacerations and to close surgical incisions. It reacts with moisture on the skin's surface to form a strong, flexible bond. DERMABOND is used topically to hold closed easily approximated skin edges of wounds from surgical incisions, including punctures from minimally invasive surgery, and simple, thoroughly cleansed, trauma-induced lacerations. *(See full Prescribing Information for use.)*

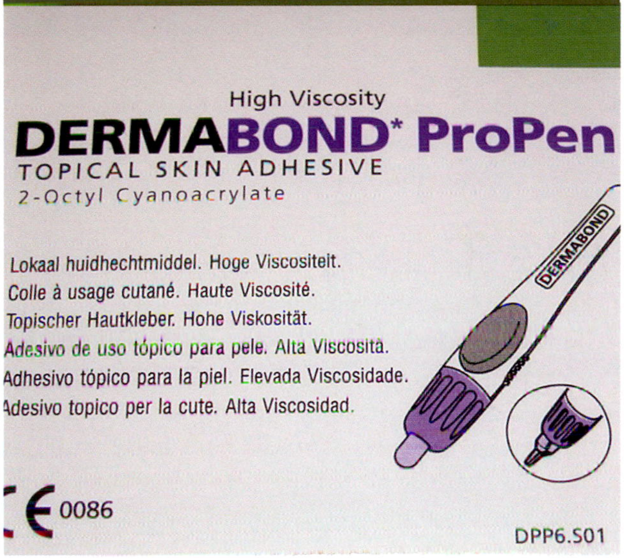

High Viscosity
DERMABOND* ProPen
TOPICAL SKIN ADHESIVE
2-Octyl Cyanoacrylate

Lokaal huidhechtmiddel. Hoge Viscositeit.
Colle à usage cutané. Haute Viscosité.
Topischer Hautkleber. Hohe Viskosität.
Adesivo de uso tópico para pele. Alta Viscosità.
Adhesivo tópico para la piel. Elevada Viscosidade.
Adesivo topico per la cute. Alta Viscosidad.

CE 0086

DPP6.S01

FIGURE 3. *2-Octyl cyanoacrylate or skin glue. Photograph: Courtesy of Ethicon, Inc, Somerville, New Jersey.*

size of the defect. This approach is best for corneal defects less than 2 mm, but it might be possible to place sutures to act as a scaffold rather than as a tension-inducing closure. The glue is then placed on this scaffold of smaller defects.

CLINICAL IMPLICATIONS

Unfortunately, penetrating injuries to the eye continue to be common in theater. Injury to the eye is found historically in 5% to 10% of all combat casualties. Treatment of these injuries requires specialized ophthalmic procedures within 24 to 48 hours. Medical personnel who provide initial treatment should note the following principles:

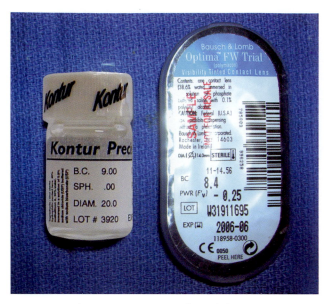

FIGURE 4. *Therapeutic contact lens* (left; *Kontur Kontac Lens Company, Richmond, California) and standard contact lens* (right; *Bausch & Lomb, Rochester, New York*).

1. Supply eye protection in the combat zone. This is mandatory and must be emphasized to soldiers and commanders by all medical personnel at all levels of care.
2. Determine the severity of ocular wounds. Personnel at level I and level II medical treatment facilities should evacuate all patients with penetrating globe injuries to a medical treatment facility with an ophthalmologist.
3. Note that loss of vision—manifested by the inability to read normal print, compared with the other eye— is suggestive of serious injury.
4. Do not apply a pressure dressing if penetrating injury is suspected. Apply a rigid eye shield instead.
5. Do not apply topical medications.
6. Start ciprofloxacin 500 mg orally or intravenously.
7. Retrieval of intraocular foreign bodies is <u>not</u> recommended in the forward surgical setting.
8. Prevent emesis.
9. Administer tetanus toxoid if indicated and evacuate the patient.
10. Triage patients with eye injuries and attend to the A–B–Cs and the life-threatening injuries first. Then treat eyesight and limb injuries.
11. Distinguish major ocular injuries from minor injuries. (This can be a difficult process.)
12. Avoid nonsteroidal antiinflammatory drugs with intraocular injuries. If evaluation to an ophthalmologist is delayed for more than 24 hours, consider treatment with a topical beta-blocker (timolol, levobunolol, etc) twice a day to help prevent intraocular pressure elevation.

> **Plain films or CT must be obtained to rule out an intraocular or intraorbital foreign body prior to performing any MRI.**

DAMAGE CONTROL

With suspected ocular injury, place a rigid dressing over the eye, start antibiotics, and evacuate to the nearest military treatment facility that has an ophthalmologist.

SUMMARY

Because of the nature of high-velocity projectiles and explosive fragmentation devices, multiple facial and ocular injuries are quite common on the battlefield. Primary fragmentation from IEDs or secondary projectiles (eg, rocks, dirt, glass, or metallic fragments) can be responsible for penetrating globe injuries, including a direct perforation of the cornea. Medical personnel must be ever vigilant about patients with eye injuries, particularly patients with suspected penetrating globe injuries. This case provides tips on the repair of a nonlinear corneal perforation.

SUGGESTED READING

Chapter 14: Ocular injuries. In: *Emergency War Surgery, Third United States Revision*. Washington, DC: Department of the Army, Office of The Surgeon General, Borden Institute; 2004.

Thach AB, ed. *Ophthalmic Care of the Combat Casualty (a Textbook of Military Medicine)*. Washington, DC: Department of the Army, Office of The Surgeon General, Borden Institute; 2003.

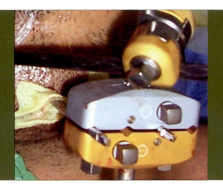

II.4
Maxillofacial Reconstruction

CASE PRESENTATION

This host nation male sustained gunshot wounds to the right side of his face. He had comminuted maxillary and mandibular fractures. Additionally, there were multiple missing and shattered teeth, fragments penetrating neck zones I to III, a shredded parotid gland, a severed Stenson's duct, and facial nerve transection. He had significant soft-tissue trauma to the right side of the face (Fig. 1). At the combat support hospital (CSH), he underwent angiography, neck and face exploration, and a tracheotomy. The ends of the parotid duct were identified and ligated. The wound was loosely approximated and dressed. Later, he was transferred to another hospital for more definitive treatment. Prior to reconstruction of the rami and arch, arch bars were placed on the patient's dentition after debridement of tooth particles and fragments. The maxilla was broken into four pieces. The patient received maxillomandibular fixation that ensured good, reproducible occlusion (Fig. 2). Titanium plates and screws were used to stabilize as many bone fragments as possible, with careful reapproximation at the Le Fort I level. Working together, the oral and maxillofacial surgeon and the cardiothoracic surgeon harvested two ribs (nos. 4 and 6) from the patient's right side. The patient's condylar head was removed, because it was completely fractured from the rest of the comminuted mandible. The zygomatic arch was extremely comminuted, with multiple fragments only several millimeters in length. One rib was used to reconstruct the patient's right mandibular condyle and ramus, and the other rib was used to reconstruct the right zygomatic arch. Titaninum plates and screws were used to secure the bone grafts to stable bones. The inferior alveolar nerve could not be repaired, because too much destruction had occurred (future reconstruction would involve a microsurgical graft repair). A parotidectomy was also perfomed. No ends of the facial nerve could be identified. The patient was released from fixation to check the occlusion, rinse and suction the oral cavity, and remove the throat pack. He was then placed back into fixation to stabilize the segmented maxilla because no palatal stent was available. Meticulous reapproximation of the soft tissues was accomplished in layers. A Penrose drain was placed. The patient was given intravenous (IV) antibiotics, and wound care was provided. Wire cutters were with the patient at all times. Maxillomandibular fixation was planned for 6 weeks to let the maxilla heal. He was extubated within the week and transferred from the CSH. Good facial symmetry was achieved (Fig.

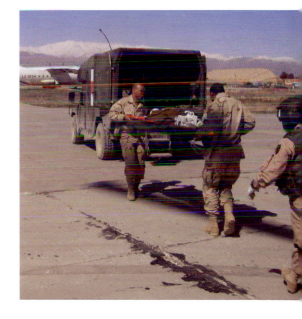

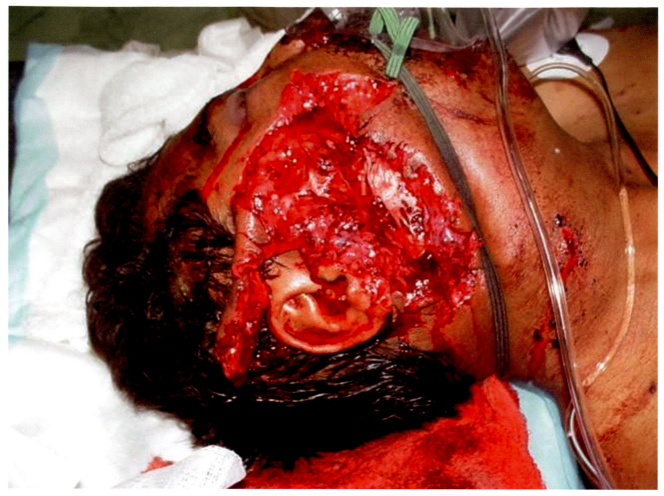

FIGURE 1. *Intraoperative exploration of wounds. Note neck wounds and soft-tissue avulsion of the face.*

3). Long-term follow-up was not available. Further microsurgical reconstruction would have been beneficial, but the overall esthetics and basic function were preserved using this technique.

TEACHING POINTS

1. This case is an example of a patient who required extensive reconstruction within the limitations of a level III medical treatment facility.

2. Facial reconstruction is tedious and time consuming. The primary goal in treating US patients is stabilization and evacuation. On the other hand, non-US patients require definitive treatment in theater. This treatment requires equipment that is not standard issue in the deployed level III medical facility. By necessity, level III facilities have acquired additional specialized equipment to handle these difficult patients.

3. Alternative approaches could have been utilized in the facial reconstruction of this patient. External fixation of reconstruction bars could also have been used. The degree of comminution and the condylar head remnant indicated that bone grafting was the logical choice to reconstruct the mandible. Costochondral grafting is a definitive treatment to replace a mandibular condylar head, whereas a reconstruction bar would be temporary. The rib graft also provided excellent contour for the reconstruction of the zygomatic arch, thus restoring the projection of the midface.

4. This case also demonstrates the need for sub-specialties within the level III medical treatment facility. Neurosurgeons, oral and maxillofacial surgeons, and ophthalmologists who are available in theater greatly enhance the capabilities of the level III medical facility. These medical pro-

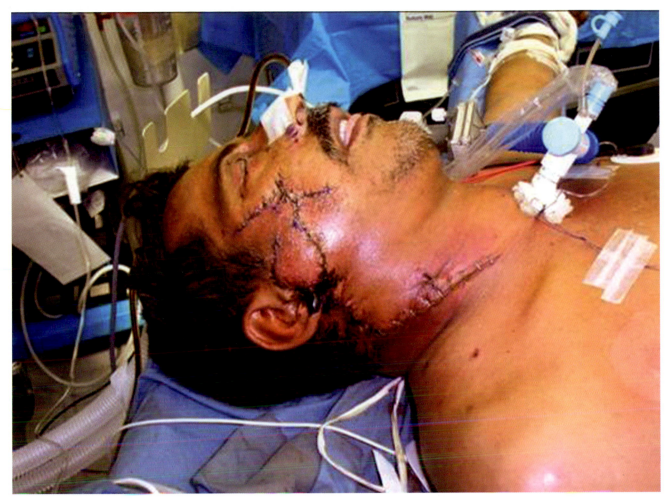

FIGURE 2. *Final closure obtained and patient placed back into maxillomandibular fixation.*

fessionals provide a higher level of expertise and patient care beyond basic stability when evacuation is not an option or when evacuation could present a greater risk of morbidity.

CLINICAL IMPLICATIONS

1. Autologous bone grafts are a useful and accepted way to reconstruct facial injuries definitively. Costochondral grafts can be used to reconstruct the mandibular ramus and the zygomatic arch. Iliac crest bone grafts or cranial bone grafts can be used to reconstruct the orbital floor.

2. Multiple surgeon teamwork expedites tedious, time-intensive reconstruction. Mission and operational tempo often mandate limiting operating time to as close to 2 hours as possible. Usually, definitive reconstruction cannot be accomplished that quickly. If teams are not available, staging of reconstruction is done.

3. A tracheotomy is an ideal airway for patients with extensive facial trauma. These patients have extensive edema and may undergo several operations for reconstruction. The tracheotomy is a definitive airway that is more easily secured and maintained.

4. Repair of Stenson's duct (not done in this case) is accomplished by cannulation with a small gauge angiocath. The duct is then reapproximated with fine absorbable sutures over the cannula to maintain patency (Fig. 4).

5. Suspected facial nerve injuries should be explored and primarily repaired if possible. Facial nerve branches that are lacerated at a site anterior to a vertical line drawn down from the lateral canthus of the eye do not need to be surgically reapproximated because these branches are very small and will spontaneously regenerate with good return of facial function (Fig. 5). If the wound

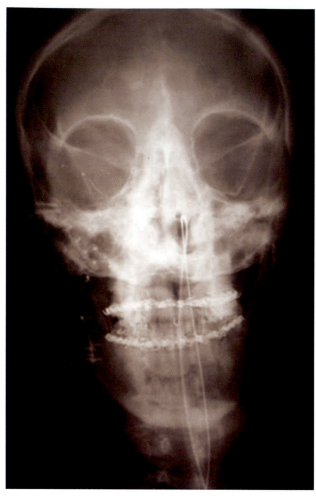

FIGURE 3. *Note symmetry obtained at mandibular ramus and zygomatic arch. Bone screws and plates are radiopaque.*

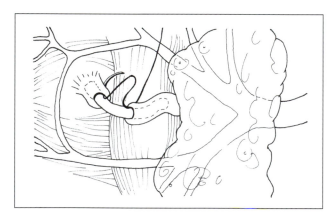

FIGURE 4. *Repair of parotid duct.*

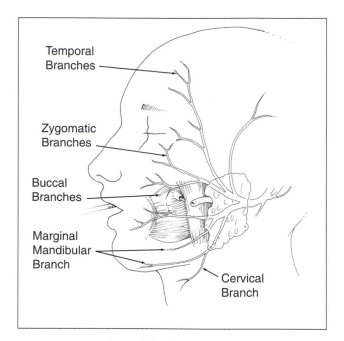

Temporal Branches

Zygomatic Branches

Buccal Branches

Marginal Mandibular Branch

Cervical Branch

FIGURE 5. *Branches of the facial nerve, parotid duct injury.*

is heavily contaminated and cannot be closed primarily, the severed ends of the nerve should be located and tagged for identification and repair at the time of wound closure.

6. Patients placed into maxillomandibular fixation must have wire cutters with them at all times in case they need to be cut loose because of airway compromise. Use umbilical tape to fashion a necklace so that the wire cutters are around the patient's neck during transport. If MEDEVAC crews are reluctant to transport a patient in wire maxillomandibular fixation, small elastics can be used to achieve maxillofacial fixation until the patient arrives at a stable location.

DAMAGE CONTROL

Damage control of oromaxillofacial injuries will center around airway and hemorrhage control. Emergency cricothyroidotomy may be necessary with unstable facial fractures where a definitive airway cannot be rapidly established. Approximation of large bony fragments with loose closure of overlying soft tissue may allow adequate hemorrhage control to get the patient out of the operating room for further resuscitation.

ERICH ARCH BAR

The Erich arch bar (also known as the Erich dental bar or the Erich arch bar meter coil)—a metal arch bar secured with soft, stainless wires—is an arch bar commonly used in the repair of mandibular fractures. The Erich arch bar is an important tool in occlusal restoration, particularly in cases of comminuted and oblique fractures and the loss of continuity of the mandible.

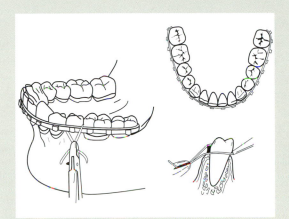

Advantages

- Rigidity.
- Maxillomandibular fixation easily applied.
- Easily adaptable to elastic traction.
- May be prefabricated or adapted.
- Continuous occlusal (superior tension band) control.

SUMMARY

This case demonstrates a method of definitive facial reconstruction and highlights the need for diverse specialties within a level III medical treatment facility. It also provides some practical advice for dealing with extensive facial trauma.

SUGGESTED READING

Chapter 4: Aeromedical evacuation. In: *Emergency War Surgery, Third United States Revision*. Washington, DC: Department of the Army, Office of The Surgeon General, Borden Institute; 2004.

Chapter 5: Airway/breathing. In: *Emergency War Surgery, Third United States Revision*. Washington, DC: Department of the Army, Office of The Surgeon General, Borden Institute; 2004.

Chapter 13: Face and neck injuries. In: *Emergency War Surgery, Third United States Revision*. Washington, DC: Department of the Army, Office of The Surgeon General, Borden Institute; 2004.

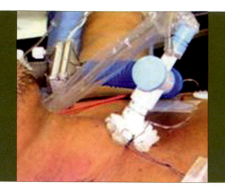

II.5
Mandible Gunshot Wound

CASE PRESENTATION

A host nation male suffered a gunshot wound to his left mandible (Fig. 1). His airway was intact, and his vital signs were stable on presentation to the emergency department. He underwent operative debridement and washout of the wound. There was no oral and maxillofacial surgeon (OMFS) nor ear, nose, and throat (ENT) surgeon assigned to the level III facility at the time. In addition, an oromaxillofacial surgery/microplate set was not available. After several days, the wound appeared clean and free of devitalized tissue and contamination (Fig. 2). After consulting with a remotely assigned OMFS, a team of general and orthopaedic surgeons took the patient to the operating room for definitive repair (Fig. 3). Using an orthopaedic handset, the major fragments were reduced and reapproximated with a single plate (Fig. 4). Other fragments were lag screwed into position. After further debridement and irrigation, the soft tissue was closed (Fig. 5). Arch bars were placed to maintain the reduction and stabilize the mandible (Fig. 6). The wounds healed well. After 5 weeks, the arch bars were removed, and the patient demonstrated normal occlusion and function.

TEACHING POINTS

1. Initial treatment of high-velocity missile injuries involves the basic principles of wound debridement and liberal irrigation to remove devitalized tissue and foreign debris, regardless of the anatomical site of injury.

2. Fixation and stabilization of fractures with soft-tissue closure (when possible) should be accomplished once the wound is cleared of dead tissue and debris. This can be accomplished within several days of wounding, dependent on the extent of soft-tissue injury and the degree of wound contamination.

3. Because this patient could not be transferred to a higher level of care, definitive repair had to be accomplished on-site. Using a multidisciplinary team of general surgeons (who deal with soft-tissue wounds regularly) and orthopaedic surgeons (who deal with plate-and-screw technology daily), after researching the surgical options and consulting with an OMFS, the patient underwent definitive reconstruction with an excellent outcome.

4. Arch bars are placed to help reduce the fracture and provide a tension band. The mandible may be reduced and internally fixed prior to

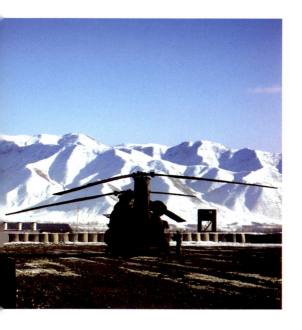

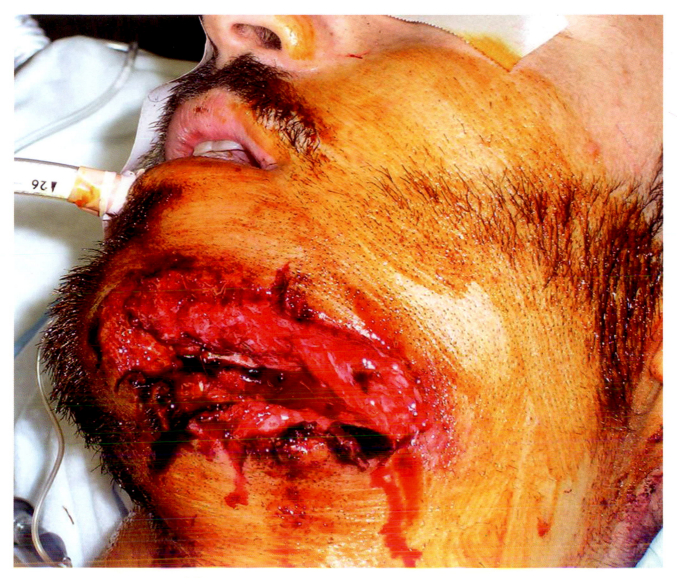

FIGURE 1. *Gunshot wound to left mandible.*

placement of the arch bars if the fracture is easily anatomically reduced. However, correct sequencing should be arch bar placement to help reduce the fracture, then internal fixation after a good reduction.

CLINICAL IMPLICATIONS

Often, in the deployed setting, surgeons may encounter clinical situations unfamiliar to them. In an emergency situation—by following Advanced Trauma Life Support (ATLS) guidelines—a patient can often be stabilized enough for transport to a higher level of care. For patients who must remain for definitive care (typically enemy prisoners of war or host nation civilians), consider the following:

1. Follow the basic principles of surgical care:
   a. Wound debridement and washout.
   b. Antibiotics as appropriate.
   c. Stabilization of fractures.
   d. Wounds left open until clean enough for closure (with either wound VACs or wet-to-dry dressings).
   e. Nutritional support.
2. Consult other surgeons/physicians if in unfamiliar territory.
   a. Often, general surgeons have widely different surgical experience.
   b. Other surgery specialists may have additional expertise that could be synergistic in a patient's care.
   c. Available specialists can be consulted remotely either by telephone or e-mail.

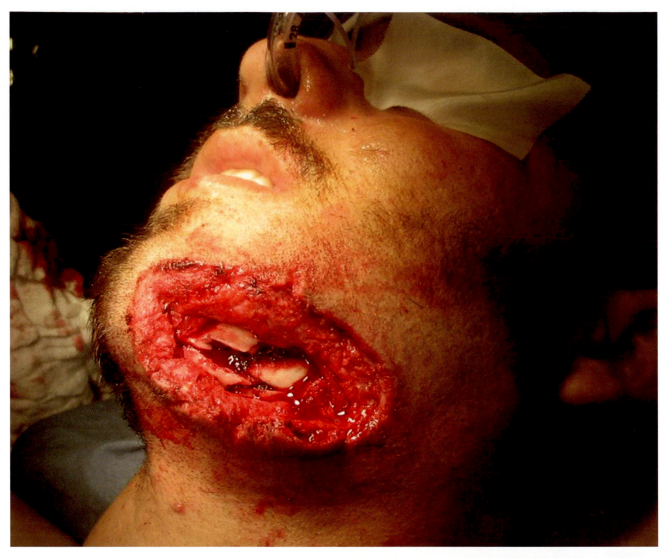

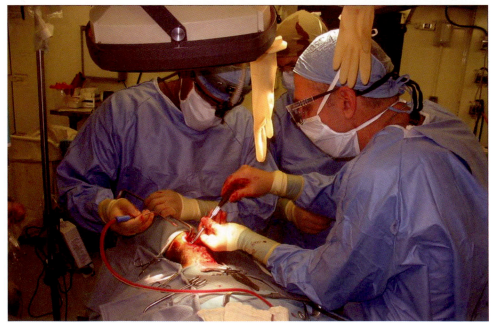

FIGURE 2. (Top) *Wound several days postinjury.*

FIGURE 3. (Bottom) *Operative repair. Sterile gloves are used to cover operating room light handles.*

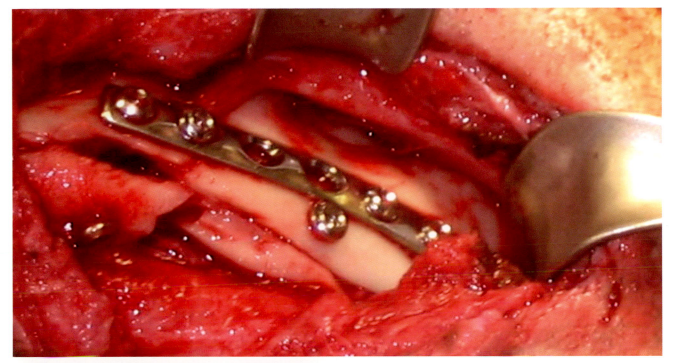

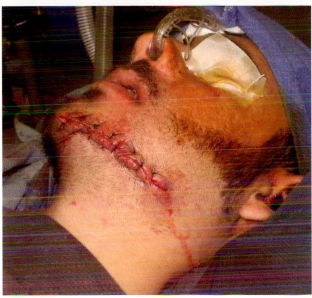

FIGURE 4. (Top) *Approximation of mandible fragments with plate.*

FIGURE 5. (Bottom Left) *Wound closure.*

FIGURE 6. (Bottom Right) *Arch bar stabilization.*

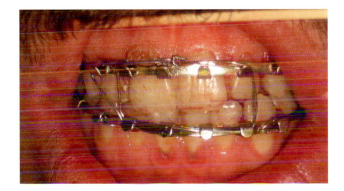

3. Consult available references and the Internet.
4. Do not try something that has little chance of success.

DAMAGE CONTROL

With extensive jaw or facial injuries, emergency cricothyroidotomy may be necessary at the outset of the resuscitation phase.

SUMMARY

Combat surgery can often challenge the most experienced surgeons to the limits of their capabilities. Nonetheless, by following basic surgical principles, by thoroughly researching surgical options, and by seeking assistance from locally available—as well as remotely assigned—specialists, a successful outcome is more probable.

SUGGESTED READING

Chapter 13: Face and neck injuries. In: *Emergency War Surgery, Third United States Revision*. Washington, DC: Department of the Army, Office of The Surgeon General, Borden Institute; 2004.

High-Energy Facial Injuries

by COL Karen M. Keith, DDS, MD

Since 2003, in the most recent conflicts of Iraq and Afghanistan, approximately one third of combat injuries involve the head and neck. Today's soldier wears more effective personal protective equipment into combat than at any other time in history. Modern body armor protects the torso, and the Kevlar helmet provides excellent protection to the head and brain. As the conflict has progressed, ballistic eyewear protection has been enforced. Consequently, nonlethal but extremely morbid wounds of exposed limbs and the facial area have increased disproportionately in the overall distribution of injuries. The oral and maxillofacial (OMF) surgeon has necessarily played a significant role in the management of these patients. The unique training of OMF surgery makes the surgeon a force multiplier in times of crisis. The OMF surgeon can provide anesthesia; perform tracheotomies; elevate cranial flaps; harvest bone grafts from the calvarium, iliac crest, tibia, and rib; and elevate the temporalis, pectoralis, and other myocutaneous flaps.

Unlike previous conflicts, a soldier can now be evacuated from theater to the United States in as little as 4 days. Thus, resuscitation and stabilization are the acute management goals for these soldiers. However, the morbidity of coalition and host nation troops not evacuated to higher echelons of care is also improved by the skills and ingenuity of the combat surgeons. Forward Surgical Teams (FSTs) provide immediate treatment, with rapid evacuation to level III echelon care at the combat support hospital (CSH). The OMF surgeon is assigned to the CSH or to a Head and Neck Team. Only in very recent years (2003) has an extensive OMF surgery set been fielded, which includes the full range of craniofacial plating sets and external fixation equipment. This greatly expands the capability of the OMF surgeon. The basic needs for stabilization and fixation, however, remain arch bars and wire, and any deploying surgeon needs to understand their proper application.

Many lessons learned regarding current injury patterns and etiologies resulted in modification of treatment protocols for injuries of the head and neck. Improvised explosive devices (IEDs) currently account for 40% to 60% of injuries to soldiers and civilians. These devices cause wounds grossly contaminated with dirt, plastic, gravel, material, and flesh. Other high-velocity projectile wounds result from gunshots and mortar blasts. Globe rupture or penetration, otological blast damage, burns, punctures, and avulsive soft-tissue wounds with extensive hard-tissue comminution represent the injury patterns that present many challenges and considerations (Figs. 1 and 2).

In any head and neck trauma, the first consideration should always be the airway. Often, the patient is intubated in the field or soon after presentation to the emergency room. Most often, patients are intubated orally because it is easier and safer in a trauma setting than placing a nasal tube. If there are no concomitant midface injuries, the patient can be extubated and reintubated nasally before addressing OMF surgery repair. If a patient has midface fractures, caution must be exercised when placing a nasal tube to avoid inadvertent entrance through a cranial base fracture, potentially causing cerebral injury. Another approach to securing an endotracheal tube is to pull an orally placed tube out through a submental incision. This provides a secure airway without hampering the surgeon's ability to wire the teeth and jaws closed. In cases of severe facial trauma, in which evacuation or prolonged intubation (oral or nasal) are anticipated because of edema, ventilator weaning difficulty, or multiple returns to the operating room, a tracheotomy is strongly advocated. Patients should also have cricothyroidotomies converted to tracheotomies prior to evacuation to the next echelon of care. This will guarantee a secure airway for transport and for the next phase of treatment.

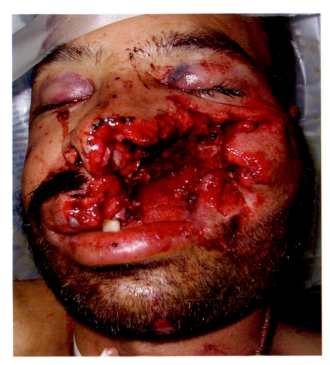

FIGURE 1. *Example of destructive, avulsive combat injuries.*

Once the airway is secured, a thorough examination must be performed to determine the extent and severity of the injury. OMF injuries are not life-threatening once the airway and bleeding are controlled. Bleeding is controlled with packing, judicious cautery, or suture ligation. Prophylactic antibiotics and tetanus prophylaxis are administered. After initial stabilization, a thorough assessment of the extent of injury and reconstructive needs are performed.

History and a focused physical examination guide the imaging. In an immature theater, plain films and clinical acumen can successfully guide surgical treatment. Clinical examination can be hampered by intubation and by the cervical collar. Fine-cut (1–3 mm) axial CT images, when available, of the patient's face help delineate the injuries and are more useful than plain radiography. If the patient's cervical spine is cleared, coronal CT images offer additional information. Three-dimensional reconstructions are particularly useful when planning the repair of complex OMF surgery injuries (Fig. 3). The surgeon evaluates all the studies and makes the diagnosis and treatment plan. The surgeon must consider the extent of comminution, avulsion, and contamination of the hard- and soft-tissue structures. Avulsive or penetrating trauma in this region can involve damage to salivary ducts, branches of the facial or trigeminal nerve, and vascular structures. The physical examination should include identifying such damage and tagging structures that cannot be handled at the current echelon of care, thereby affording a greater chance for future successful repair at the next echelon of care.

Consideration must be given to the overall condition of the patient. Definitive repair is time-consuming and can involve multiple, lengthy procedures. If the patient cannot tolerate prolonged surgeries, the surgeon can consider washouts and shorter staged procedures based on patient progress and stability. For US soldiers, definitive reconstruction will not usually be performed at the level III echelon of care.

Copious irrigation and careful, serial debridement are essential to minimize the potential for infection and future esthetic concerns of OMF wounds. It is important not to overlook seemingly inconsequential puncture wounds. Careful exploration of wound cavities can reveal an extensive radius of damage and foreign debris, such as plastic, dirt and small glass particles, and occult fractures secondary to the impact of the fragmentation. Pulse lavage is an excellent adjunct when available. Copious irrigation with a surgical scrub assists in overall cleansing. Small

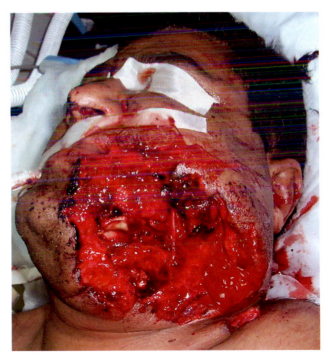

FIGURE 2. *Example of destructive, avulsive combat injuries in another patient.*

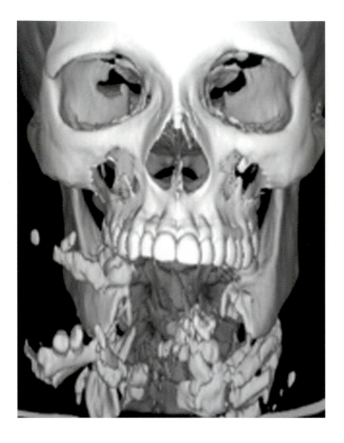

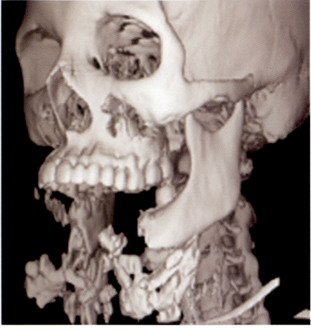

FIGURE 3. *Three-dimensional CT reconstructions in AP (Left) and oblique (Right) views of facial trauma. Note comminuted mandible fracture and maxillary Le Fort level injury.*

punctate wounds on the face that are easily debrided should be closed primarily for esthetic concerns rather than allowed to heal by secondary intention.

With fractures that involve the midface or mandible, arch bars and maxillomandibular fixation (MMF; Fig. 4) need to be placed prior to reduction and fixation. Immediate reduction of the fracture and improvement of occlusion can be obtained with a bridle wire (24 or 25 gauge) placed around at least two teeth on either side of the fracture. If the patient has a nondisplaced subcondylar fracture and normal occlusion, he can be treated with a soft diet and proscriptions on wearing a helmet and protective ("gas") mask. Occlusion is something that the OMF surgeon remains particularly attentive to because it can guide final reapproximation and fixation of hard tissue. Wiring the patient's teeth closed establishes the correct occlusion, which may be especially problematic with avulsion of bony fragments. Note that teeth in the line of fracture can be maintained if stable and not interfering with establishing the occlusion. If fractured with exposed pulp, or very loose, teeth should be removed. Only using an anatomical reduction, without MMF, to reduce fractures can risk giving the patient a postoperative malocclusion that can then necessitate additional extensive surgery

to rectify. Once the fracture is fixated, the MMF is released. The arch bars usually remain in place until the fracture is healed (6 weeks) in case elastics or additional manipulation is required.

Any patient who will remain in MMF (closed reduction) should have wire cutters available at all times. Umbilical tape is used to hang them around the neck. Wire cutters are for the provider assisting the patient to release the MMF if necessary for airway issues. This is a very rare occurrence. Emesis is not usually itself an indication for release. If the patient is evacuated, elastics (6-ounce

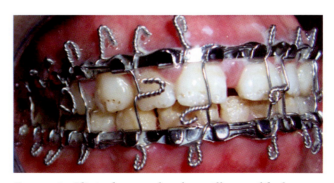

FIGURE 4. *Clinical example of maxillomandibular fixation with arch bars and wire loops.*

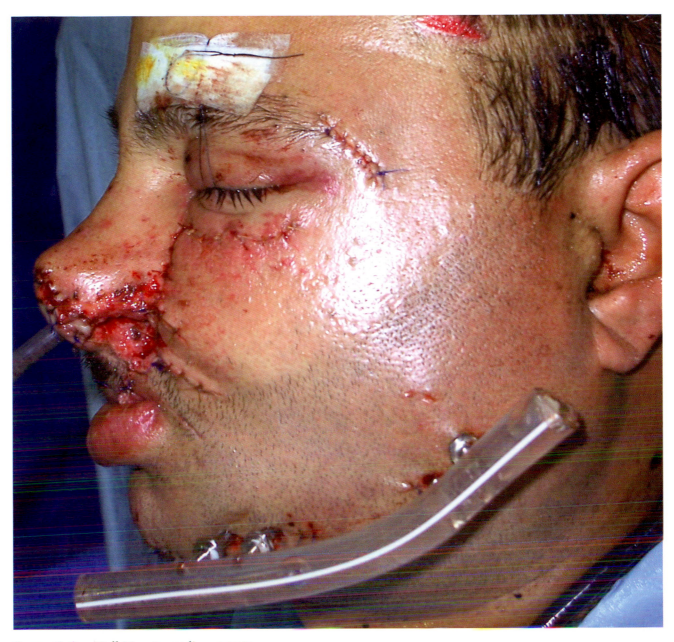

FIGURE 5. *Joe Hall Morris appliance system.*

JOE HALL MORRIS DEVICE

The Joe Hall Morris device (or the biphasic system) is an example of an external-pin fixation appliance. It allows fixation of a mandibular fracture with no major incisions. This technique is ideal for areas with significant soft-tissue loss or infection. This biphasic device serves as the patient's mandible until the fracture site has completely healed. The Joe Hall Morris device was used extensively in World War II, but it is not used so widely any more. Surgeons, however, should be familiar with this technique and include it as part of their surgical armamentarium. It is particularly useful in edentulous patients with comminuted fractures.

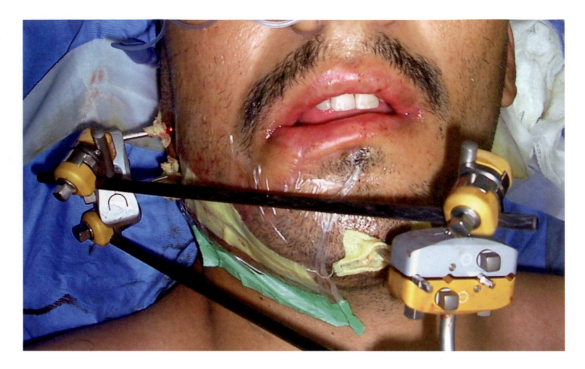

FIGURE 6.
Wrist external pin fixation system.

orthodontic elastics) can be used instead of wire for closed reduction. This minimizes patient discomfort until the next echelon of care is reached, but is more suitable for patient management during evacuation. Remember to discuss fixation with the evacuation team.

Comminuted, avulsed, and contaminated fractures are often best treated initially with external fixation rather than with open reduction and internal fixation. The biphasic system, known as the Joe Hall Morris device (Fig. 5), is the most common and familiar device to the OMF surgeon. However, the orthopaedic hand and wrist external fixation device works effectively and is a simpler system that requires less time to place (Fig. 6). This is ideal in areas of significant soft-tissue loss or infection (Fig. 7). It is also particularly beneficial in an edentulous mandible with comminuted fractures (Fig. 8). The surgeon can also elect to place a reconstruction plate across a comminuted mandible fracture (Figs. 9 and 10). The site must be thoroughly irrigated and debrided, and the plate must be covered with soft tissue (Fig. 11). If there is an inadequate soft-tissue envelope, a soft-tissue flap can be rotated to cover the defect (Figs. 12 and 13), or the surgeon can choose to convert to external pin fixation.

Burns need to be evaluated for airway concerns with fiberoptic intubation or early tracheotomy if edema or inhalation injury causes respiratory distress. Associated tracheal or laryngeal injury needs to be assessed. Orbital compartment syndrome requires lateral canthotomy and cantholysis. Silvadene should be avoided on the face because of its caustic nature.

In combat, the OMF surgeon can be confronted with many challenging and complex injury patterns in a less than optimal environment. The goals of facial bone fracture repair are realignment and fixation of the fragments in the correct anatomical position with the proper occlusion. MMF (closed reduction with wire) is inferior, but often easier and most readily available. Plates and screws, reconstruction plates, and external pin fixation are also part of the armamentarium. Depending on the extent of injury, several staged procedures will be required to definitively reconstruct a patient. Planning should be done after three-dimensional reconstruction of CT scans and stereolithography model fabrication. The ability to preserve soft tissue enhances the esthetics, psychological recovery, and function of the overall reconstruction. Flaps, bone grafts, and alloplastic materials can be used to provide the best reconstructive efforts to improve the patient's quality of life. Training in myocutaneous flaps and adjunctive procedures with other surgeons has resulted in many creative and versatile reconstruction techniques. Therefore, the surgeon must consider the patient's status, support systems, available technology in theater, and the long-term goals for reconstruction and develop the best course of action for all assessed patients.

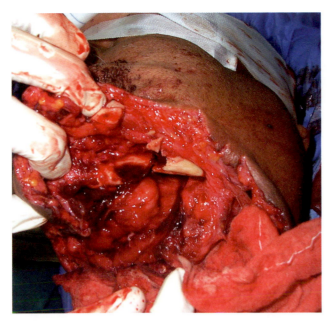

FIGURE 7. *Comminuted mandible fractures with avulsion of hard and soft tissues.*

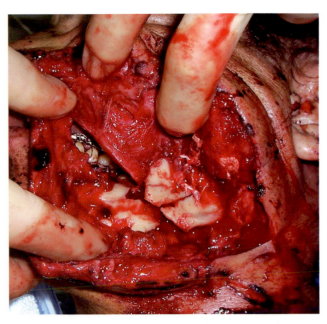

FIGURE 8. *Comminuted mandible fractures with avulsion of hard and soft tissues in another patient.*

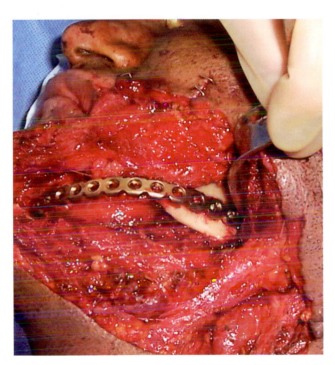

FIGURE 9. *Clinical example of an open reduction with internal fixation during initial surgery.*

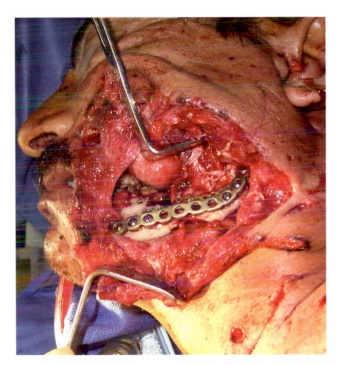

FIGURE 10. *Open reduction with internal fixation during initial surgery in another patient.*

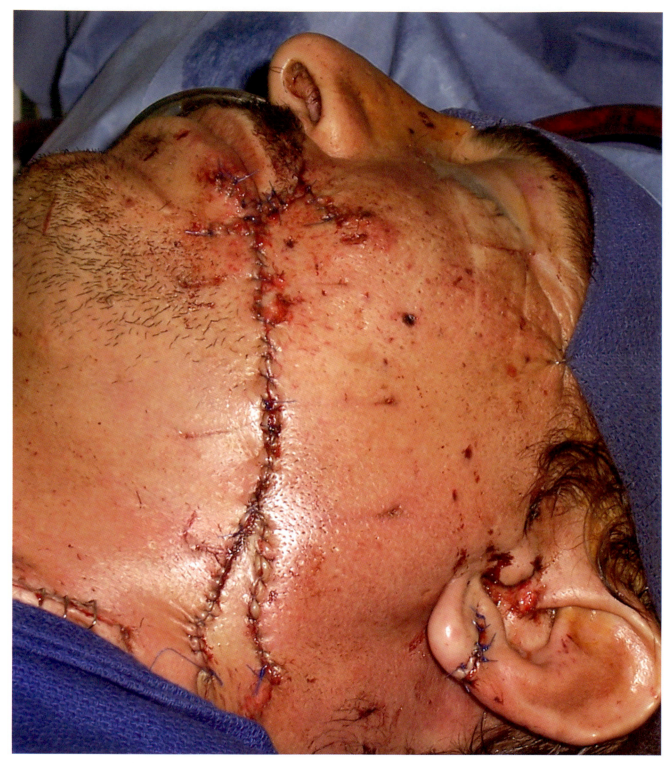

FIGURE 11. *Primary closure established over hardware using available local soft tissue.*

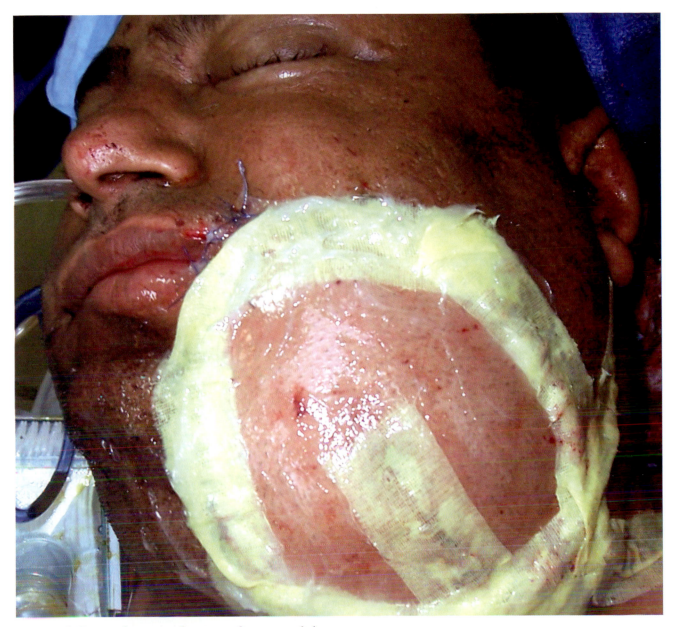

FIGURE 12. *Pectoralis major flap is used to cover defect.*

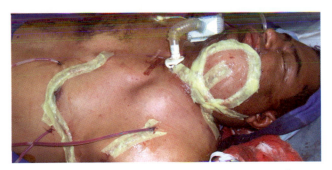

FIGURE 13. *Pectoralis major musculocutaneous flap.*

SUGGESTED READING

Chapter 13: Face and neck injuries. In: *Emergency War Surgery, Third United States Revision.* Washington, DC: Department of the Army, Office of The Surgeon General, Borden Institute; 2004.

Powers DB, Haug RH. The role of the oral and maxillofacial surgeon in wartime, emergencies and terrorist attacks. *Oral Maxil Surg Clin North Am.* 2005;17:xi–xii (preface).

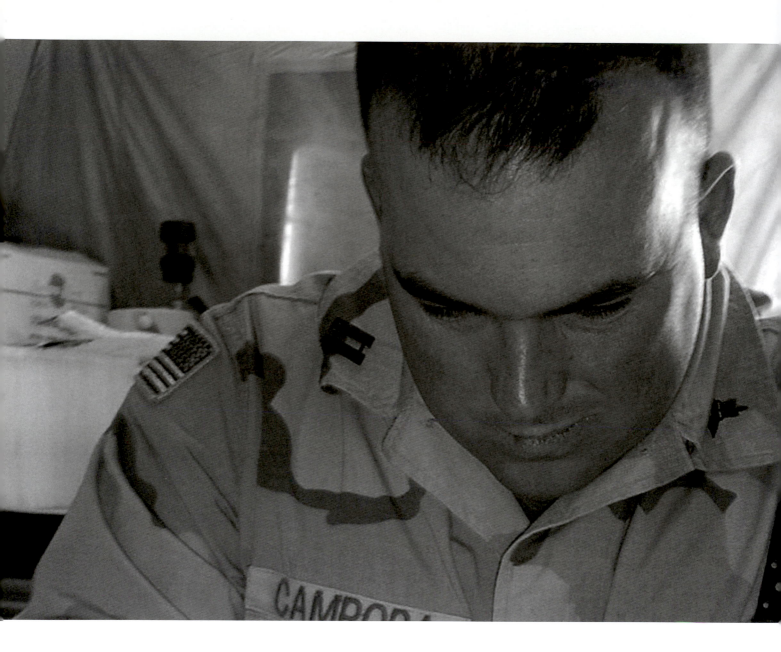

Chapter III
HEAD AND SPINE TRAUMA

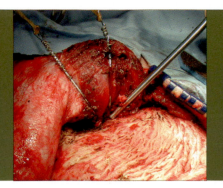

III.1
Penetrating Head Injury With Subdural Hematoma

CASE PRESENTATION

This male soldier suffered a penetrating gunshot wound to the head. The patient arrived at the combat support hospital (CSH) intubated. He failed to open his eyes, and he withdrew upper and lower extremities symmetrically to pain. His pupils were equal in size, midpoint, and reactive. A single entrance wound was identified in the right temporal region (Fig. 1). Skull images showed the tip of a large bullet (Fig. 2). CT showed the bullet embedded in the skull base at the right temporal tip, as well as a right subdural hematoma with midline shift (Fig. 3). No other injuries were identified. The patient was taken to the operating room for emergent craniotomy. The entire right hemisphere of the skull was exposed by reflecting the scalp and temporalis muscle anteriorly (Fig. 4). A trauma craniectomy was fashioned and the bone elevated from the underlying dura mater (Fig. 5). The dura was opened in parallel strips to expose and aspirate an acute subdural clot while preventing malignant swelling of the brain (Fig. 6). The bullet was not visible, and no attempt was made to recover it. Closure was performed without replacement of the bone flap. Duraplasty was performed by sewing ellipses of bovine pericardium into the dural openings using 4-0 braided nylon suture. After achieving a watertight closure, the scalp was approximated over an epidural drain and an intracranial pressure (ICP) monitor was placed on the uninjured side. Empiric broad-spectrum antibiotics and phenytoin were administered. The patient was left intubated postoperatively and evacuated to a level IV medical treatment facility. After prolonged intensive care, he recovered to independent living.

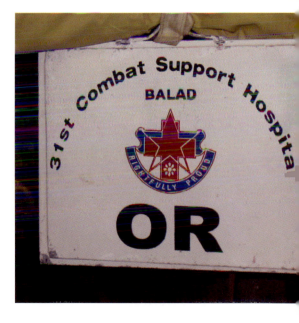

TEACHING POINTS

1. During the primary and secondary surveys, attention should be placed on a complete examination of the scalp and neck. Fragments that enter the cranial vault with a transtemporal, transorbital, or cross-midline trajectory should be suspected of having associated neurovascular injuries. Multiple wounds are typically involved in combat-related brain injuries, and these injuries generally involve the face, neck, and orbit. Entry wounds may be through the upper neck, face, orbit, or temple (Fig. 7). Scalp hemorrhage should be initially controlled using rapid, simple techniques. After addressing the patient's airway, breathing, and circulation, the level of consciousness should be determined.

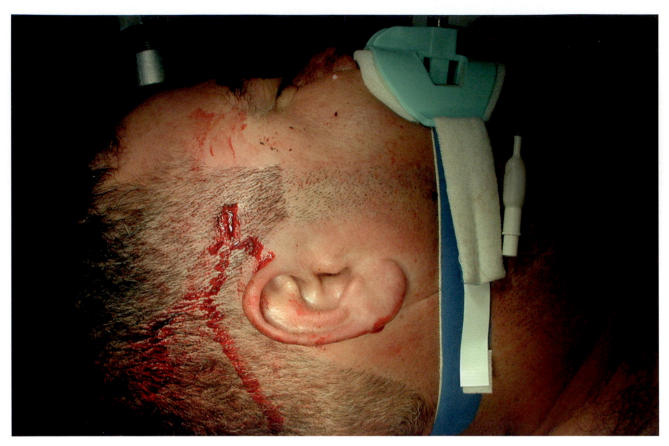

FIGURE 1. *Entrance wound in the right temporal region.*

2. The level of intact neurological function is best assessed by determining the Glasgow Coma Scale (GCS; see Appendix C) score and pupillary function. A GCS score of 8 or greater indicates a good prognosis. The finding of unilateral acute pupillary dilation should raise immediate concern of ipsilateral brain herniation. Patients exposed to explosive blasts may experience iridoplegia (paralysis of the pupil), which is not indicative of herniation.

3. Acute intervention has the greatest effect on casualties with a GCS score of 6 to 8, if ICP can be controlled and cerebral blood flow maintained until the patient receives the required neurosurgical management. Casualties with a GCS score of 5 or less do poorly, and expectant management may be considered.

4. A single, dilated or nonreactive pupil adds urgency and implies the presence of a unilateral (usually ipsilateral), space-occupying lesion with secondary brain shift. Immediate surgery is indicated.

5. Any attempt to retrieve intracranial missiles must be made on a case-by-case basis, weighing the risk of further neurological injury.

CLINICAL IMPLICATIONS

If the determination has been made that emergency surgery is needed because of a space-occupying lesion with neurological changes, an intracranial hematoma producing a greater than 5-mm midline shift or similar depression of cortex, a compound depressed fracture with neurological changes, or penetrating injuries with neurological deterioration, the following principles apply:

1. The GCS score and pupils should be evaluated as soon as tactically possible. Both should be regularly reassessed thereafter. The finding of acute pupillary dilation should raise immediate concern of brain herniation.

2. Intracranial hypertension should be relieved with hemicraniectomy, duraplasty, and ventriculostomy. A large craniectomy flap for wide exposure is recommended. A series of 1- to 2-cm parallel slits in the dura is a technique for relieving dural tension and removing a subdural hematoma.

3. Broad-spectrum antibiotics should be administered.

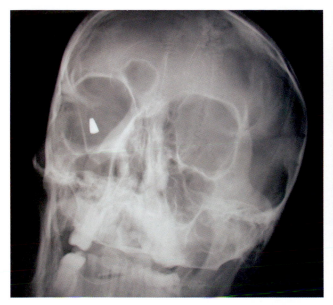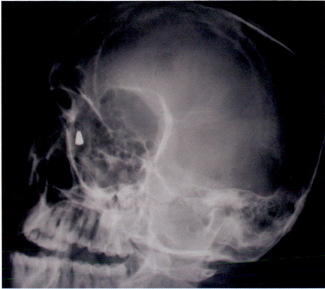

FIGURE 2. *Skull radiographs (PA and oblique) show the tip of a large bullet.*

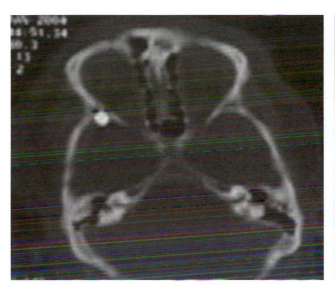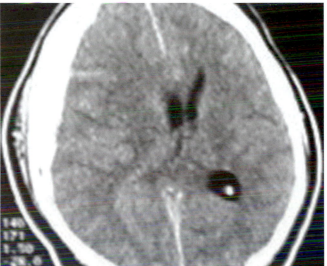

FIGURE 3. *CT image showing the bullet embedded in the skull base at the right temporal tip* (Left), *as well as a right subdural hematoma with midline shift* (Right).

4. Hematoma should be evacuated and bleeding controlled.

5. For penetrating injury, remove devitalized brain and accessible foreign bodies, and irrigate with antibiotic solution.

6. A watertight closure of the dura should be attempted. If duraplasty is required, pericranium, temporalis fascia, or tensor fascia lata may be used.

7. The galea of the scalp should be closed.

8. Tension-free closure of the scalp should also be performed.

9. If the bone flap cannot be replaced, it may be discarded or preserved in an abdominal wall pocket. If the bone flap is unsalvageable, it can be replaced later by a polyetheretherketone (PEEK) cranioplasty.

10. Meticulous debridement of the scalp and subcutaneous tissues is important to prevent infection.

11. A decision to attempt retrieval of intracranial missiles has to be individualized, weighing the serious risk of increasing neurological injury. Sequelae due solely to bullet migration are uncommon.

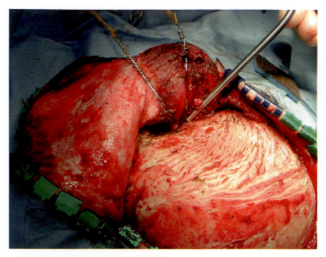

FIGURE 4. *The entire right hemisphere of the skull was exposed by reflecting the scalp and temporalis muscle anteriorly.*

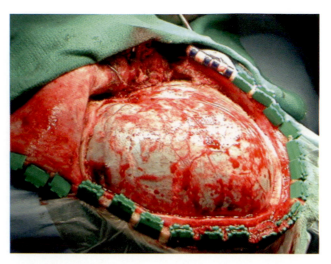

FIGURE 5. *Trauma craniectomy. Bone removed from the underlying dura mater.*

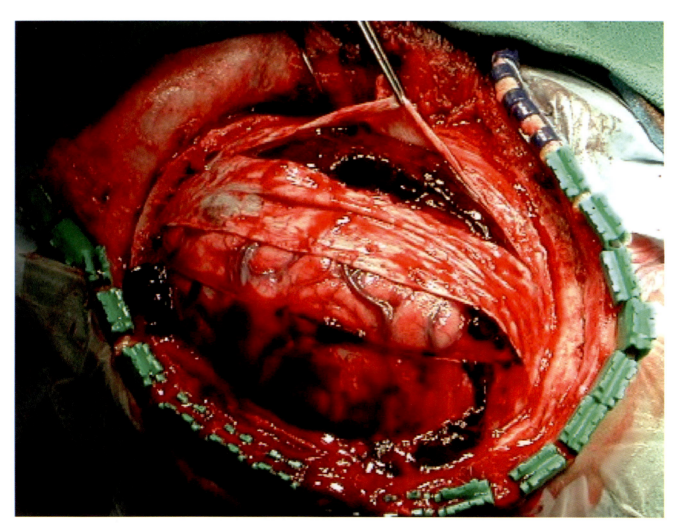

FIGURE 6. *Dura mater opened in parallel strips exposing acute subdural clot.*

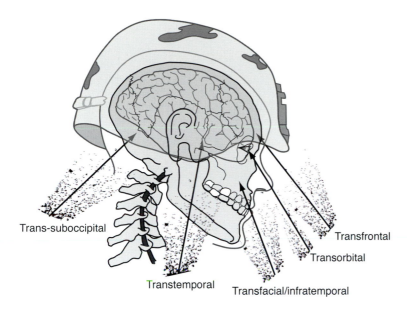

Trans-suboccipital

Transfrontal

Transorbital

Transtemporal

Transfacial/infratemporal

FIGURE 7. *Common vectors of penetrating injury in which the projectile has not traversed the helmet.*

INTRACRANIAL PRESSURE (ICP)

Elevation of the pressure within the skull is often a common complication of serious neurological conditions. The average ICP in adults ranges from 0 to 10 mm Hg. The maximal upper limit of desirable ICP is 20 mm Hg. Pressures more than 40 mm Hg are considered extremely elevated. ICP may be high because of:

- A rise in the cerebrospinal fluid (known as *hydrocephalus*).
- Brain swelling caused by fluid leaking into the brain (known as *cerebral edema*).
- Intracranial hemorrhage.

Regardless of the underlying cause, elevated ICP is a severe medical problem that should be treated immediately. Classic symptoms of ICP include Cushing's triad (named after Harvey Williams Cushing [1869–1939], an American neurosurgeon):

- Hypertension.
- Bradycardia.
- Irregular respirations.

12. Tension-free scalp closure is essential, but replacement of multiple skull fragments in an attempt to reconstruct the skull defect is not appropriate in the battlefield setting.

DAMAGE CONTROL

If CT is not available—and the patient has neurological injury and a deteriorating neurological examination without localizing signs—burr holes may be of diagnostic utility, but are usually inadequate to treat acute hematomas. Neurosurgical damage control includes early ICP control, cerebral blood flow preservation, and prevention of secondary cerebral injury from hypoxia, hypotension, and hyperthermia.

SUMMARY

This case demonstrates large craniectomy exposure of the cerebral hemisphere and evacuation of a subdural hematoma. Although duraplasty and watertight closure of the dura are ideal, a gel foam or gel-film barrier may be laid in the subdural and epidural planes if primary closure of the meninges is technically impossible. The bone flap may be discarded or stored in a subcutaneous abdominal pouch for replacement after 30 days. A large craniectomy exposure of the cerebral hemisphere for evacuation of a subdural hematoma is demonstrated. A dural opening using the entire expanse of the cranial opening should be created.

SUGGESTED READING

Brain Trauma Foundation. *Summary of the Guidelines for Field Management of Combat-Related Head Trauma.* New York, NY: Brain Trauma Foundation; 2005.

Chapter 15: Head injuries. In: *Emergency War Surgery, Third United States Revision.* Washington, DC: Department of the Army, Office of The Surgeon General, Borden Institute; 2004.

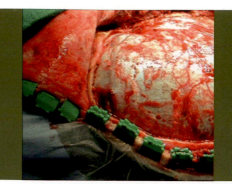

III.2
Basilar Skull Fracture With Pneumocephaly

CASE PRESENTATION

This 21-year-old male sustained a traumatic head injury from a mortar attack. He was initially comatose and during transport, he was bag-ventilated with a face mask. The patient presented to the combat support hospital (CSH) alert but confused, with a Glasgow Coma Scale (GCS) score of 14. His chief complaint was nausea, and he vomited twice. He was intubated for airway protection and bag-ventilated. His physical examination revealed a blood-tinged, clear fluid discharge from his left ear, and his neurological examination was significant for confusion. Cranial nerve exam was normal, as were his gross motor and sensory exams. CT of his head revealed a basilar skull fracture and severe pneumocephaly (Fig. 1). The discharge from his ear had a high glucose content consistent with cerebrospinal fluid (CSF). The patient was placed on 100% oxygen continuous positive airway pressure and seated in an upright position. Four hours later, there was marked improvement in his pneumocephaly. He was extubated and continued treatment with a 100% oxygen face mask. The following day, his mental status was normal. Over the next 2 days, he was encouraged to sit upright and, when sleeping, place his right ear down. His CSF leak improved and resolved spontaneously by the time the patient was evacuated.

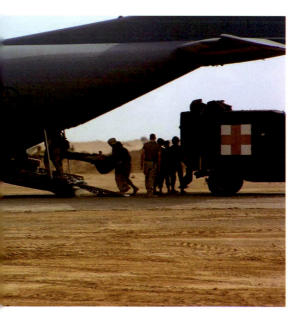

TEACHING POINTS

1. Pneumocephaly is a condition in which air enters the cranial vault. This finding on neuroimaging is indicative of a violation of the skull integrity. Most often, it is seen following craniotomy. However, in this case, the diffuse extent suggests air entrance through the basilar skull fracture exacerbated by vigorous bag ventilation through a face mask during transport.

2. Basilar skull fracture results from closed-head injury and high-velocity penetrating head injury when a force applied to the skull causes a transient dysmorphic change in skull shape. The most common clinical signs include CSF otorrhea and Battle's sign for petrous bone fractures, and CSF rhinorrhea and raccoon eyes for anterior cranial vault fractures.

3. There can be fractures through the wing of the sphenoid bone, the sella, sphenoid sinuses, the clivus, and ethmoid air cells—all of which can contribute to pneumocephalus and a CSF leak. A fracture through the posterior wall of the frontal sinus, although not classically a skull base fracture, can also lead to the same clinical presentation.

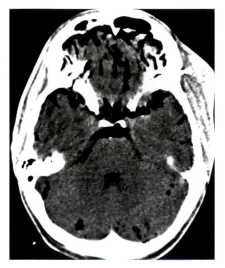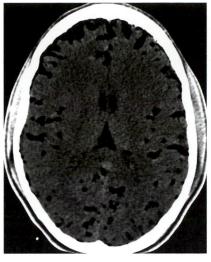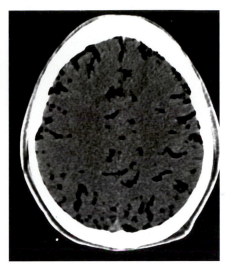

FIGURE 1. *Selected axial CT images demonstrating diffuse pneumocephaly from the skull base to the apex.*

4. Generally, pneumocephaly is asymptomatic and does not require treatment. However, if there is a sufficient burden of air, it can cause increased intracranial pressure as it adds volume to the confined space of the intracranial vault. Typically, the presenting symptoms include headache, nausea, and vomiting. This condition can also lead to mental status changes and focal neurological deficits (eg, motor paresis).

5. Treatment for pneumocephaly is inhaled oxygen. By placing the patient on 100% oxygen, nitrogen in the intracranial air will exchange with oxygen. The oxygen will, in turn, be consumed metabolically by the neurons and glial cells of the brain. In this way, the free gas inside the skull will be absorbed. This treatment can be simply the use of a 100% oxygen face mask. With proper treatment, recovery will be full and complete.

6. A CSF leak is a high-risk factor for subsequent infection. With head elevation and time, most traumatic CSF leaks will resolve spontaneously. However, if this condition persists, other treatment modalities should be considered, including the following:

   a. Ventricular or lumbar drainage.
   b. Packing of the middle ear, mastoid air cells, or eustation tube.
   c. Endoscopically packing the leak through the sinuses.
   d. Direct intracranial repair.

CLINICAL IMPLICATIONS

1. Triage decisions in the patient with craniocerebral trauma should be based on the admission GCS score and pupillary exam.

2. A basilar skull fracture can be caused by penetrating or blunt trauma mechanisms. The most common clinical signs include the following:

   a. CSF otorrhea, often associated with Battle's sign.
   b. CSF rhinorrhea, often associated with raccoon eyes.
   c. Pneumocephalus.
   d. Headache.
   e. Nausea and vomiting.

BATTLE'S SIGN

Named after William Henry Battle (1855–1936), an English surgeon, this sign suggests fracture at the base of the posterior portion of the skull (fractura basis cranii) and may also suggest underlying brain trauma. It consists of bruising immediately behind the ears. Another common sign of a skull injury is **raccoon eyes**, a purplish discoloration around the eyes following fracture of the frontal portion of the skull base. Battle's sign is seen several days after a basilar skull fracture.

3. CT is the definitive radiographic study in the evaluation of head trauma and should be used liberally. Deployable CT scanners in standard ISO (International Organization for Standardization) shelters are increasingly available in the field environment.

DAMAGE CONTROL

Initial treatment of basilar skull fracture with pneumocephalus consists of the following actions:

1. Head elevation.
2. 100% oxygen delivery.
3. Use of antibiotics when evacuating the patient to a medical facility (with a neurosurgeon) for further treatment.

SUMMARY

This is a case in which trauma resulted in a basilar skull fracture with a CSF leak. This injury, combined with aggressive bag ventilation, produced severe pneumocephaly associated with confusion, nausea, and emesis. Treatment with 100% oxygen and head elevation resulted in rapid improvement of symptoms and pneumocephaly. Upon discharge of the patient, the CSF leak had resolved.

SUGGESTED READING

Chapter 13: Face and neck injuries. In: *Emergency War Surgery, Third United States Revision.* Washington, DC: Department of the Army, Office of The Surgeon General, Borden Institute; 2004.

Chapter 15: Head injuries. In: *Emergency War Surgery, Third United States Revision.* Washington, DC: Department of the Army, Office of The Surgeon General, Borden Institute; 2004.

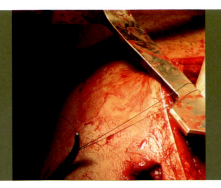

III.3
Right Hemisphere Fragment Wound

CASE PRESENTATION

This middle-aged, host nation male presented to the combat support hospital (CSH) with a severe brain injury. Neurological examination was significant for eyes that opened to noxious stimuli and pupils that were equal and reactive. He had a left hemiparesis and was localizing to pain with his right upper extremity. Examination of the scalp was significant for a right frontal entrance wound (Fig. 1) and a parietal exit wound. He was intubated. A lateral skull film showed retained fragments (Fig. 2) and a CT of the brain revealed a right frontal extracranial fragment, traumatic subarachnoid hemorrhage, and a right parietal parenchymal fragment (Fig. 3). He was taken to the operating room. The head was positioned in Mayfield pins to expose the right hemisphere. A trauma flap was fashioned by reflecting the scalp and temporalis muscle anteriorly. The dura mater was reflected forward, and parenchymal bleeding was stopped using bipolar electrocautery and topical fibrillar (Figs. 4–7). Because there was little swelling, the dura was reflected back and closed primarily over a subdural drain. The bone was secured using microplates and screws, and the temporalis fascia was closed with 0-VICRYL suture, followed by 2-0 VICRYL for the galea aponeurotica. Scalp edges were approximated with surgical staples, and an intracranial pressure (ICP) monitor was placed opposite the injured side. The patient was extubated within a week and recovered with residual left hemiparesis and no speech deficits.

TEACHING POINTS

1. Patients who present with nondominant hemisphere brain injury have a better prognosis than patients who have dominant brain injury. This case emphasizes the often better prognosis seen in nondominant hemisphere injuries.

2. Other presenting signs and symptoms that indicate a favorable prognosis in this case include the following:

   a. The admission CT showed no midline shift.
   b. The ventricles were not penetrated.
   c. There was no injury to deep structures of the brain.

CLINICAL IMPLICATIONS

Brain injury is common in combat environments and may occur secondary to penetrating blast or blunt mechanisms. Initial medical management

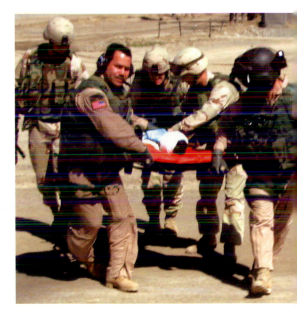

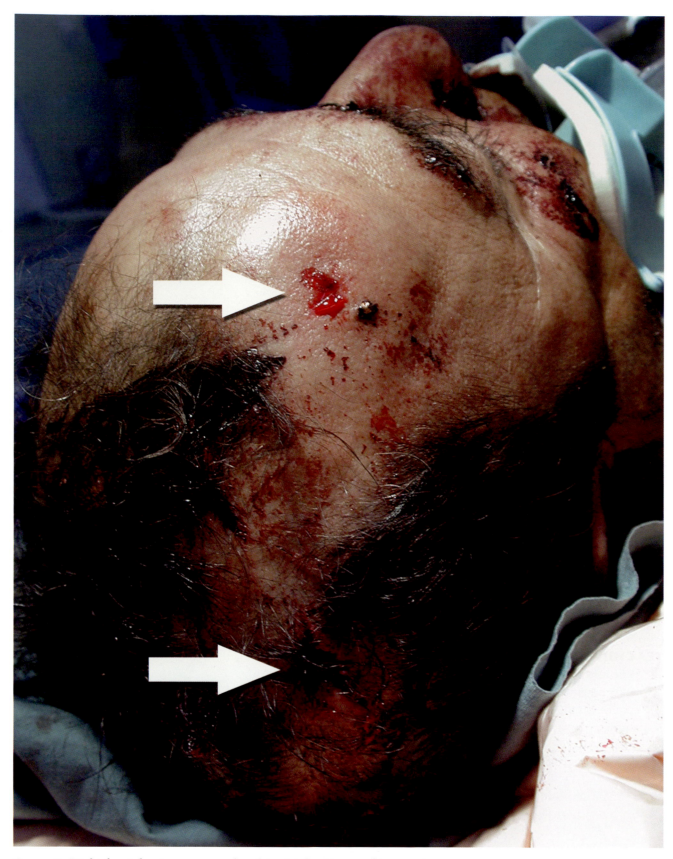

FIGURE 1. *Right frontal entrance wound and parietal exit wound* (arrows).

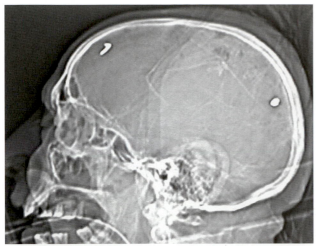

FIGURE 2. (Left) *Lateral skull radiograph showing metallic fragments in the frontal and parietal regions of the skull.*

FIGURE 3. (Bottom) *Series of axial CT images demonstrate a right frontal extracranial fragment, traumatic subarachnoid hemorrhage, and a right parietal lobe parenchymal fragment.*

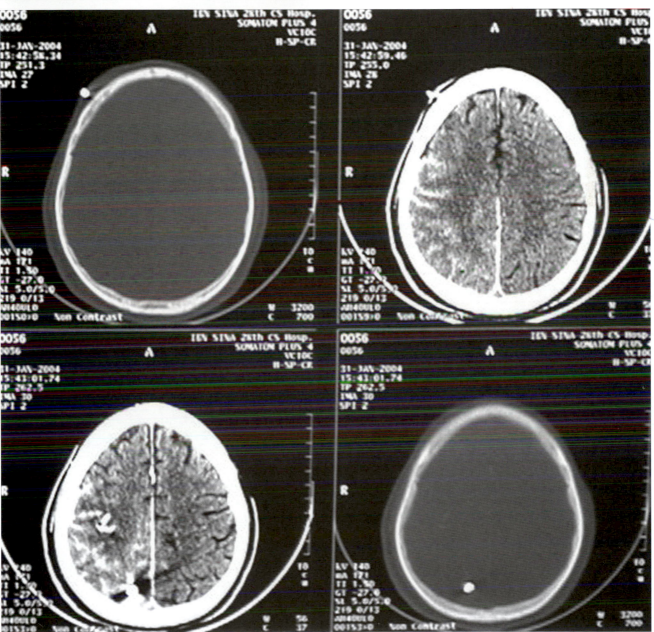

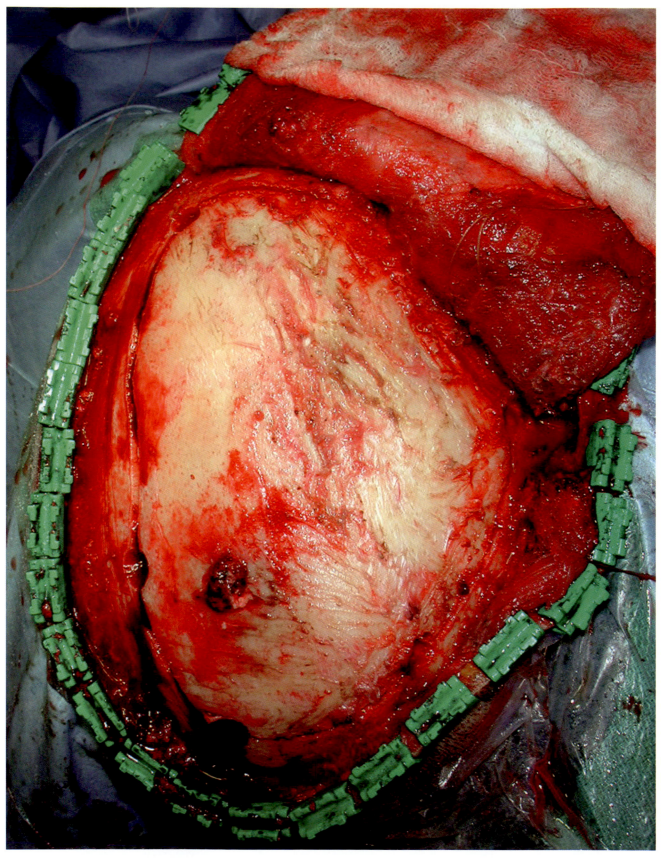

Figure 4. *A trauma flap was fashioned by reflecting the scalp and temporalis muscle anteriorly. The bone flap was fashioned using multiple burr holes and a craniotomy footplate high-speed drill attachment.*

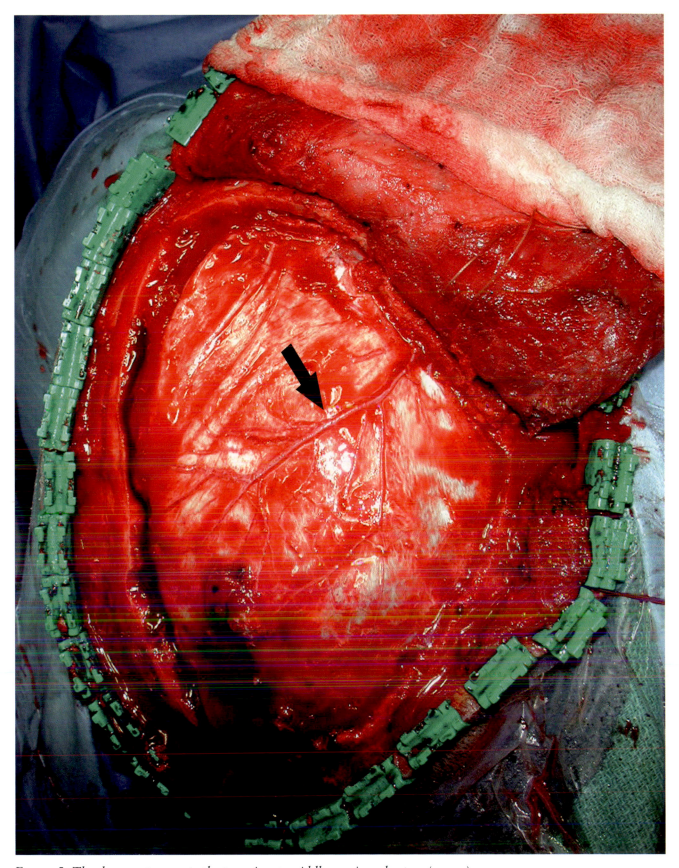

FIGURE 5. *The dura mater—note the prominent, middle meningeal artery* (arrow).

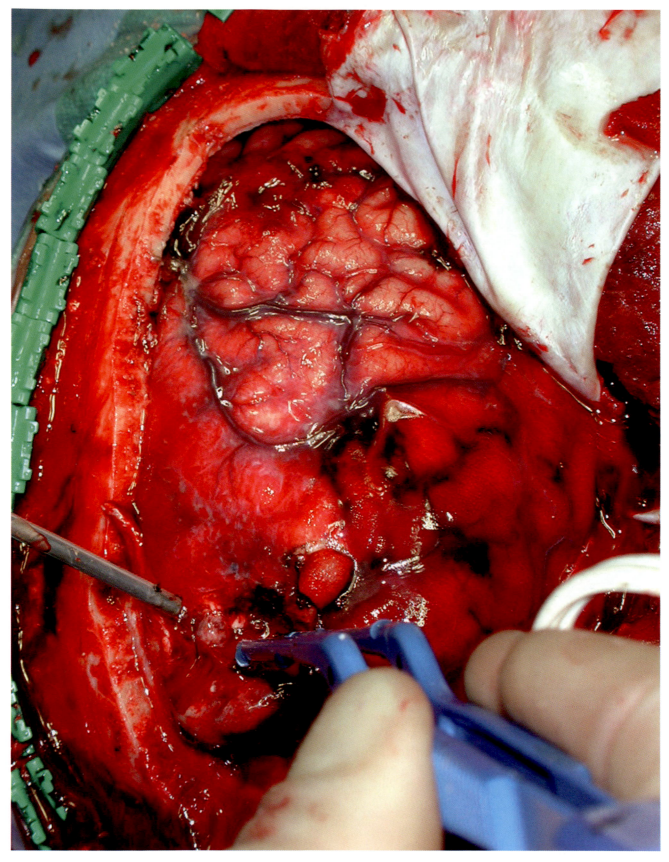

FIGURE 6. *The dura mater was reflected forward, and parenchymal bleeding was stopped using bipolar electrocautery.*

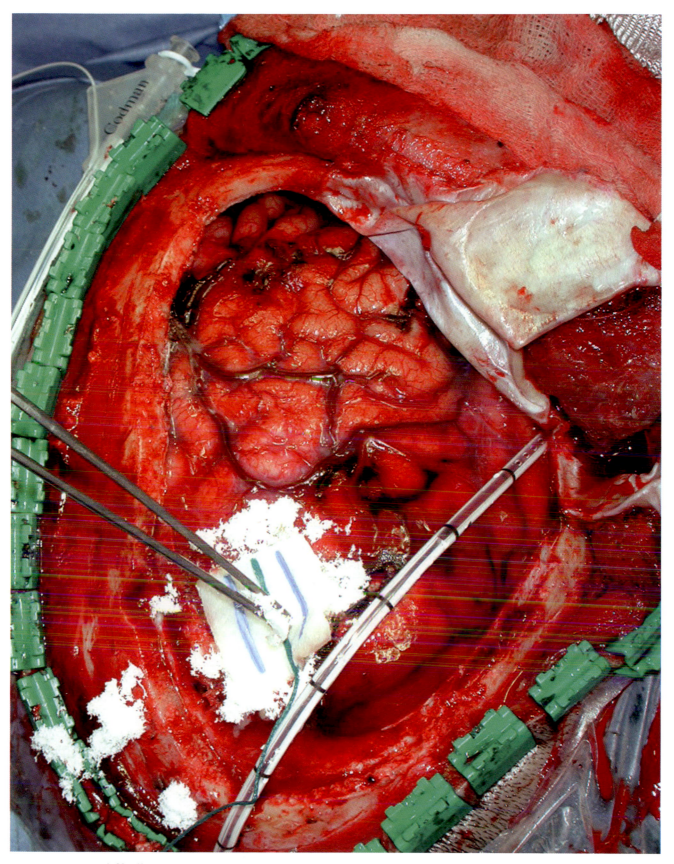

Figure 7. *Topical fibrillar was placed inside the bullet tract and tamponaded with a cottonoid patty.*

is critical to prevent secondary brain injury due to physiological derangement and includes:

1. Managing patients with a Glasgow Coma Scale score of 12 or less in an intensive care unit, if available.
2. Avoiding hypoxia and maintaining a PaO_2 of 100 mm Hg or greater.
3. Maintaining the PCO_2 between 35 to 40 mm Hg.
4. Elevating the head of the bed to about 30 degrees.
5. Sedating (or pharmacologically paralyzing) intubated patients.
6. Administering broad-spectrum antibiotics to patients with penetrating injuries.
7. Administering phenytoin to prevent seizures.
8. Administering mannitol to patients with a deteriorating neurological examination and suspicion of herniation.
9. Treating hypovolemia to help maintain cerebral perfusion pressure.
10. Evacuating the patient to a facility with a neurosurgeon as soon as possible.

DAMAGE CONTROL

Neurosurgical damage control includes early ICP control, cerebral blood flow preservation, and prevention of secondary cerebral injury from hypoxia, hypotension, and hyperthermia. Intubation with adequate ventilation and control of hemorrhage with adequate resuscitation, followed by immediate evacuation to the nearest neurosurgeon, are critical. Unnecessary diagnostic delays must be avoided.

SUMMARY

This case demonstrates a patient with severe primary brain injury due to a penetrating mechanism. In this case, secondary injury was minimized by appropriate neurosurgical intervention, resulting in an excellent, functional outcome for the patient.

SUGGESTED READING

Chapter 15: Head injuries. In: *Emergency War Surgery, Third United States Revision*. Washington, DC: Department of the Army, Office of The Surgeon General, Borden Institute; 2004.

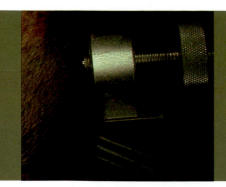

III.4
Manual Craniotomy for Penetrating Head Injury

CASE PRESENTATION

A 22-year-old helmeted soldier suffered a forehead injury during the explosion of an improvised explosive device (IED). He was the front-seat passenger in a HMMWV (high-mobility multipurposed wheeled vehicle or "Humvee") when debris from the blast struck him. He arrived at the combat support hospital (CSH) fully awake, with a Glasgow Coma Scale score of 15 and no focal neurological deficits. Physical examination revealed a laceration on the right frontal region of the scalp (Fig. 1). CT showed depressed right frontal bone fragments and a 3-cm hematoma with minimal mass effect (Fig. 2). No other significant injuries were noted on secondary survey. The patient was taken to the operating room. He was positioned in Mayfield pins to expose the right frontal region of the head. Then the scalp and temporalis muscle were elevated together after incision just behind the hairline from the sideburn to the midline. A brace and bit were used to fashion a burr hole just anterior to the site of skull penetration (Fig. 3), and then two more burr holes were created to place the penetration site in the center of a triangle (Fig. 4). After developing the epidural plane with a no. 3 Penfield dissector, a Gigli saw guide was passed from one burr hole to another (Fig. 5). The Gigli saw blade was then drawn through the epidural plane and used to cut the bone edges on all three sides of the triangle (Fig. 6). The bone flap was removed to expose the underlying dural laceration, which was enlarged in stellate fashion. After irrigation, the acute hematoma was spontaneously expressed by the swollen surrounding brain. After removal of the hematoma, the cavity was irrigated and visible bleeding stopped with bipolar electrocautery (Fig. 7). Hemostasis was then completed using fibrillar hemostatic agent. After hemostasis, a pledget of gel foam was laid in the epidural plane to create a barrier above the unclosed dura mater (Fig. 8). The bone flap was replaced using burr hole covers and screws to maximize his cosmetic outcome (Fig. 9). The galea aponeurotica was reapproximated using 2-0 VICRYL in inverted interrupted fashion, and the scalp edges were approximated with staples (Fig. 10). The forehead laceration was closed with 5-0 monofilament nylon. The patient was extubated at the end of the case, ambulated that evening, and ate a regular breakfast the following day. He was evacuated to a level IV medical treatment facility shortly thereafter and recovered without neurological deficit.

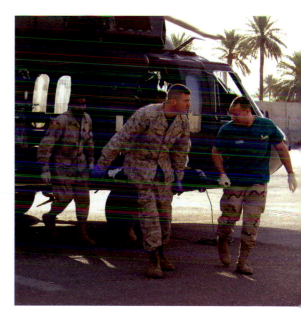

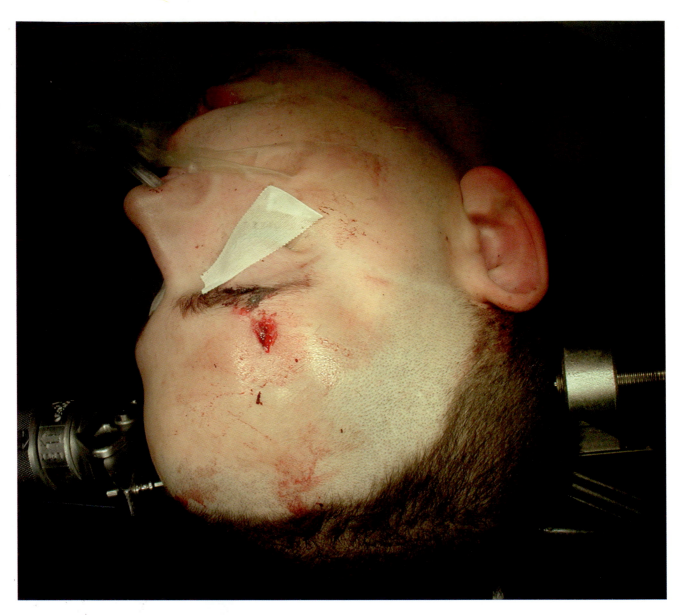

FIGURE 1. (Top) *Right frontal scalp laceration.*

FIGURE 2. (Bottom) *These images show right frontal bone fragments and a 3-cm hematoma with minimal mass effect. There is overlying soft-tissue edema.*

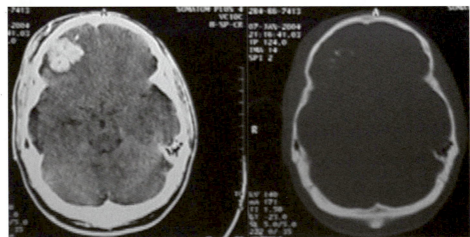

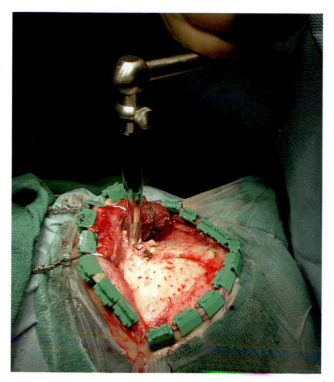

FIGURE 3. *A brace and bit were used to fashion a burr hole just anterior to the site of skull penetration.*

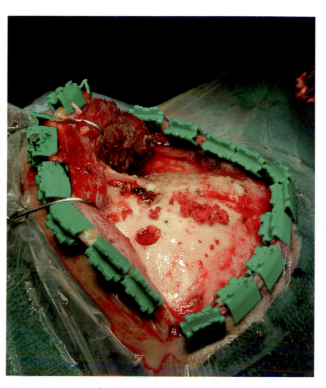

FIGURE 4. *Three burr holes have been created, with the entrance wound centered between them.*

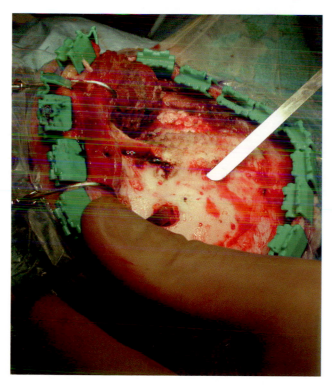

FIGURE 5. *A Gigli saw guide has been passed between two burr holes.*

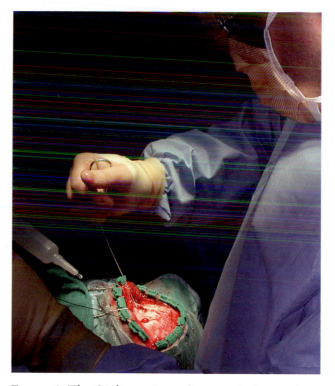

FIGURE 6. *The Gigli saw is used to cut the bone edges between burr holes.*

MEDICAL RAPID PROTOTYPING IN COMBAT CASUALTY CARE
Using Duplicate Anatomical Structures in Orthopaedic Reconstructions

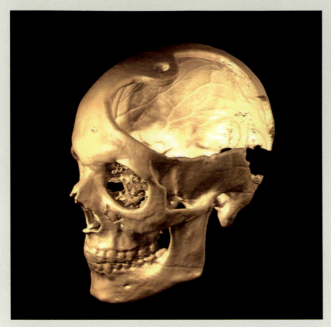

FIGURE 1. *Three-dimensional CT of patient s/p craniectomy.*

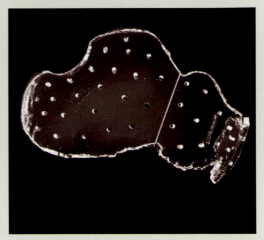

FIGURE 2. PMMA *cranial plate (implant).*

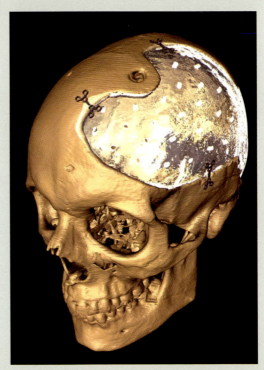

FIGURE 3. *Craniectomy model with implant in place.*

Modeling of craniofacial and other orthopaedic injuries (see Heterotopic Ossification sidebar on page 294), and the creation of custom implants and fixation devices are accomplished at Walter Reed Army Medical Center's 3D Medical Applications Center. Presurgical models are produced by a process known as stereolithography and delivered within 48 hours of receipt of appropriate CT scans. These duplicate anatomical structures are made available to any military medical center where they are used in preoperative planning, as well as in prosthetic fabrication. Custom cranial implants are also produced in-house at Walter Reed and sterilized, ready for implantation. Approximately 45% of models fashioned at Walter Reed are craniofacial.[1]

Case Presentation

A soldier on foot patrol in Iraq was struck by a sniper's bullet punching through his helmet just above the left ear. Fragments of Kevlar, bullet, and bone were driven into his brain and through the torcula. An initial craniotomy and debridement were performed at a deployed Combat Support Hospital (CSH). A second operation at another CSH was required to expand the craniectomy due to increases in intracranial pressure. After the patient was stable, he was medevaced to the level IV medical facility in Landstuhl, Germany, and, subsequently, to the National Naval Medical Center in Bethesda, Maryland. Two months after the

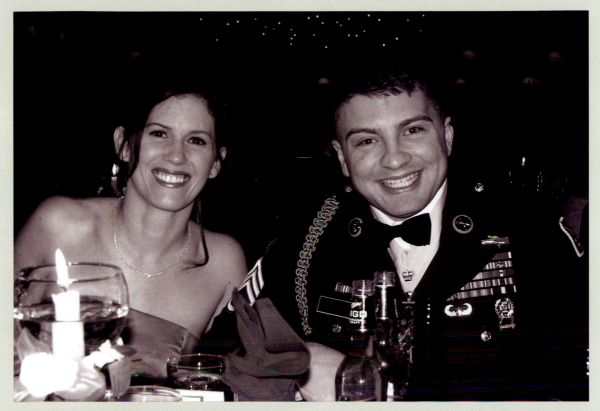

FIGURE 4. *Patient and his wife 5 months post-op.*

injury, extensive rehabilitation therapy was begun. Approximately 5 months from injury, a custom-made, two-piece, polymethyl methacrylate (PMMA) cranial plate was prepared and surgically implanted (Figs. 1–3). The plate was retained by small titanium fixation plates and screws. The patient was discharged postoperatively to continue rehabilitation therapy that included physical and cognitive functions. He shows minimal physical evidence of the injury and has demonstrated significant improvement in all neurological functions (Fig. 4).

—STEPHEN L. ROUSE, DDS

1. Walter Reed Army Medical Center 3D Medical Applications Center Web site. Available at: http://www.wramc. amedd.army.mil/Patients/healthcare/3dapp/. Accessed November 13, 2007.

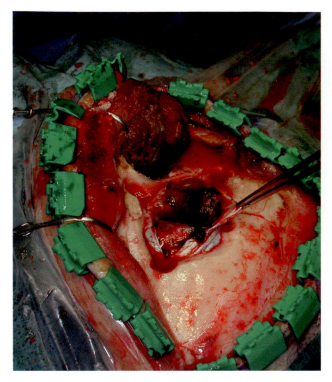

FIGURE 7. *Wound after the dura mater has been opened and the hematoma evacuated.*

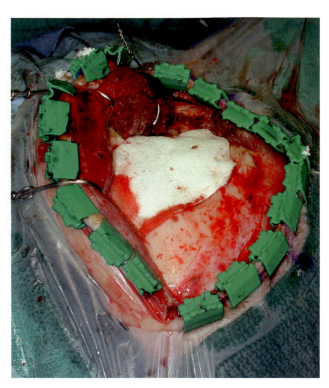

FIGURE 8. *A pledget of gel foam was laid in the epidural plane to create a barrier above the unclosed dura mater.*

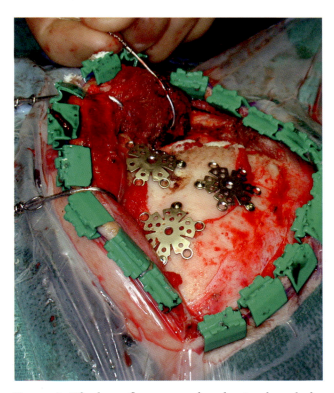

FIGURE 9. *The bone flap was replaced using burr hole covers and screws to maximize the patient's cosmetic outcome.*

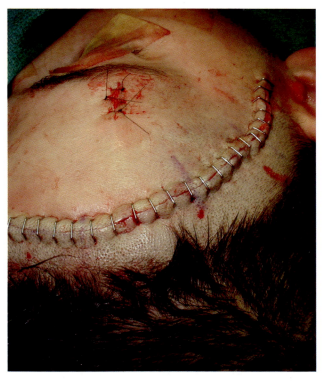

FIGURE 10. *After closure of the galea aponeurotica, surgical and entrance wounds are closed.*

TEACHING POINTS

1. In general, patients should not decline neurologically during surgery of the brain. Outcomes are closely associated with presenting neurological examination.
2. This case shows the manual technique of fashioning a bone flap when a high-speed drill is unavailable. A brace, bit, and Gigli saw kit require no external power source and are extremely portable in a single, small sterilization tray.
3. Standard closure techniques are also shown. In this case, the dura mater was not reapproximated and a drain was unnecessary. In general, primary closure of the dura mater should be performed if technically possible. A patch may be fashioned from pericranium, which can be harvested during elevation of the scalp.

CLINICAL IMPLICATIONS

In the combat environment, neurosurgeons may not be available or circumstances may prevent evacuation of patients to facilities with neurosurgical capability. If a neurosurgeon is not available, general surgeons may need to perform this surgery. Indications for emergent surgical management include the following:

1. Space-occupying lesions with neurological changes:

   a. Acute subdural hematoma.
   b. Acute epidural hematoma.
   c. Abscess.

2. Intracranial hematoma producing a greater than 5-mm midline shift or similar depression of the cortex.
3. Compound depressed fracture with neurological changes.
4. Penetrating injuries with neurological changes.

DAMAGE CONTROL

Severe head injuries are often seen in combination with significant chest, abdomen, and extremity injuries. Hemorrhage control and damage control techniques should be used to treat the cranial injury as soon as possible. It is often possible to operate in a major body cavity and on the brain simultaneously.

SUMMARY

This case is an example of an excellent outcome in a patient with a penetrating brain injury using a manual craniotomy technique. This technique can be used in austere environments when faced with a deteriorating patient with penetrating brain injury and should be studied by all deploying general surgeons.

SUGGESTED READING

Chapter 11: Critical care. In: *Emergency War Surgery, Third United States Revision*. Washington, DC: Department of the Army, Office of The Surgeon General, Borden Institute; 2004.

Chapter 15: Head injuries. In: *Emergency War Surgery, Third United States Revision*. Washington, DC: Department of the Army, Office of The Surgeon General, Borden Institute; 2004.

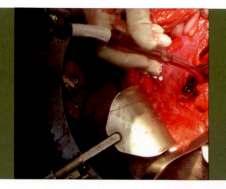

III.5
Spinal Cord Injury Without Paralysis

CASE PRESENTATION

This 5-year-old host nation male sustained injuries after multiple weapons were discharged into a vehicle that was attempting to run a checkpoint. His vital signs were stable. However, he was persistently tachycardic despite fluid resuscitation. The patient complained of persistent, severe abdominal pain. His neurological motor examination was intact. A large entrance wound was apparent on his lower back. He was taken to the operating room (OR) where exploratory laparotomy revealed a small bowel laceration, which was repaired. No other abdominal injuries were found. The patient was placed in the prone position to determine the extent of dorsal damage. He had an exposed spinal cord (at the L3 level) with a cerebrospinal fluid leak (Fig. 1). The spine was stable, with only posterior spinal column involvement. Because of extensive tissue damage around the spinal cord, a gluteal flap was created and rotated over the spinal canal to prevent cerebrospinal fluid leakage and infection (Fig. 2). A wound vacuum-assisted closure (VAC) device was placed over the wound, and the patient was taken to the intensive care unit (ICU) for continued resuscitation. His postoperative course was unremarkable, and he returned to the OR on subsequent occasions for tissue debridement, wound VAC placement, and eventual wound closure. After prolonged rehabilitation, the patient was discharged and able to walk without assistance.

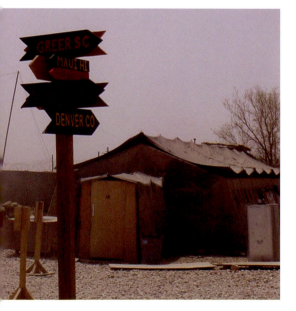
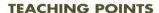

TEACHING POINTS

1. Wounds to the back may involve any anterior body compartment. High-velocity fragments may travel to any part of the body. It is imperative that a full-body radiological evaluation be performed to rule out injuries distant from the obvious entry wounds.
2. ICUs must have the equipment necessary to provide care to pediatric patients. It is essential that the deployed level II and level III medical treatment facilities (combat support hospital [CSH]/ Forward Surgical Team [FST]) have the necessary equipment and trained personnel to manage pediatric surgery patients.
3. Wound VAC dressings have proven useful in sealing cerebrospinal fluid leaks.

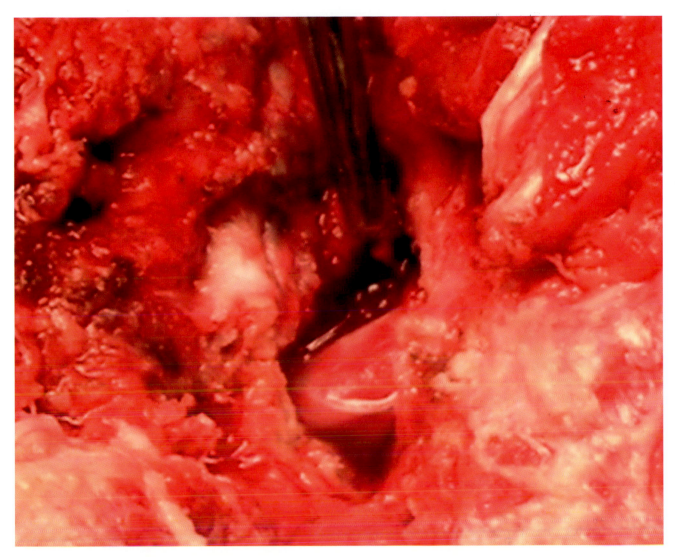

FIGURE 1. *Close-up of the exposed spinal cord.*

CLINICAL IMPLICATIONS

1. When complex wounds involving the head, thorax, abdomen, or extremities coexist with vertebral column injuries, lifesaving measures take precedence over the definitive diagnosis and management of the spinal column and spinal cord. The spine must be immobilized to prevent neurological deterioration until the extent of spinal stability is determined. However, unlike blunt force mechanisms, penetrating spinal trauma often results in no spinal column instability. Removal of fragments from the spinal canal is indicated in patients with neurological deterioration.

2. Combat injuries of the spinal column, with or without associated cord injury, differ from those routinely encountered in civilian practice. They are often open, contaminated, and associated with other organ injuries.

DAMAGE CONTROL

1. Emergent spine surgery for penetrating or closed injuries of the spinal cord is only indicated in the presence of neurological deterioration.

2. In neurologically stable patients with fragments in the cervical canal, delaying surgery for 7 to 10 days reduces problems with dural leak and makes repair easier.

SUMMARY

This case demonstrates the association of hollow viscus injury associated with penetrating back injury. Remarkably, this patient made a good, functional

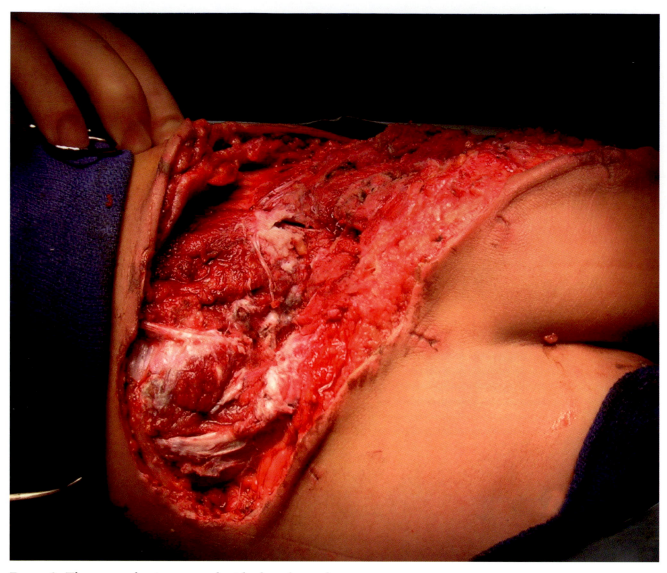

FIGURE 2. *The exposed spine covered with gluteal muscle.*

recovery because trauma tenets were rigorously followed. Specifically, the patient was appropriately resuscitated, intraabdominal injuries were repaired, and the exposed spinal cord was then covered with a muscle flap and wound VAC. Bony structures in this penetrating injury remained stable. It is imperative that all treatment team members understand the likelihood of providing care to individuals of all ages. In addition, high-velocity wounds can travel throughout the body.

SUGGESTED READING

Chapter 17: Abdominal injuries. In: *Emergency War Surgery, Third United States Revision.* Washington, DC: Department of the Army, Office of The Surgeon General, Borden Institute; 2004.

Chapter 20: Wounds and injuries of the spinal column and cord. In: *Emergency War Surgery, Third United States Revision.* Washington, DC: Department of the Army, Office of The Surgeon General, Borden Institute; 2004.

Chapter 33: Pediatric care. In: *Emergency War Surgery, Third United States Revision.* Washington, DC: Department of the Army, Office of The Surgeon General, Borden Institute; 2004.

COMMENTARY
Hemicraniectomy

by LTC Rocco A. Armonda, MD

A major paradigm shift has occurred in the far-forward treatment of neurotrauma patients. Prior historical practices of radical debridement and minimal decompression have been replaced by minimal debridement and radical decompression (Fig. 1). This is especially true in the presence of blast-induced penetrating brain injury or under body armor injury. Because of the combination of improved body armor, advanced combat casualty care at the site of wounding, and rapid evacuation, a higher proportion of neurotrauma casualties benefit from early neurosurgical intervention. Theoretically, the far-forward neurosurgeon has modern imaging capability, electric drills, and all the equipment necessary for cranial-spinal decompression and resuscitation. In some cases, the deployed neurosurgeon may receive casualties in less than an hour after injury, due to the heroic efforts of the tactical MEDEVAC. On arrival, these patients may have already been intubated, chemically paralyzed, and without a sensorimotor examination. In such cases, the neurosurgeon is dependent on the axial CT imaging of the brain to determine if the casualty will benefit from aggressive cranial-spinal decompression; invasive cranial monitoring with medical management; or compassionate, nonheroic palliative care. Those penetrating injuries that course through the diencephalon (hypothalamus/thalamus) or brain stem (known as the central core of the brain or in some cases "zona fatalis") uniformly do poorly. Patients are more likely to survive in a minimally responsive state, without the ability to interact with their environment. They eventually succumb to delayed infections and the morbidity of a dependent, bedridden life. However, this is not the case for those patients with focal mass lesions, localized or hemispheric edema, or penetrating trauma above the diencephalon or above the ventricular level, with a motor examination demonstrating withdrawal or localization to stimuli. These patients may benefit greatly from a decompressive hemicraniectomy and hematoma evacuation. The focus of a far-forward neurosurgeon is to decompress the brain stem, obtain hemostasis, and stabilize the patient for a 7,000+ mile transport to the United States. Given this mission, the neurosurgeon seeks to avoid complications associated with delayed hydrocephalus, diffuse cerebral edema, or delayed hematoma formation. Preferably, this is done by placing a ventriculostomy when indicated in theater prior to transport; performing a large (12 cm or more) hemicraniectomy when delayed swelling is suspected (ie, postblast injury); and ensuring hemostasis, as confirmed by a postoperative, pre-MEDEVAC CT scan before transport to the continental United States. A summary of the typical complications and respective treatment during the first 6 months is listed in Table 1.

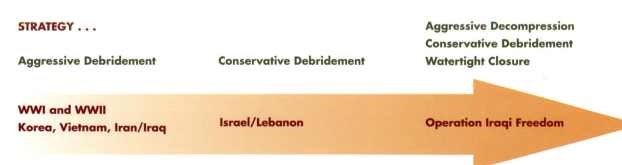

FIGURE 1. *Historical evolution of treatment paradigms for penetrating brain injury.*

TABLE 1. *Complications of Wartime Penetrating Brain Injury*

TIME	TYPE OF COMPLICATIONS	TREATMENT	TYPICAL LOCATION

0–24 hours	ICP increased
	Hematoma
	Ischemia
	
	Anatomical defect
	Hypoxia
	
	Hypotension
		Hemicraniectomy
		Evac/coag correction
		Decompression/identity occlusion
		  (angiography)
		Anatomical closure
		Airway/pulmonary correction
		Overt or occult EBL
		PRBCs/FFP/PLTs vs whole
		  blood vs hypertonic saline
			Level III
			(FST/CSH)

24–48 hours	ICP increased Hematoma Hydrocephalus Edema Seizures	Hemicraniectomy Evac/coag correction Ventriculostomy Decompression Antiepileptics/EEG monitoring	Level III (CSH)
72 hours–1st week	Edema ICH (contusion) Hydrocephalus CSF leak Ischemia Pseudoaneurysm Seizures	Medical/surgical decompression Correct coagulopathy Ventriculostomy Repair/CSF diversion Medical/endovascular Tx Surgical/endovascular Tx Antiepileptics/EEG monitoring	Level IV/V (LRMC)

2nd–3rd week	Infection
	Vasospasm
	
	Pseudoaneurysm
	Seizures
	Delayed hydrocephalus
		R/O abscess, repair CSF leak
		Multimodal monitoring (transcranial
		  Doppler, brain tissue oxygen, EEG,
		  CBF monitoring)
		Treatment: microballoon angioplasty
		  intraarterial nicardipine
		Endovascular vs microsurgery Tx
		Antiepileptics
		VP shunt (low-pressure; consider use
		  of a programmable valve)
			Level V
			(NNMC, WRAMC)

1–6 months	Infection
	Low-pressure hydrocephalus
	Syndrome of the Trephine
	Seizures
	Cranioplasty complications:
	  Temporalis atrophy
	  Infection
	  Hydrocephalus
	  Epidural/subgaleal
	    hygroma/hematoma
	  ICH
	  Scalp necrosis
		R/O abscess, meningitis, and ventriculitis
		VP shunt (programmable valve)
		Reconstructive cranioplasty
		Antiepileptics
		
		Resuspension/implant/fat graft
		Prosthesis removal
		VP shunt
		Drainage
		
		Evacuation
		Free flap
			Level V
			VA-civilian rehabilitation,
			polytrauma center

CBF: *cerebral blood flow*; coag: *coagulopathy*; CSF: *cerebrospinal fluid*; CSH: *combat support hospital*; EBL: *estimated blood loss*; EEG: *electroencephalogram*; evac: *evacuation*; FFP: *fresh frozen plasma*; FST: *Forward Surgical Team*; ICH: *intracranial hemorrhage*; ICP: *intracranial pressure*; LRMC: *Landstuhl Regional Medical Center*; NNMC: *National Naval Medical Center*; PLTs: *platelets*; PRBCs: *packed red blood cells*; R/O: *rule out*; TCD: *transcranial Doppler*; Tx: *treatment*; VA: *Veterans Administration*; VP: *ventriculoperitoneal*; WRAMC: Walter Reed Army Medical Center.*

Traumatic Brain Injury

by Katherine M. Helmick, MS, CNRN, CRNP, and Deborah L. Warden, MD

Traumatic brain injury (TBI) has been called the signature injury of the current conflicts in Afghanistan and Iraq.[1] TBI can be subclassified into blunt (closed) injury and penetrating brain injury. Troops with penetrating brain injury are usually identified and cared for immediately because of the overt nature of their intracranial lesions, as exemplified in the case studies in Chapter III. Neurosurgical intervention was necessary in all cases, and excellent recovery outcomes were also reported. Historically, in times of military conflict, penetrating brain injury has been well reported. However, in the context of the current conflict, closed-brain injury (specifically mild TBI) has emerged as a real concern and potentially threatening healthcare problem. Approximately 29% of Operation Iraqi Freedom/Operation Enduring Freedom battle-injured casualties, who were medically evacuated through Walter Reed Army Medical Center, sustained at least a mild TBI.[2] Several peacetime military studies have helped to elucidate the physical and cognitive sequelae occurring after mild TBI or concussion. Delays in reaction time and declines in arithmetic calculation abilities have been shown to affect concussed cadets up to 7 days after injury.[3,4] In addition, neurocognitive impairment has been found in athletes who did not lose consciousness while sustaining a concussion.[5] For these reasons, there is concern that a soldier who has sustained a mild TBI may become sufficiently impaired as to affect personal and unit readiness. A concussion is suspected in anyone exposed to or involved in a blast, fall, vehicle crash, or direct head impact who becomes dazed, confused, or loses consciousness, even momentarily.

The operational setting provides a unique set of circumstances that prompts special considerations in the assessment and management of mild TBI in order to arrive at an optimal plan for both the injured and the mission. Certain variables that are present in current theater operations make the identification of mild TBI even more critical. Many troops experience numerous deployments that increase their risk of sustaining more than one concussion. In addition, the unconventional nature of current operations has translated into an increased likelihood of exposure to blast during a tour of duty. In Operation Iraqi Freedom, blast-induced brain injury is the primary mechanism that produces TBI. Blast injury may cause TBI through multiple mechanisms, including injury from energized debris that may cause blunt or penetrating brain injury, as well as displacement of the person that may result in a closed-brain injury pattern. The potential to cause brain injury from primary blast is under current study.

The assessment and management of implications from mild TBI differ from the neurosurgical patients portrayed in the case studies. In these patients, the Glasgow Coma Scale (GCS) score was assessed and influenced the management process to include neurosurgical intervention. Unfortunately, the GCS is not a sensitive assessment tool for mild TBI because many individuals score 15 and appear uninjured; however, they may have significant physical or neurocognitive signs and symptoms. A brief, yet valuable, tool that can be used to assess deficits after mild TBI is the Military Acute Concussion Evaluation (MACE). Embedded within MACE is the Standardized Assessment of Concussion[6] (SAC), a validated tool used extensively in the sports realm to assess neurocognitive functioning.

Concussion management guidelines have been developed and disseminated for field operational use.[7] These guidelines specifically address the assessment and management of mild TBI occurring in the context of a military operational setting. Assessment is based on

4							
5	2945	1358	GSW CHEST	X	X	③—	
6			GSW Abd	X	X	③—	
7		1570	SYNCOPE				
8	2946	1358	GSW: ① FLANK	X		①—	
9	2944	1358	② LE INJ.	X	X	X	ORTHO
1C	2947		② LE INJ.	X	X		ORTHO
OB	2942	1333	BURNS ® ARM		X		

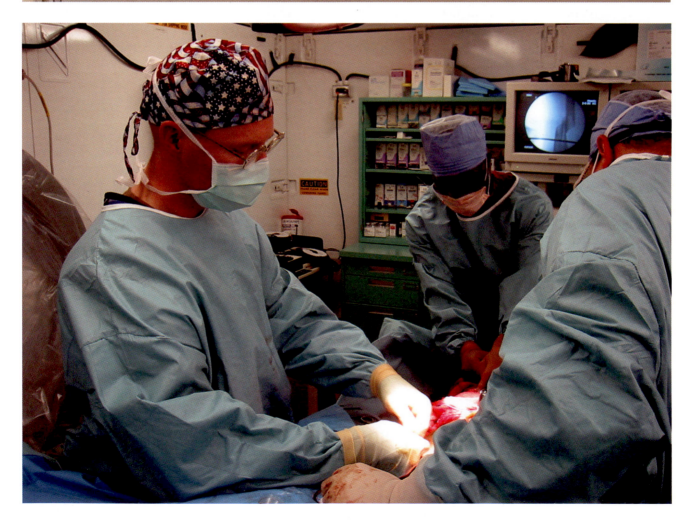

utilizing MACE, as well as identifying red flags that would prompt an urgent evacuation to a higher echelon of care. Treatment algorithms are based on symptomatic relief, as well as protection of the soldier until asymptomatic. An educational intervention emphasizing the anticipated course of recovery has been demonstrated to reduce morbidity.[8] Various cognitive tests may be utilized to gain more objective information with regard to cognitive deficits after TBI. Prior to return to duty, troops are exertionally tested (eg, running in place for 5 minutes, doing sit-ups for 5 minutes, etc) to evaluate them for a possible return of TBI symptoms. (See Appendix D for the MACE form.)

REFERENCES

1. Okie S. Traumatic brain injury in the war zone. *N Engl J Med*. 2005;352:2043–2047.

2. Warden D. Military TBI during the Iraq and Afghanistan wars. *J Head Trauma Rehabil*. 2006;21:398–402.

3. Warden DL, Bleiberg J, et al. Persistent prolongation of simple reaction time in sports concussion. *Neurology*. 2001;57:524–526.

4. Bleiberg J, Cernich AN, et al. Duration of cognitive impairment after sports concussion. *Neurosurgery*. 2004;54:1073–1080.

5. McCrea M, Kelly JP, et al. Immediate neurocognitive effects of concussion. *Neurosurgery*. 2002;50:1032–1040.

6. McCrea M, Kelly JP, Randolph C. *Standardized Assessment of Concussion (SAC): Manual for Administration, Scoring and Interpretation*. 2nd ed. Waukesha, WI: Authors; 2000.

7. Defense and Veterans Brain Injury Center Working Group on the Acute Management of Mild Traumatic Brain Injury in Military Operational Settings. *Clinical Practice Guidelines and Recommendations*. Available at: http://www.pdhealth.mil/downloads/comprehensive_program_for_traumatic_brain_injury.pdf. Accessed September 4, 2007.

8. Ponsford J, Willmott C, et al. Impact of early intervention on outcome following mild head injury in adults. *J Neural Neurosurg Psychiatry*. 2002;73:330–332.

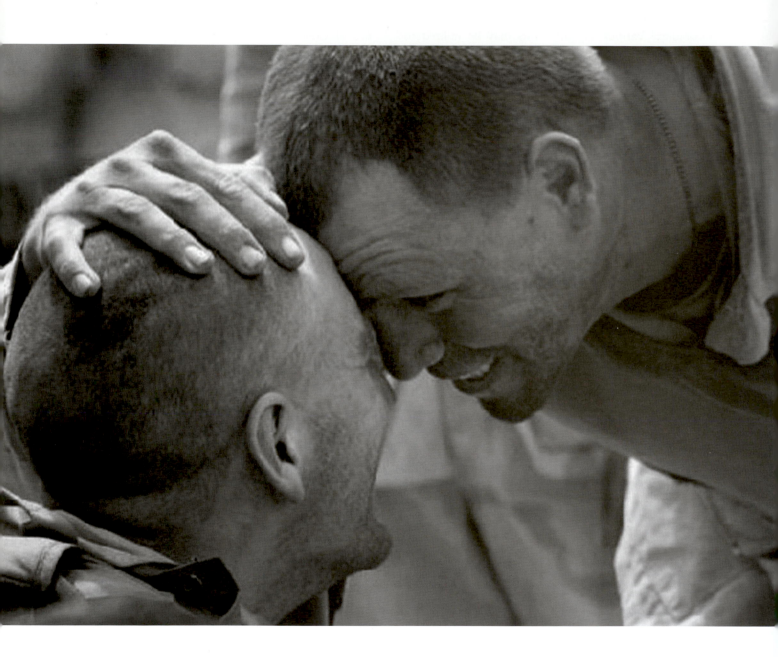

Chapter IV
THORACIC TRAUMA

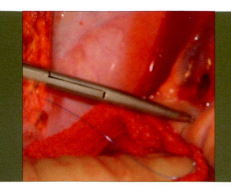

IV.1
Penetrating Thoraco-Abdominal Trauma, I

CASE PRESENTATION

This 20-year-old host nation male was riding his donkey and got caught in a mortar barrage. He presented with hypotension and multiple fragment entry wounds to his chest and abdomen (Fig. 1). A FAST exam revealed a pericardial effusion (Fig. 2). At laparotomy, a large liver laceration was discovered (Fig. 3). This was rapidly packed to control bleeding. A median sternotomy was performed. A penetrating injury near the right atrial appendage, in the groove of the right coronary artery, was identified (Fig. 4). This was repaired using 3-0 Prolene suture with pledgets fashioned from the patient's pericardium. A horizontal mattress suture was used to avoid occluding the right coronary artery (Fig. 5 [also see Fig. 8]). Continued bleeding from the right chest necessitated a right thoracotomy where several lung lacerations were controlled. Further abdominal exploration revealed several small bowel lacerations that were repaired. A temporary abdominal closure was performed (Fig. 6). After 36 hours, the patient was returned to the operating room for reexploration. The liver laceration was not bleeding, and bowel edema had resolved. The patient's abdomen was closed, and his recovery was uneventful (Fig. 7).

TEACHING POINTS

1. This case demonstrates the relatively common combat scenario in which a patient presents with multiple truncal wounds and hypotension, posing the dilemma of which body cavity to open first. In this case, although the FAST exam revealed a pericardial effusion, the patient's relative stability allowed exploratory laparotomy with control of bleeding prior to sternotomy.

2. It is important to be aware of the coronary arteries when repairing cardiac injuries. In this case, a horizontal mattress suture was used to avoid occlusion of the coronary artery.

3. It is critical for the surgeon faced with a multiply wounded patient to approach each injury systematically. The importance of a well-trained team able to keep the patient stable and warm during this process cannot be overstated. Ongoing resuscitation and patient warming are fundamental.

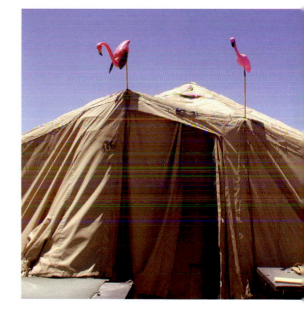

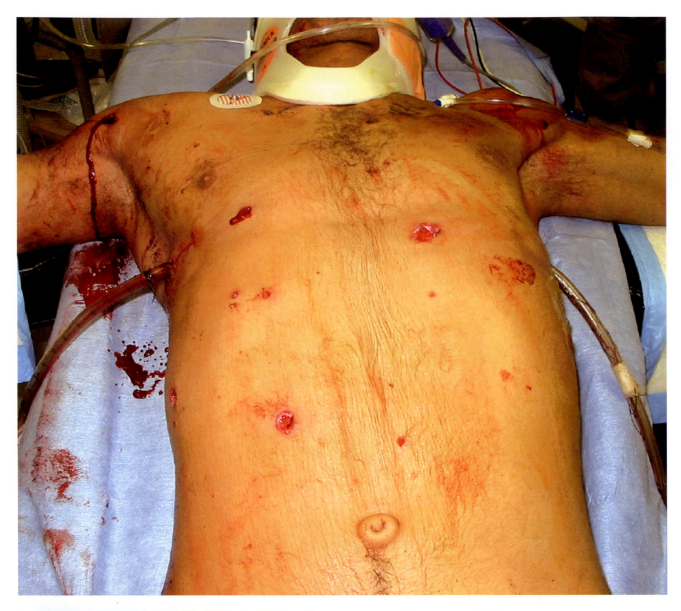

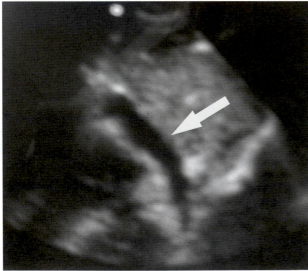

FIGURE 1. (Top, page 120) *Patient on admission to the CSH. Note penetrating wounds of the chest and abdomen.*

FIGURE 2. (Bottom, page 120) *Ultrasound (FAST) shows pericardial effusion* (arrow).

FIGURE 3. (Top, page 121) *Laparotomy revealing large liver laceration.*

FIGURE 4. (Bottom, page 121) *Median sternotomy exposure. Note right atrial penetrating wound* (arrow).

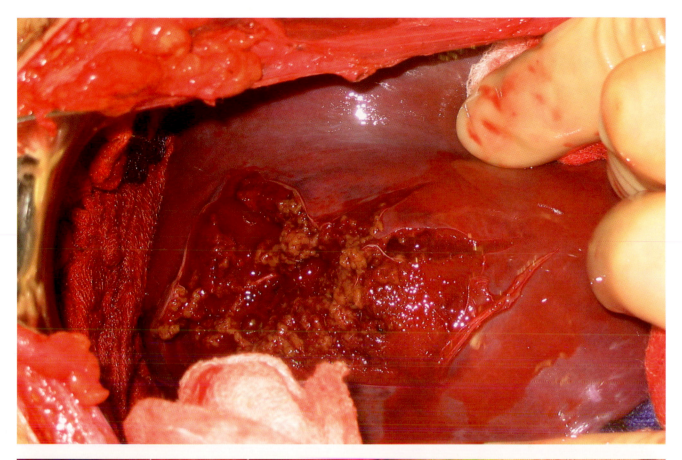

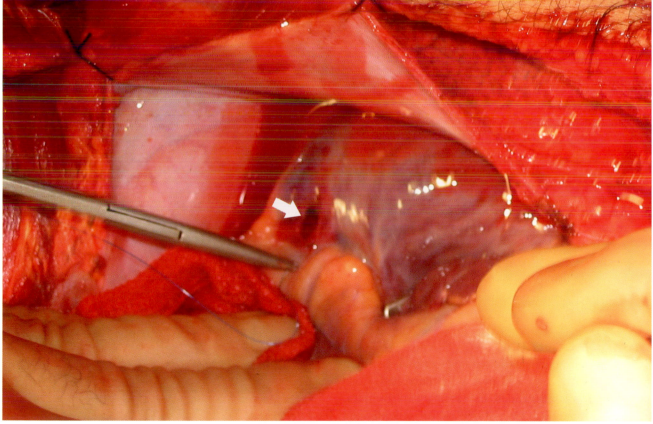

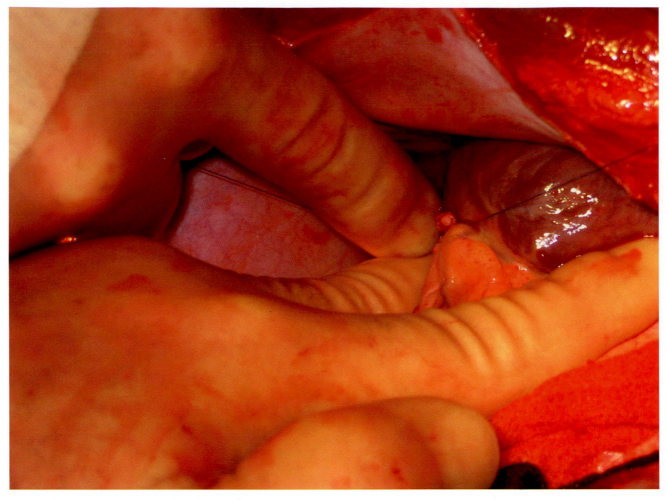

Figure 5. *The cardiac injury has been repaired.*

CLINICAL IMPLICATIONS

1. Isolated punctures of the heart should be exposed by opening the pericardium and occluding the injury with finger pressure. Other methods include the use of a Foley catheter or skin staples.
2. Use pledgeted horizontal mattress sutures (2-0 or 3-0 Prolene) on a tapered needle for definitive repair. Care must be taken to avoid injury to the coronary artery and muscle (Fig. 8). Simple figure-of-eight suture repair may be used if there is no risk of coronary artery occlusion.
3. Atrial repairs may include simple ligature, stapled repair, or running suture closure.

DAMAGE CONTROL

This case represents classic damage control. Bleeding from the heart, lung, and liver was controlled. Contamination was controlled by closing enterotomies, and the abdomen was temporarily closed with planned reoperation.

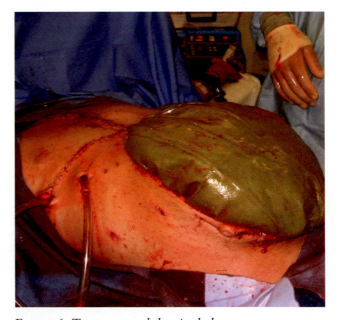

Figure 6. *Temporary abdominal closure.*

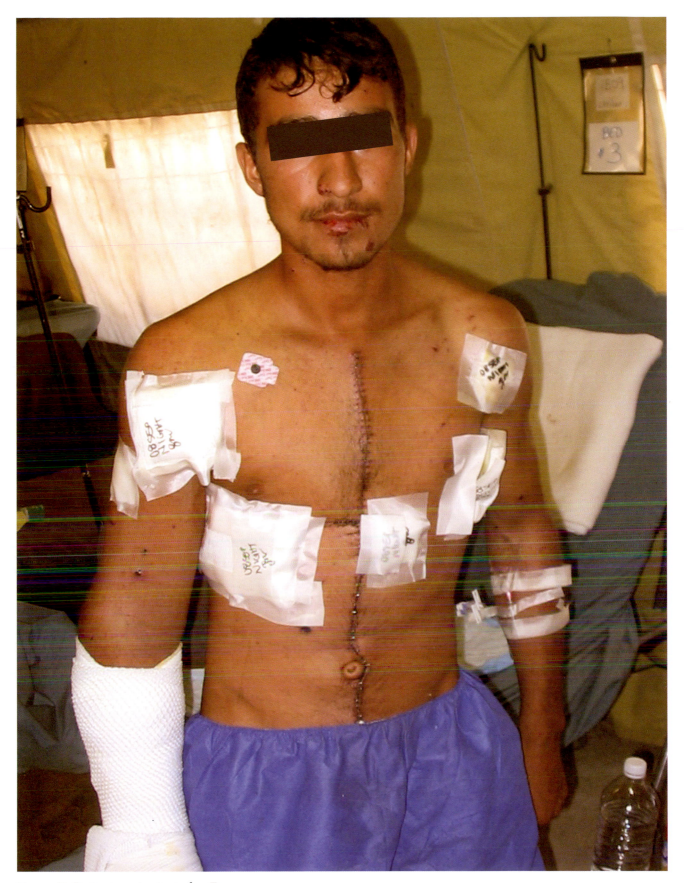

FIGURE 7. *Patient on post-op day 7.*

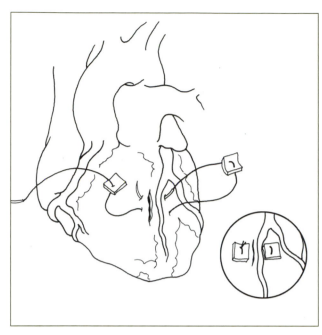

FIGURE 8. *Repair of penetrating cardiac injury.*

SUMMARY

This case demonstrates an appropriate approach to a patient with multiple penetrating injuries to the thorax and abdomen. Using damage control techniques and a systematic approach with ongoing appropriate resuscitation, the patient made a full recovery.

SUGGESTED READING

Chapter 12: Damage control surgery. In: *Emergency War Surgery, Third United States Revision*. Washington, DC: Department of the Army, Office of The Surgeon General, Borden Institute; 2004.

Chapter 16: Thoracic injuries. In: *Emergency War Surgery, Third United States Revision*. Washington, DC: Department of the Army, Office of The Surgeon General, Borden Institute; 2004.

Chapter 17: Abdominal injuries. In: *Emergency War Surgery, Third United States Revision*. Washington, DC: Department of the Army, Office of The Surgeon General, Borden Institute; 2004.

Chapter 22: Soft-tissue injuries. In: *Emergency War Surgery, Third United States Revision*. Washington, DC: Department of the Army, Office of The Surgeon General, Borden Institute; 2004.

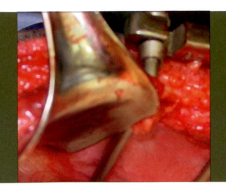

IV.2
Penetrating Thoraco-Abdominal Trauma, II

CASE PRESENTATION

A 40-year-old host nation male arrived at the Forward Surgical Team (FST) 30 minutes after sustaining multiple gunshot wounds from an AK-47. He was conscious. There were multiple entry and exit wounds to the left upper extremity, as well as two entry wounds to the left thorax, which entered lateral to the nipple at the nipple line. Vital signs showed a blood pressure of 100/60 mm Hg and a heart rate of 120 beats per minute. A chest tube was placed in the left hemithorax with a return of 250 cc of blood. A FAST scan was negative for intraabdominal blood and negative for pericardial blood. Abdominal examination was negative for signs of peritonitis, and the abdomen was flat without distention. An initial chest X-ray, taken after chest tube placement, showed a moderate-sized left hemothorax and adequate chest tube placement. There were two bullet fragments that were apparently in the lower ipsilateral thorax. No abdominal films were taken, and resuscitation was performed according to Advanced Trauma Life Support (ATLS) protocol. The patient was taken to the operating room (OR) to address the extremity wounds after initial resuscitation with crystalloid and 2 units of packed red blood cells (PRBCs). He required washout of the multiple gunshot wounds and open reduction of a forearm fracture. Total time in the OR was 90 minutes. During this time, chest tube output was followed closely. Drainage for the next hour was 200 cc. He continued to receive resuscitation in the OR with crystalloid, and his blood pressure remained stable. The patient was then transferred to the intensive care unit (ICU), where chest tube output continued to be monitored. He became hypotensive and responded to boluses of crystalloid and packed RBCs. Chest tube output increased to 300 cc for the next hour. A repeat chest X-ray showed adequate drainage of the hemothorax. Abdominal examination revealed a distended abdomen. Repeat FAST scan was positive for intraperitoneal fluid. He was returned to the OR for urgent laparotomy. The patient was placed supine with a bump under the left hemithorax in preparation for a left thoracotomy. On entering the abdomen, a large amount of blood was evacuated immediately. A splenic laceration (Fig. 1) and a left colon perforation at the splenic flexure were encountered. There was gross fecal soilage of the peritoneal cavity, with an approximately 2-cm diaphragm defect. Splenectomy was performed and damage control principles followed. The left hemithorax was inspected through the

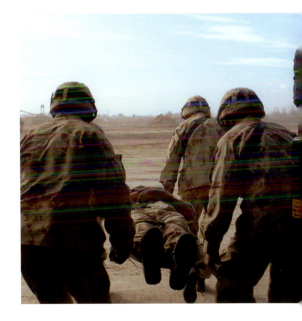

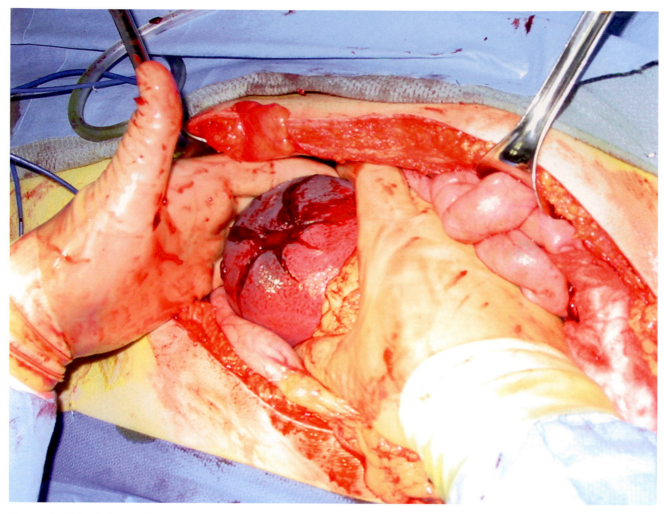

Figure 1. *Splenic laceration.*

diaphragmatic defect (Fig. 2), and there was no active hemorrhage from the left hemithorax. Postoperatively, there was no further significant hemorrhage from the chest tube. The patient was urgently evacuated to a level III medical treatment facility, where definitive surgery was performed.

TEACHING POINTS

1. Thoracoabdominal injuries, especially at the level of the nipple line or below, carry a high incidence of intraperitoneal injury. As demonstrated in this case, a high index of suspicion must accompany such injuries and immediate laparotomy considered, even without definitive evidence of intraperitoneal injury.

2. After placing the chest tube on the affected side, this patient's condition stabilized, allowing further studies to fully evaluate his injury. Lacking sensitivity, a FAST scan performed early after penetrating trauma may be negative. If plain X-rays (chest X-rays, KUB [kidneys, ureters, and bladder]) with radiopaque markers for the entry and exit wounds reveal that the trajectory of the fragment likely passed through the peritoneal cavity, then laparotomy should be performed.

3. When it is unclear to the surgeon which body cavity is likely the source of bleeding, position the patient supine with the affected hemithorax "bumped up" to a 30- to 45-degree angle. This will allow access to both the abdomen and the chest. By rotating the OR table up to 30 degrees, the chest will essentially be in the lateral decubitus position, easily allowing a thoracotomy incision to be made (Fig. 3).

CLINICAL IMPLICATIONS

1. When the patient presents with a penetrating truncal injury, proceed with ATLS protocol. If the patient does not have an indication for an emergency

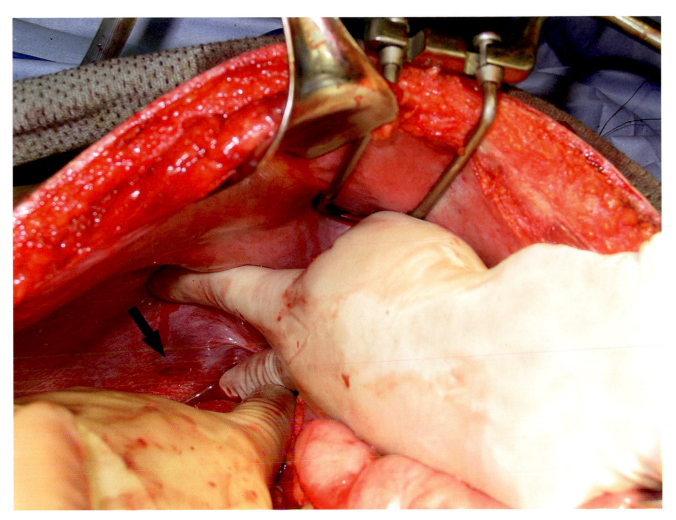

FIGURE 2. *Small diaphragmatic injury.*

department (ED) thoracotomy (ie, loss of vital signs or refractory hypotension with a penetrating thoracic wound), then proceed with a plain chest X-ray and abdominal films. Mark the entry and exit wounds with a radiopaque marker. This can help determine the trajectory of the missile (ie, does it cross the diaphragm?; Fig. 4). Obvious signs—such as free air under the diaphragm or a hemopneumothorax—will help guide the surgeon to the next step. **If the patient loses vital signs in the ED, he will require an immediate thoracotomy for resuscitation.**

2. Patients hypotensive with penetrating chest injuries should undergo immediate tube thoracostomy with airway control. Rapid evaluation with chest X-ray and a FAST scan will help guide the surgeon as to which body cavity should be entered first, but neither study should overrule clinical judgment. Should the patient remain unstable, the amount of chest tube output may mandate immediate thoracotomy. Specifically, if greater than 1,500 cc of blood are recovered immediately, then immediate thoracotomy is indicated. With lesser amounts of initial chest tube output (less than 1,500 cc), urgent operation may be necessary based on the time elapsed after injury, the patient's clinical condition, or the surgeon's judgment.

3. The pitfalls and limited sensitivity of chest X-ray, FAST scan, chest tube output, and diagnostic peritoneal lavage (DPL) are many and well known.[1–5] Nonetheless, initial evaluation of a stable patient with a gunshot wound to the chest should include a chest X-ray with entry and exit markers, as well as a FAST scan. The FAST scan can be helpful in determining priorities. If a patient with a gunshot wound to the chest is hypotensive and an initial chest X-ray reveals no significant hemothorax or pneumothorax, a nega-

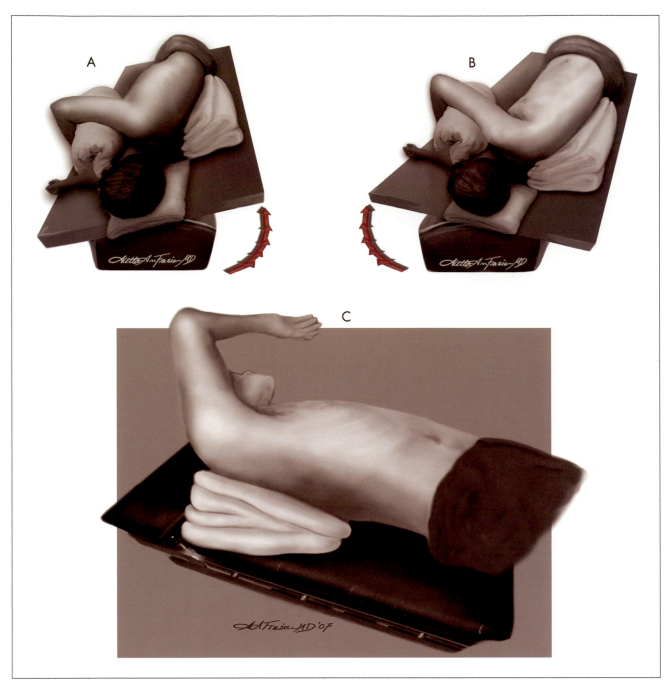

FIGURE 3. *Bent table.*

tive FAST scan for pericardial blood will guide the surgeon toward performing a laparotomy as the initial procedure. The chest wound can be managed with a simple tube thoracostomy.

4. However, if the patient has a significant hemothorax and the chest tube is placed first, this may not actually reflect an intrathoracic injury. Even if such an injury is present, a transthoracic intraabdominal

injury cannot be excluded. If there is a diaphragmatic injury, the chest tube output may actually reflect intraabdominal bleeding. In this situation, a DPL could be helpful, using 15,000 RBCs/mm^3 as the threshold for a positive result. With a negative DPL, the initial procedure should be a thoracotomy.

5. A CT image of the chest and abdomen may also provide clues as to the location of the injury. A CT

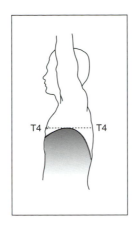

FIGURE 4. *Penetrating thoracic injuries below the T4 level (nipple line) have a high probability of involving abdominal structures.*

image is more sensitive and specific for diagnosing intraabdominal and intrathoracic hemorrhage. In the field environment, CT imaging may not be available. With an unstable patient, CT imaging is not an option.

6. A helpful maneuver when performing a laparotomy is to look for significant hemorrhage through the diaphragm into the hemithorax. If there is a diaphragmatic defect with gross fecal soilage, it is also prudent to do a lavage through the defect to reduce the risk of postoperative empyema. Enlarge the defect as necessary and close with a running Prolene suture. In addition, the best clues will come from the anesthesiologist. Elevated peak airway pressures, persistent hypotension, or hypoxia suggest that there is a problem in the thorax rather than in the abdomen.

DAMAGE CONTROL

With massive intraperitoneal and thoracic injuries, the priority is hemorrhage control. This may be accomplished with packing of the abdomen after bleeding has been controlled. The thoracic cavity can also be packed once hemorrhage control has been achieved. Temporary closure of both cavities can be used and the patient returned to the ICU for further resuscitation and warming prior to return to the OR for definitive repair.

SUMMARY

Managing thoracoabdominal injuries requires a high index of suspicion for injuries in both the thorax and abdomen. In the unstable patient, tube thoracostomy and X-rays with radiopaque markers will assist the surgeon in determining where to intervene. Adjunctive studies that include the FAST scan and CT imaging may prove helpful in the appropriate clinical situation. Despite all

the best efforts at diagnosis, the wrong cavity is entered about 23% to 44% of the time.[4,5] The best course of action is to maintain intraoperative flexibility and be prepared to change course rapidly and enter another body cavity. The best position for these cases is supine, arms extended, with a bump under the relevant thorax. Prep the patient widely, from neck to knees. A Foley catheter should be in place. This positioning allows the surgeon to perform a laparotomy, thoracotomy, or a median sternotomy without the need to reposition the patient.

REFERENCES

1. Murray JA, Berne J, Asensio JA. Penetrating thoracoabdominal trauma. *Emerg Med Clin North Am.* 1998;16(1):107–128.
2. Boulanger BR, Kearney PA, et al. The routine use of sonography in penetrating torso injury is beneficial. *J Trauma.* 2001;51(2):320–325.
3. Thal E, May RA, Beesinger D. Peritoneal lavage. Its unreliability in gunshot wounds of the lower chest and abdomen. *Arch Surg.* 1980;115(4):430–433.
4. Asensio JA, Arroyo H Jr, et al. Penetrating thoracoabdominal injuries: Ongoing dilemma—Which cavity and when? *World J Surg.* 2002; 26(5):539–543.
5. Hirshberg A, Wall MJ Jr, et al. Double jeopardy: Thoracoabdominal injuries requiring surgical intervention in both chest and abdomen. *J Trauma.* 1995; 39(2):225–229.

SUGGESTED READING

Chapter 16: Thoracic injuries. In: *Emergency War Surgery, Third United States Revision.* Washington, DC: Department of the Army, Office of The Surgeon General, Borden Institute; 2004.

Chapter 17: Abdominal injuries. In: *Emergency War Surgery, Third United States Revision.* Washington, DC: Department of the Army, Office of The Surgeon General, Borden Institute; 2004.

Merlotti GJ, Dillon BC, et al. Peritoneal lavage in penetrating thoracoabdominal trauma. *J Trauma.* 1988;28(1):17–23.

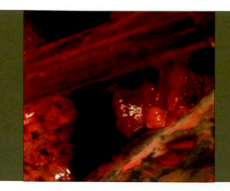

IV.3
Thoracotomy for Massive Hemothorax

CASE PRESENTATION

This 27-year-old male presented about 90 minutes after sustaining penetrating injuries to the right chest and left thigh. The patient was hypotensive. Immediate right tube thoracostomy resulted in 1,700 cc of blood output. He was hypothermic, with a temperature of 93.9°F and a pH of 7.09. The international normalized ratio was 1.7. A whole blood drive was initiated. Transfusion in combination with recombinant Factor VIIa corrected his coagulopathy. Right anterolateral thoracotomy was performed. The right internal mammary artery was transected and ligated immediately. The inferior pulmonary ligament was divided, and the entire lung was mobilized. The bullet tract was in the vicinity of the pulmonary hilum. The pulmonary hilum was dissected enough to allow vascular control. The bullet tract included all three lobes, and bleeding from this wound was heavy. The lung was consequently twisted around the hilum, resulting in some hemorrhage control and allowed assessment of the wounds (Fig. 1). Injuries to the inferior and middle lobes were more peripheral and were stapled across with a gastrointestinal anastomosis (GIA) stapler using a few reloads. This controlled the bleeding. Injury to the upper lobe was more central and bleeding continued. A tractotomy with a GIA stapler was performed, with oversewing of the bleeders and air leak that produced excellent results. The hemithorax was washed out, the lung was returned to its correct anatomical position, and the chest was closed with two large thoracostomy tubes in place. The femur fracture and wound were addressed with washout and external fixation as the patient was warmed and resuscitated at the end of the thoracotomy.

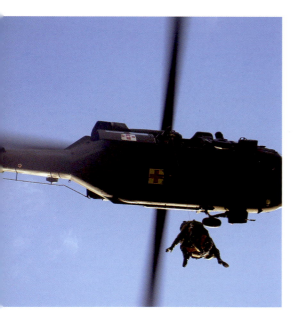

TEACHING POINTS

1. Patients presenting in hypovolemic shock with the triad of hypothermia, coagulopathy, and acidosis have a mortality rate as high as 90%.[1] They must be warmed and resuscitated rapidly. The patient in this case was given whole blood, packed red blood cells, recombinant Factor VIIa, and fresh frozen plasma, in addition to crystalloid. Military medical personnel must be expert in the use of all of these products to save patients in extremis.

2. Thoracotomy is indicated for massive hemothorax usually defined as 1,500 cc of output with initial tube thoracostomy or 200 cc of output per hour for 4 hours.

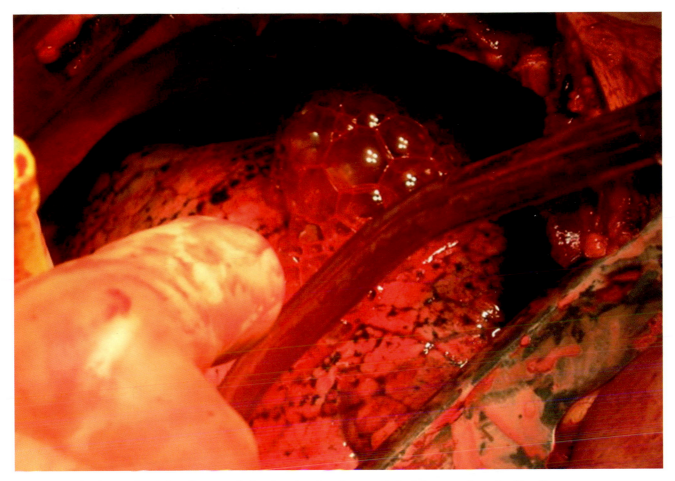

FIGURE 1. *The lung after it has been mobilized and twisted around the hilum to slow the bleeding.*

CLINICAL IMPLICATIONS

1. Tube thoracostomy alone is adequate treatment for most simple lung parenchymal injuries.
2. Large air leaks not responding to thoracostomy will require open repair.
3. Simple bleeding should be controlled with absorbable sutures on a tapered needle or with staples (eg, TA-90 staples).
4. Bleeding tracts should be opened with a GIA stapler, and bleeding points should be ligated. To avoid an air embolism produced by positive pressure ventilation, simple closure of the entrance and exit wounds of the lung parenchyma is contraindicated. Remember: The more central the injury, the higher the risk of air embolism.
5. Resection of the bleeding area of the lung may be necessary. Avoid anatomical resection in favor of a simple wedge resection.
6. Uncontrolled parenchymal or hilar bleeding, or complex hilar injuries with massive air leaks, should be controlled with hilar clamping (or a "hilar twist";

Fig. 2) and attempted repair. Pneumonectomy should be performed as a last resort because it is associated with a 90% mortality rate.[1]

DAMAGE CONTROL

In patients with exsanguinating hemorrhage from thoracic injury, the goal is to stop the bleeding and restore a stable physiological status. The following principles apply:

1. Large lung staplers should be used to perform nonanatomical wedge resections to achieve hemostasis and control of air leaks rapidly.
2. In pulmonary tractotomy (Fig. 3), the lung bridging the wound tract is opened between long clamps or with a stapler, the wound is inspected, bleeding points are ligated, and air leaks are controlled.
3. If the patient continues to bleed despite the above measures, packing and temporary chest closure may be necessary to allow further resuscitation.

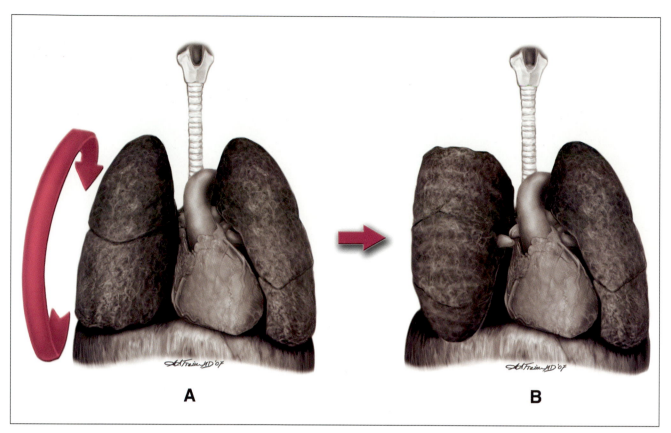

FIGURE 2. *Hilar clamping or "hilar twist."*

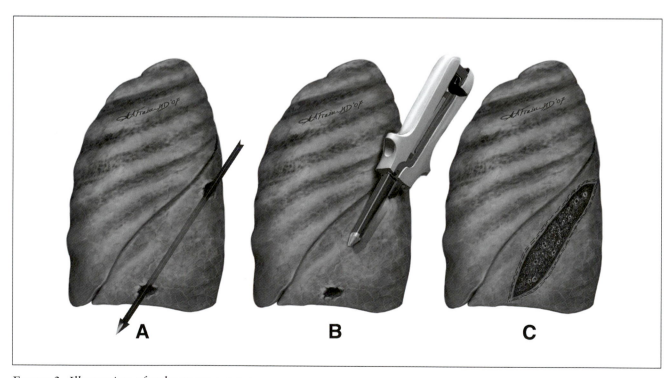

FIGURE 3. *Illustration of pulmonary tractotomy.*

SUMMARY

This case demonstrates a successful approach to massive hemothorax in a hypotensive, coagulopathic, and cold patient. The combination of expert resuscitation with damage control thoracotomy resulted in this patient's survival.

REFERENCE

1. Deb S, Fonseca P. Respiratory distress following pneumonectomy. *Chest*. 1999;116:1461–1463.

SUGGESTED READING

Chapter 16: Thoracic injuries. In: *Emergency War Surgery, Third United States Revision*. Washington, DC: Department of the Army, Office of The Surgeon General, Borden Institute; 2004.

Chapter 17: Abdominal injuries. In: *Emergency War Surgery, Third United States Revision*. Washington, DC: Department of the Army, Office of The Surgeon General, Borden Institute; 2004.

Chapter 23: Extremity fractures. In: *Emergency War Surgery, Third United States Revision*. Washington, DC: Department of the Army, Office of The Surgeon General, Borden Institute; 2004

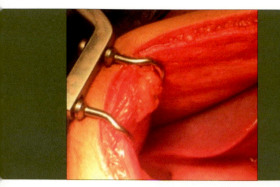

IV.4
Spinal Injury With Penetrating Thoracoabdominal Injuries

CASE PRESENTATION

A 25-year-old male presented with a single gunshot wound that entered through the back and traversed the midthoracic spine. The patient was paraplegic with no sensation or motor function below a midthoracic level (T5). He complained of mild abdominal pain. The initial chest radiograph was unremarkable, as was the FAST exam. The patient was taken to the operating room (OR) for abdominal exploration. Shortly after intubation, he developed symptoms consistent with a tension pneumothorax, and a right chest tube was placed with resolution of symptoms. Intraoperatively, the patient was found to have a large injury of the anterior duodenum that extended from the first portion of the duodenum to the body of the stomach and a smaller posterior injury of the second portion of the duodenum (Fig. 1). The anterior duodenum was repaired using a Heineke-Mikulicz repair, opening it horizontally and closing it vertically to ensure that the lumen was not narrowed. A right medial visceral rotation was performed to ensure that there was no injury to the inferior vena cava. Injury to the pancreas, ampulla, porta hepatitis, and diaphragm were specifically ruled out, as well as small bowel and colon injuries. A small injury to the liver was packed. Bowel edema precluded closure of the abdomen, and a sterile bag was sewn to the skin (Fig. 2).

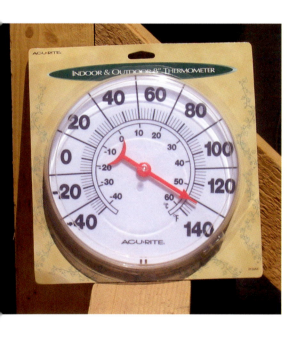

TEACHING POINTS

This case demonstrates the destructive power of a high-velocity missile entering the back and traversing the abdomen and chest with injury to multiple organs. The following points deserve emphasis:

1. Penetrating injuries to the back—especially gunshot wounds—should undergo exploratory laparotomy, particularly when CT imaging is not available.
2. Duodenal repairs should be liberally drained.
3. To prevent abdominal compartment syndrome, the abdomen should not be closed under tension.
4. When thoracic injury is suspected, tube thoracostomy should be performed, especially if the patient cannot be observed continuously.
5. Spine immobilization should be maintained in patients with spinal cord injury until they have been evaluated by a neurosurgeon, if one is available.

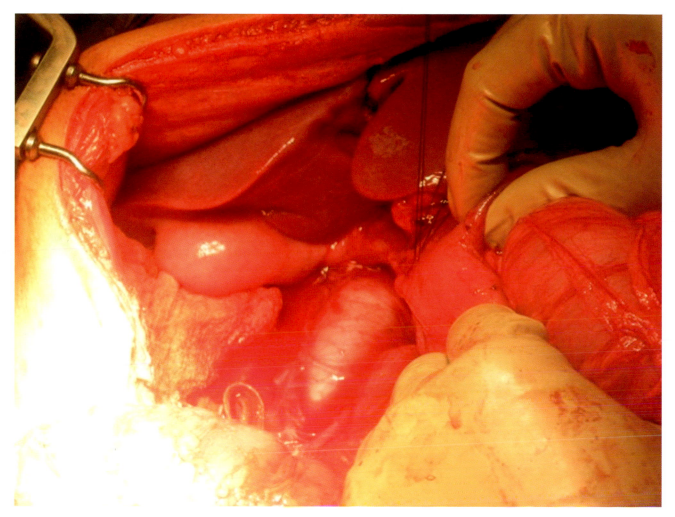

FIGURE 1. *Intraoperative view of duodenal injury.*

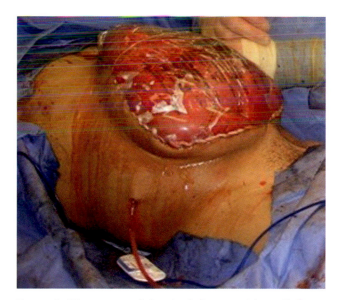

FIGURE 2. *Temporary abdominal closure with sterile bag.*

CLINICAL IMPLICATIONS

1. Posterior truncal penetrating injuries from the tip of the scapula to the sacrum (Figs. 3 and 4) may have caused retroperitoneal and intraabdominal injuries. A low threshold for exploratory laparotomy is warranted in these patients.

2. Injuries to the duodenum are frequently associated with injury to other organs. Damage control techniques should be considered early. Do not close the abdominal fascia under tension. Leave the skin open.

3. Minor injuries of the duodenum can be repaired primarily, and large injuries should be repaired if the lumen will not be narrowed by more than 50%.[1] If the lumen will be narrowed by more than 50%, consider the following options:

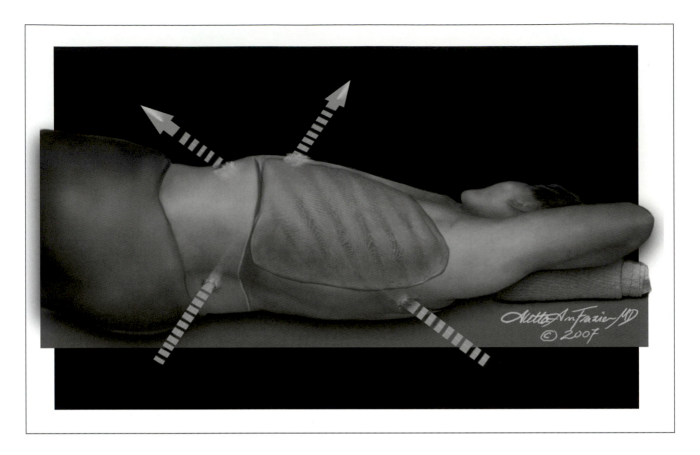

FIGURE 3. (Top) *Trajectory of missiles may include both chest and abdomen.*

FIGURE 4. (Bottom Left) *Penetrating thoracic injuries below the T4 level (nipple line) have a high probability of involving abdominal structures.*

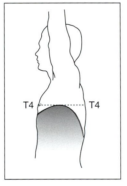

FIGURE 5. (Bottom Right) *(A) Duodenal injury. (B) Gastrojejunostomy. (C) Ligation of the pylorus. Alternate method of closing the pylorus is stapling across it with a TA stapler.*

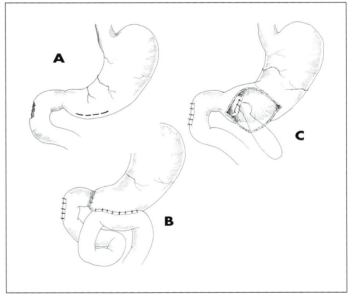

a. For major injuries, close the pylorus temporarily and divert the gastric stream with a gastrojejunostomy (Fig. 5).

b. Use a Heineke-Mikulicz repair (as in this case) for the first portion of the duodenum extending to the stomach.

c. Create an anastomosis between the injury and a Roux-en-Y limb.

d. Consider draining the injured area and transferring the patient to a facility equipped for large procedures, if pancreaticoduodenectomy is required.

e. Close the injury around a tube duodenostomy using 2-0 VICRYL suture with a Malecot catheter, if available.

DAMAGE CONTROL

Injuries of the duodenum are frequently associated with injuries to other organ systems and hemorrhage. When repair of duodenal injuries cannot be performed using relatively simple techniques, damage control should be considered, specifically:

1. Control hemorrhage and contamination.
2. Pack and close the patient temporarily.
3. Resuscitate the patient to normal physiology.
4. Plan for future reoperation and definitive repair.
5. Note that emergent spine surgery for penetrating injuries of the spinal cord is indicated only in the presence of neurological deterioration.

SUMMARY

Penetrating spine injuries associated with hollow viscus injuries should undergo appropriate treatment of the viscus trauma without extensive debridement of the spinal injury, followed by appropriate broad-spectrum antibiotics. This patient presented with a penetrating back injury and paraplegia. Exploratory laparotomy revealed injuries to multiple organs. The patient's abdomen was temporarily closed to prevent abdominal compartment syndrome, as is often necessary with these types of injuries.

REFERENCE

1. Chapter 17: Abdominal injuries. In: *Emergency War Surgery, Third United States Revision*. Washington, DC: Department of the Army, Office of The Surgeon General, Borden Institute; 2004.

SUGGESTED READING

Chapter 16: Thoracic injuries. In: *Emergency War Surgery, Third United States Revision*. Washington, DC: Department of the Army, Office of The Surgeon General, Borden Institute; 2004.

Chapter 20: Wounds and injuries of the spinal column and cord. In: *Emergency War Surgery, Third United States Revision*. Washington, DC: Department of the Army, Office of The Surgeon General, Borden Institute; 2004.

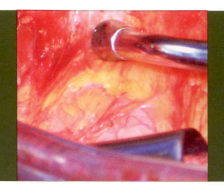

IV.5
Traumatic Pericardial Tamponade

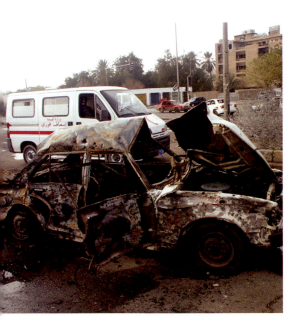

CASE PRESENTATION

A 40-year-old civilian contractor was wounded when a mortar struck in the vicinity of his sleep trailer. The patient was brought to the Emergency Medical Treatment (EMT) section of the combat support hospital (CSH) where he was alert, oriented, and complaining of a little pain in the right groin and left chest. His vital signs on arrival were a heart rate of 110 beats per minute and a blood pressure of 80/60 mm Hg. The initial survey revealed a superficial wound below the left nipple, a penetrating wound of the right groin, and what appeared to be a penetrating wound of the chest above the left nipple (Fig. 1). His abdomen was soft without tenderness. A left chest tube was placed with minimal recovery of intrathoracic blood. FAST examination was negative for intraperitoneal and pericardial fluids. A chest X-ray (CXR) revealed a metallic fragment in the left chest (Fig. 2). Despite fluid resuscitation and no obvious bleeding source, the patient's blood pressure remained below 100 mm Hg systolic. A CT scan of the chest revealed pericardial blood (Fig. 3), and the patient was taken to the operating room where he underwent an urgent median sternotomy (Fig. 4). The pericardium was open with immediate extrusion of clotted blood (Fig. 5). The patient's vital signs normalized after pericardial tamponade was relieved. The pericardium was fully opened, and a penetrating injury to the apex of the heart was found (Fig. 6). This was repaired with a single horizontal mattress suture using pericardium for pledgets (Figs. 7 and 8). The patient's chest was closed, and he was evacuated from theater the following day. He had an uneventful recovery.

TEACHING POINTS

1. Patients presenting with penetrating chest trauma and hypotension require rapid evaluation and treatment of their injuries. Immediate needle chest decompression or rapid insertion of a chest tube on the affected side will either treat or rule out tension pneumothorax or massive intrathoracic bleeding as the cause of hypotension. FAST scan should also rule out massive intraperitoneal blood, as well as pericardial blood or tamponade. Other sources of significant blood loss (retroperitoneal, pelvic or long bone fractures, or external bleeding from large, soft tissue or scalp wounds) should be sought to explain hypotension. A high index of suspicion for

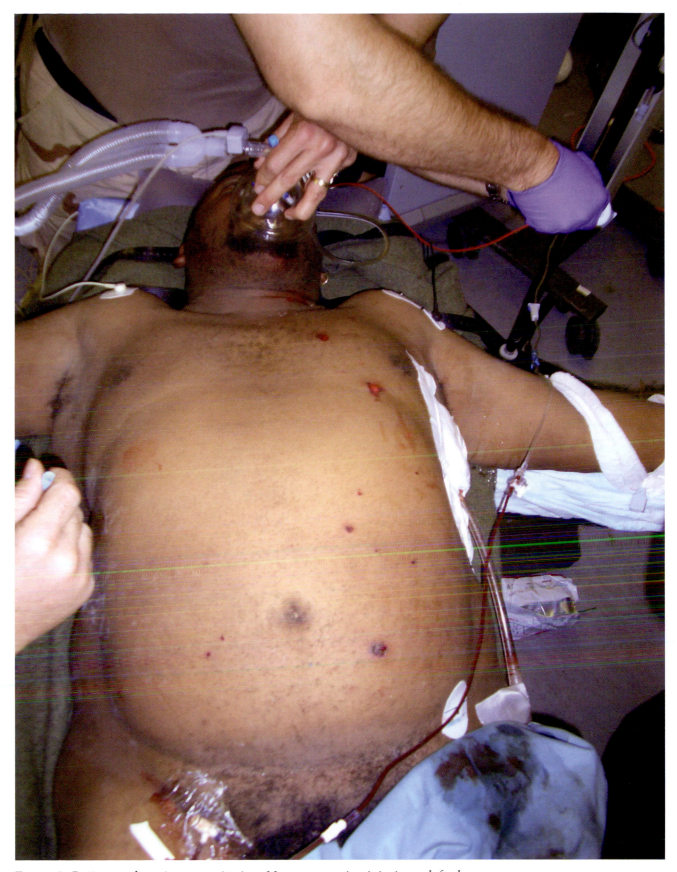

FIGURE 1. *Patient undergoing resuscitation. Note penetrating injuries to left chest.*

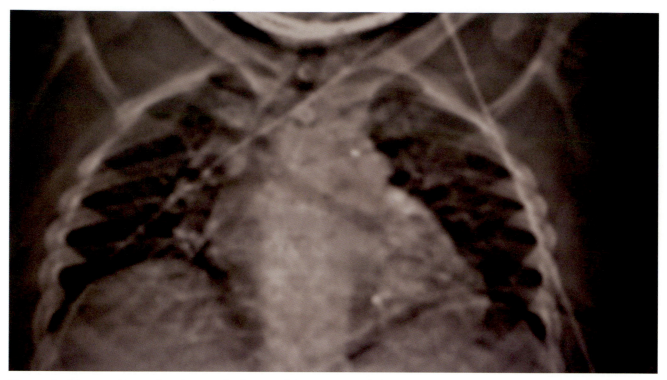

FIGURE 2. *Chest radiograph. Note multiple metal fragments in left chest.*

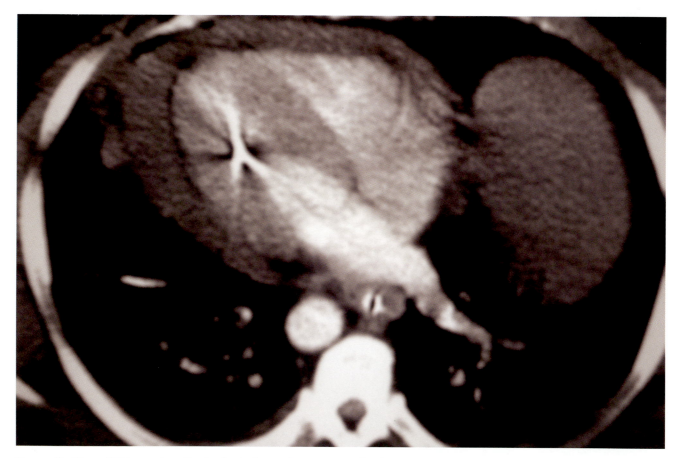

FIGURE 3. *Chest CT image* (mediastinal window) *showing metallic fragment in the heart with surrounding pericardial effusion.*

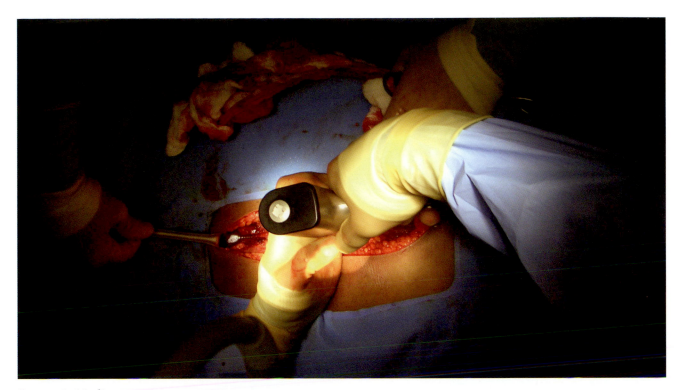

FIGURE 4. *Median sternotomy.*

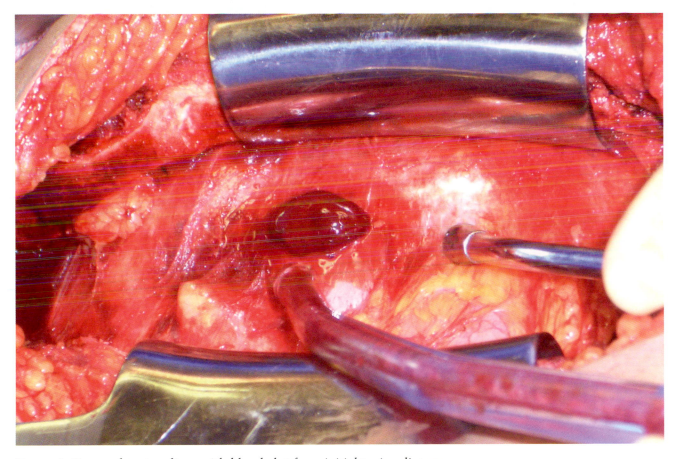

FIGURE 5. *Exposed pericardium with blood clot from initial pericardiotomy.*

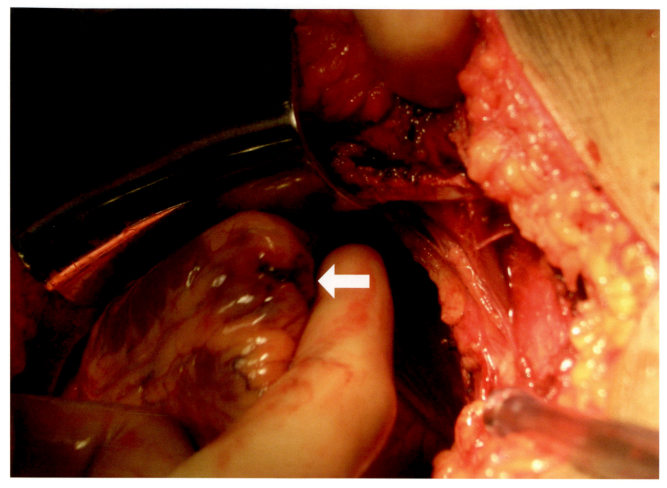

FIGURE 6. *Penetrating injury to the apex of the heart* (arrow).

pericardial tamponade should be maintained for patients with penetrating chest injuries and no other source of blood loss. This patient's large size may have decreased the sensitivity of our FAST examination. With a CT available, a chest scan readily revealed pericardial blood. If CT is unavailable and the FAST is negative, a subxiphoid pericardial window is indicated with penetrating chest trauma and ongoing hypotension with no obvious source of bleeding. A trial of pericardiocentesis may be diagnostic (as well as therapeutic), but aspiration may be falsely negative in the presence of an organized clot.

2. When suturing cardiac injuries, pericardium for the pledgets is readily available and an excellent choice. Although figure-of-eight sutures may be used, avoid compressing or compromising coronary vessels by using horizontal mattress sutures if the vessel will be crossed by the repairing suture (Fig. 9).

CLINICAL IMPLICATIONS

1. Patients presenting with penetrating chest trauma and who are hypotensive require rapid evaluation. After ensuring the patient has an adequate airway and is breathing, hypotension mandates rapid chest decompression (needle or chest tube) to rule out tension pneumothorax. If discovered by needle decompression (as evidenced by a rush of air or improvement of the patient's hemodynamics), a chest tube should be immediately inserted. There is no time to wait for a CXR to confirm the diagnosis of tension pneumothorax.

2. With ongoing hypotension, despite chest decompression, massive hemothorax should be revealed by chest tube placement or CXR. If a large amount of blood is drained immediately at chest tube insertion, urgent thoracotomy should quickly follow. Although Advanced Trauma Life Support (ATLS) guidelines suggest 1,500 cc of blood as the initial amount drained that mandates immediate

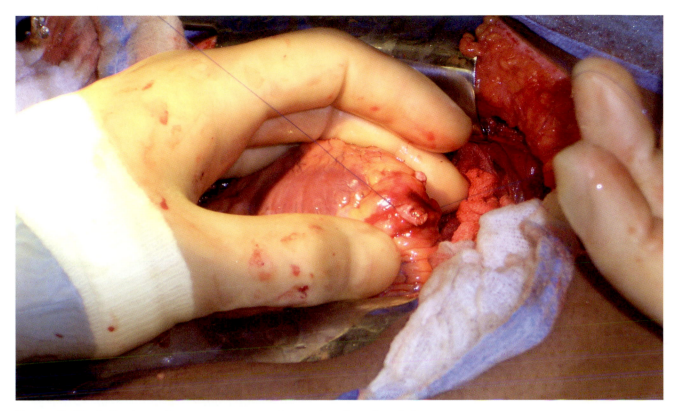

FIGURE 7. *Single horizontal mattress suture using pericardium for pledgets.*

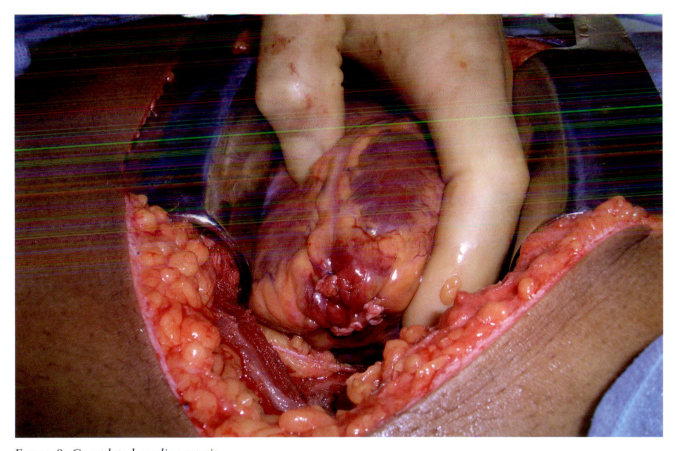

FIGURE 8. *Completed cardiac repair.*

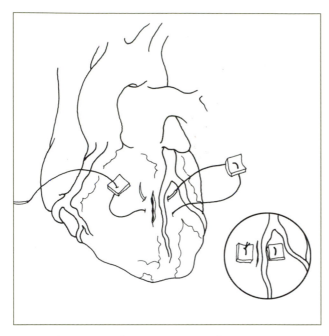

FIGURE 9. *Repair of penetrating cardiac injury.*

thoracotomy, this number should be mitigated by the type of injury (large penetrating fragment), the patient's clinical condition, as well as the length of time from injury to chest tube insertion. Patients may present to the CSH only minutes after injury. A patient in shock with 500 cc of blood in the chest within a few minutes of wounding who remains hypotensive despite initial resuscitative efforts may need urgent thoracotomy.

DAMAGE CONTROL

Although inserting a percutaneous pericardial catheter may temporarily alleviate tamponade for penetrating heart injuries, definitive repair cannot be delayed without a prohibitive risk of retamponade and cardiac arrest. Large cardiac injuries can be temporarily controlled after sternotomy with the insertion of a Foley or Fogarty catheter (depending on the size of the injury) and inflating the balloon to control bleeding. Skin staples may also be used to close a cardiac injury rapidly.

SUMMARY

Patients with penetrating chest injuries who present in shock require expeditious evaluation and management to locate the cause and quickly manage it. Tension pneumothorax, massive hemothorax, and pericardial tamponade should be rapidly investigated and treated. With ongoing hypotension and other sources of shock eliminated, a high index of suspicion for pericardial tamponade—despite a negative FAST—should be maintained and a subxiphoid pericardial window performed to definitively rule out this injury.

SUGGESTED READING

Asensio JA, Arroyo H Jr, et al. Penetrating thoracoabdominal injuries: Ongoing dilemma—Which cavity and when? *World J Surg.* 2002;26(5):539–543.

Boulanger BR, Kearney PA, et al. The routine use of sonography in penetrating torso injury is beneficial. *J Trauma.* 2001;51(2):320–325.

Chapter 16: Thoracic injuries. In: *Emergency War Surgery, Third United States Revision.* Washington, DC: Department of the Army, Office of The Surgeon General, Borden Institute; 2004.

Chapter 17: Abdominal injuries. In: *Emergency War Surgery, Third United States Revision.* Washington, DC: Department of the Army, Office of The Surgeon General, Borden Institute; 2004.

Hirshberg A, Wall MJ Jr, et al. Double jeopardy: Thoracoabdominal injuries requiring surgical intervention in both chest and abdomen. *J Trauma.* 1995; 39(2):225–229.

Merlotti GJ, Dillon BC, et al. Peritoneal lavage in penetrating thoracoabdominal trauma. *J Trauma.* 1988;28(1):17–23.

Murray JA, Berne J, Asensio JA. Penetrating thoracoabdominal trauma. *Emerg Med Clin North Am.* 1998;16(1):107–128.

Thal E, May RA, Beesinger D. Peritoneal lavage. Its unreliability in gunshot wounds of the lower chest and abdomen. *Arch Surg.* 1980;115(4):430–433.

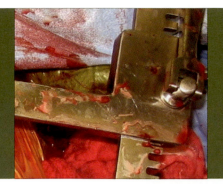

IV.6
Penetrating Right Chest Injury

CASE PRESENTATION

This male soldier sustained a penetrating right chest injury from a mortar round. He was immediately transported to the combat support hospital (CSH). On arrival in the Emergency Medical Treatment (EMT) area, he was mildly tachycardic and hypotensive. During the patient's resuscitation, a right chest tube was placed yielding the immediate return of 800 cc of blood with continued output. He was rapidly moved to the operating room (OR) and an urgent right posterolateral thoracotomy performed (Fig. 1). Hilar bleeding and air leak were apparent, and a linear stapler was used to open the fragment tract. In conjunction with the injury, this maneuver essentially resulted in a right upper lobectomy. Once the right upper lobe was removed, continued bleeding was noted from the hilum of the middle lobe. The patient had a complete middle lobe fissure, and a linear stapler was placed at the middle lobe hilum and fired, completing a middle lobectomy (Figs. 2 and 3). This completely controlled the bleeding (Fig. 4). The chest was thoroughly irrigated with warm saline, the entrance wound debrided, and the chest closed with right angle and apical chest tubes in place. The patient was evacuated in stable condition to a level IV medical treatment facility the following day.

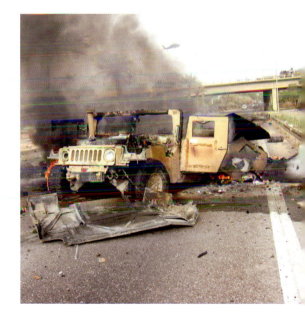

TEACHING POINTS

1. Although Advanced Trauma Life Support (ATLS) guidelines recommend urgent thoracotomy when either 1,500 cc of blood is recovered immediately on placing a chest tube or the rate of chest tube output is greater than 200 cc/hr for 4 hours, some clinical circumstances require more aggressive treatment. In this case, the close proximity of the wounded soldier to the resuscitation site resulted in a chest tube being placed within minutes of the penetrating injury. The immediate recovery of 800 cc of blood, with ongoing bleeding, indicated the likelihood of surgical bleeding. The patient also presented in shock. Taken together, urgent thoracotomy was the appropriate course of action.

2. Massive chest bleeding may make pinpointing the specific injury difficult. In this case, palpating the lung revealed the fragment tract, which allowed rapid exposure of the wound tract with a linear stapler. Once the tract is opened, locating the specific site of bleeding becomes possible (see Case IV.3, Fig. 3).

BEHIND ARMOR BLUNT TRAUMA (BABT)

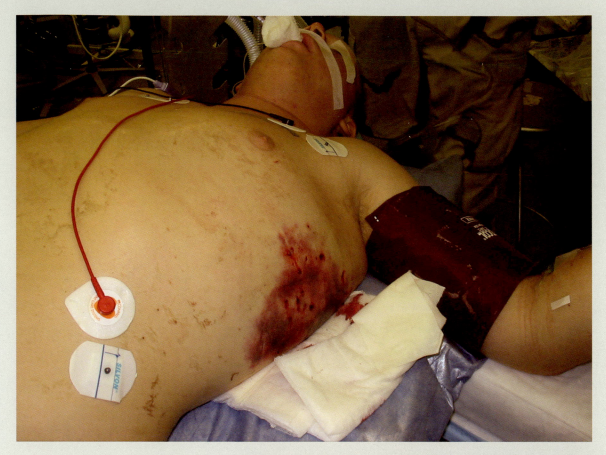

All types of body armor and helmets are designed to prevent missiles from entering the part of the body protected by the armor, and, at the same time, to dissipate the kinetic energy created by the missile. However well the armor performs, some kinetic energy is still transferred to the individual. If penetration is prevented, the mechanism of injury is converted to "behind armor blunt trauma" (BABT).[1] The severity of the injury to the patient depends on:

- missile velocity
- energy transfer produced by the defeated missile
- energy dissipated by the armor
- area of the body that absorbs the remaining energy.

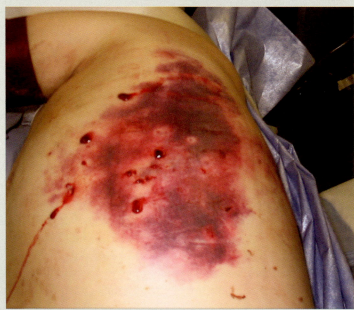

FIGURE 1. *Left-lateral chest wall injury from BABT.*

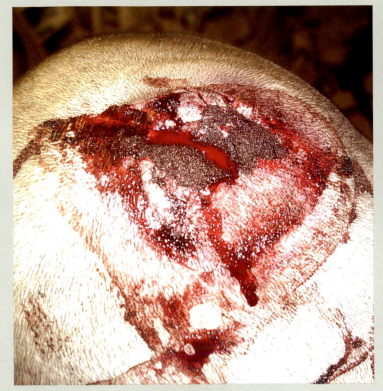

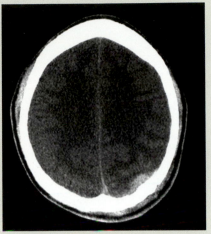

FIGURE 2. *Soldier struck by a fragment from a close proximity explosion. The fragment did not penetrate his Kevlar helmet. Note the scalp laceration as well as the underlying left occipital contusion injury. No skull fracture occurred and the soldier recovered.*

Energy transfer with resulting body wall deformation and visceral conduction can produce significant injury and death. BABT is a common mechanism of battlefield blunt trauma. Injuries produced by this mechanism include:

- fractures
- pneumothorax
- pulmonary contusion
- cardiac contusion and/or arrhythmia (commotio cordis)
- liver and spleen lacerations
- bowel injury
- traumatic brain injuries.

Invariably, skin abrasions and hematomas are evident at the point of impact (Figs. 1 and 2). Contralateral cutaneous injuries may also be present. Victims of blunt trauma mechanisms in combat must be systematically evaluated according to ATLS (Advanced Trauma Life Support) protocols. In the case of thoracic injuries, chest CT is sensitive and superior to standard chest X-ray in visualizing lung contusion, pneumothorax, and hemothorax.[2]

1. Cannon L. Behind armor blunt trauma—An emerging problem. *J R Army Med Corps.* 2001;147(1):87–96.
2. Trupka A, Waydhas C, et al. Value of thoracic computed tomography in the first assessment of severely injured patients with blunt chest trauma: Results of a prospective study. *J Trauma.* 1997;43(3):405–412.

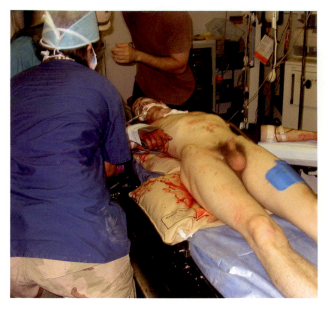

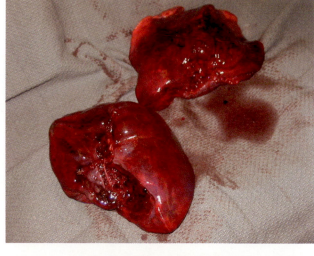

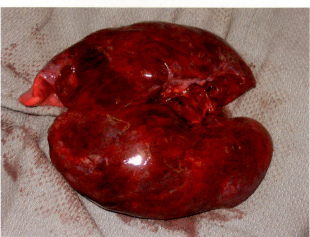

FIGURE 1. (Top Left)
Patient in OR preoperatively.

FIGURE 2. (Top Right)
Separately resected lobes.

FIGURE 3. (Bottom Right)
*Reconstructing the hilar injury
with the lobes together.*

3. Preserving viable lung tissue is certainly an important aspect of emergent thoracotomy for bleeding. Unfortunately, adequate exposure and control of massive bleeding may require resection of otherwise normal lung. Nonetheless, every effort to preserve undamaged lung should be made.

CLINICAL IMPLICATIONS

1. High-velocity penetrating lung injuries carry a high potential for life-threatening intrathoracic injuries (chest wall, lung, heart, and great vessels), as well as the possibility of peritoneal penetration. If the patient's clinical condition allows, radiological studies with radiopaque markers for the entrance and exit wounds—along with a FAST scan to evaluate for pericardial or intraperitoneal blood—should be performed.
2. If a patient presents without obtainable vital signs with recent signs of life, proceeding with an emergent (in the EMT area) thoracotomy in the combat zone should be considered only under the most favorable circumstances (minimal associated injuries, small penetrating chest injury, few or no other urgent patients, abundant resources, surgeons, and OR availability, to name just a few considerations). In general, such a patient should be triaged as expectant.
3. Patients presenting in shock should be rapidly transported to the OR for urgent thoracotomy. Simultaneous resuscitation while locating and controlling the source of bleeding should occur.

DAMAGE CONTROL

1. On entering the chest, if massive hemorrhage or air leak does not allow for rapid visualization and control of the specific injury, immediately freeing the inferior pulmonary ligament (may be accomplished bluntly) and twisting the lung around the hilum may achieve temporary control. During this time, the surgeon can catch up and

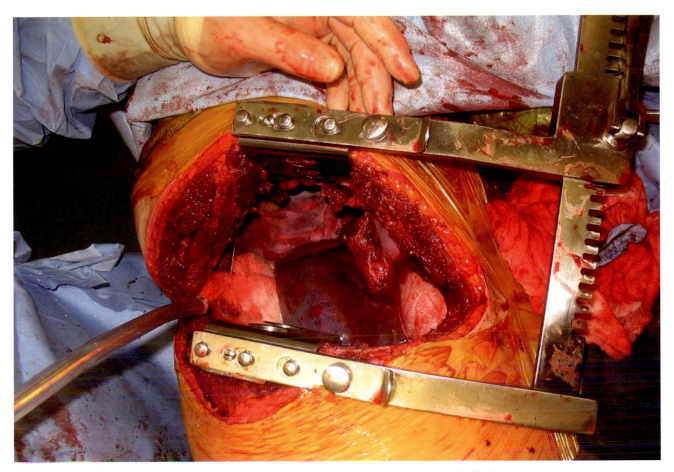

FIGURE 4. *Open right chest with intact lower lobe and stapled upper and middle lobe vessels.*

resuscitate the patient with fluid, blood, and other appropriate products. This may also allow adequate exposure for the surgeon to obtain control of the hilum with a large vascular clamp, ultimately permitting exposure of the injury and appropriate repair.

2. Pneumonectomy for lung injury (specifically for a large hilar injury) should be used only if hilar structures are irreparably damaged or as a procedure of last resort, given the high mortality of this operation.

3. If surgical bleeding is controlled, but the patient has multiple sites of oozing and is slipping toward the lethal triad (hypothermia, coagulopathy, and acidosis), packing the chest and temporary closure (similar to the temporary abdominal closure) should be used until the patient can be adequately resuscitated to allow a return to the OR for definitive repairs.

SUMMARY

High-velocity missiles (bullets and fragments) that pentrate the chest have a high potential for intrathoracic injury that may require urgent thoracotomy and/or laparotomy. Rapid evaluation and assessment of these injuries are essential so that patients will receive the appropriate initial treatment (thoracotomy, laparotomy, and chest tube), resulting in the best possible outcome.

SUGGESTED READING

Chapter 6: Hemorrhage control. In: *Emergency War Surgery, Third United States Revision*. Washington, DC: Department of the Army, Office of The Surgeon General, Borden Institute; 2004.

Chapter 12: Damage control surgery. In: *Emergency War Surgery, Third United States Revision*. Washington, DC: Department of the Army, Office of The Surgeon General, Borden Institute; 2004.

Chapter 16: Thoracic injuries. In: *Emergency War Surgery, Third United States Revision*. Washington, DC: Department of the Army, Office of The Surgeon General, Borden Institute; 2004.

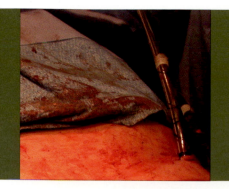

IV.7
Transmediastinal Gunshot Wound

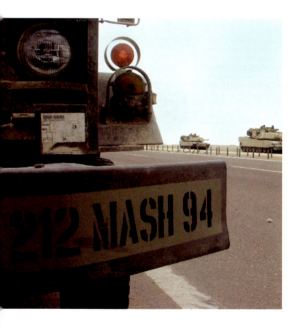

CASE PRESENTATION

A 27-year-old male soldier on routine foot patrol encountered small arms fire. All members of his patrol were wearing torso ballistic protection. The soldier sustained a direct hit to the torso, entering the left chest along the anterior axillary line just above the nipple and eventually exiting the torso through the right midaxillary line at the nipple. The 7.62-mm round was recovered by the treating medic after it exited the right chest. It was not deformed (Fig. 1). Needle chest decompression was performed in the field. Rapid transport from the point of injury to the Forward Surgical Team (FST) was accomplished within 15 minutes. On arrival, the patient was hypotensive, hypoxic, and hypothermic. Bilateral tube thoracostomies were performed, and a large hemopneumothorax (1,500 cc) was evacuated from the left chest. Refractory hypotension continued. A left thoracotomy was performed through the fifth intercostal space revealing a large laceration of the left upper lobe with active hemorrhage from segmental pulmonary vessels that were controlled with tractotomy and ligation. The bullet had traversed the anterior mediastinum. An upper anterior mediastinal hematoma was noted, and extension of the left thoracotomy across the sternum was performed with the intent of exploring the hematoma for major vascular injury (Fig. 2). A proximal injury of the left internal mammary artery/ vein and a fracture of the upper sternum were encountered from the round. The left internal mammary vessels were ligated and the sternum fracture packed. The patient was coagulopathic, and the mediastinum was gently packed and the chest covered with Ioban (antimicrobial incise drapes). A whole blood drive was instituted by the co-located battalion aid station personnel, as previously rehearsed. Blood was transfused and the coagulopathy quickly reversed. The patient was transferred to a level III intensive care unit, and further resuscitation was continued. He was reexplored the following morning, and the chest was definitively closed (Fig. 3). The patient remained hemodynamically stable and was evacuated to a combat support hospital (CSH) and eventually to Walter Reed Army Medical Center.

TEACHING POINTS

1. Contemporary management of transmediastinal gunshot wounds remains controversial. Many patients die from major vascular or cardiac injuries as a result of missiles. Those individuals who

TABLE 1. *Approaches to the Chest*

EXPOSURE	ADVANTAGES	DISADVANTAGES
Median sternotomy	Excellent exposure of heart Excellent exposure of great vessels Excellent exposure of pulmonary hilum	Posterior mediastinum difficult to expose May require separate thoracotomy for repair of tracheal or esophageal injuries
"Clamshell" thoracotomy	Excellent exposure of heart Excellent exposure of great vessels Wide exposure of pulmonary hilum, lung, and posterior mediastinum in both thoracic cavities	Exposure to heart and great vessels inferior to median sternotomy Incisional discomfort/morbidity

survive to definitive surgical care in the civilian world and remain hemodynamically stable may undergo a less invasive workup to evaluate these injuries, with definitive care planned based on the findings. Those patients who present hemodynamically unstable require prompt surgical exploration. Injuries to the mediastinum can be explored either via a median sternotomy or "clamshell" thoracotomy. Each procedure has its advantages and disadvantages, and is listed in Table 1. Regardless of the method of exploration, a thorough evaluation of all mediastinal structures (cardiac, vascular, pulmonary hilum, tracheal, and esophageal) is prudent, because any injury left undiscovered may result in death.

2. Detailed data from the US Department of Defense studies outline the basics of wound ballistics. Specific information regarding the particular missile has significant impact on the potential extent of the injury. Missiles with less deformation or yaw in tissue will characteristically produce less cavitation and smaller wound cavities independent of the tissue encountered, but with greater tissue penetration. However, specific tissues are more prone to the transfer of kinetic energy (eg, the heart and great vessels) relative to tissues less prone (eg, lung). In this case, the wound cavity was relatively small and required pulmonary tractotomy to control hemorrhage, but the resulting transgression across the mediastinum put the heart and great vessels at significant risk from both the primary and secondary ballistic cavities produced. Exploration was warranted to rule out injury despite the projected path of the bullet.

3. In this case, utilization of whole blood was critical

in rapidly correcting the patient's coagulopathy. Prior instruction of and rehearsal by the co-located battalion aid station personnel allowed surgical personnel to dedicate themselves wholly

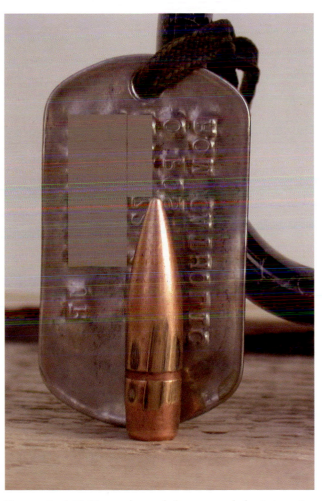

FIGURE 1. *A 7.62-mm round that caused the injury in this case.*

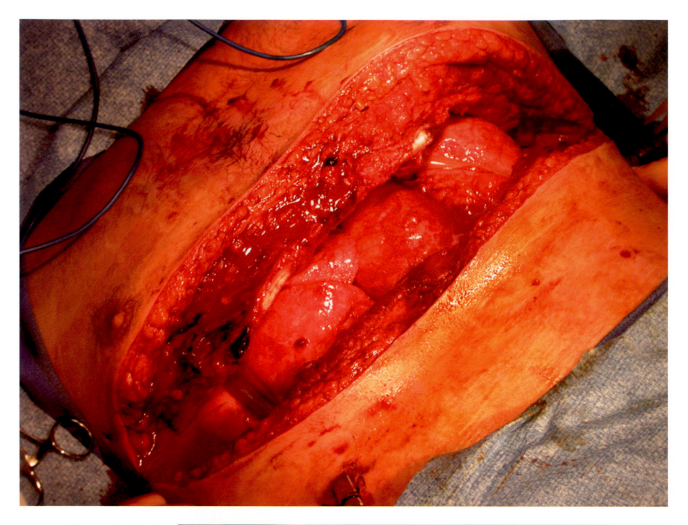

FIGURE 2. (Top) *Mediastinum exposed after transfer incision and sternotomy.*

FIGURE 3. (Bottom) *Definitive closure of the chest.*

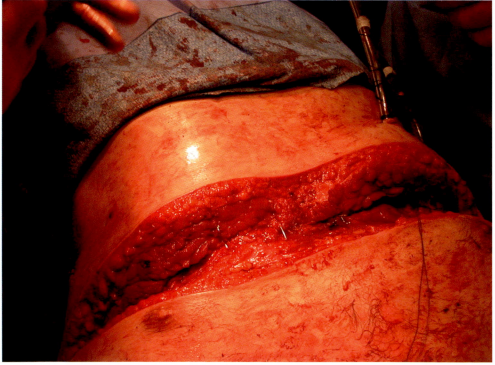

to the care of the patient, allowing the blood drive to function independently of the surgical staff.

CLINICAL IMPLICATIONS

1. Transthoracic missile injuries are often catastrophic. Acute intervention and management of penetrating thoracic trauma require the surgeon to anticipate a spectrum of injuries that includes the following:

   a. Thoracic vascular injuries.
   b. Pulmonary tractotomy and control of pulmonary hemorrhage.
   c. Pulmonary hilar injuries.
   d. Thoracic aerodigestive injuries.
   e. Penetrating cardiac injuries.

2. Exposure of these injuries necessarily defers to surgeon preference, but should incorporate some knowledge of the ballistics, as well as the potential injuries caused by these missiles.

DAMAGE CONTROL

Damage control procedures are less well tolerated in the thoracic cavity because of restrictions on pulmonary and vascular dynamics. Chest wall bleeding can be managed with packing and expected reexploration, but careful awareness of the effects of packing on hemodynamics, pulmonary compliance, and ventilation must be weighed carefully.

SUMMARY

Survival of transmediastinal ballistic injuries to a surgical facility is rare, and survival following exploration has high mortality and high morbidity rates. Battlefield environments do not allow complex diagnostic workups prior to exploration. In this case, the patient underwent acute aggressive intervention with a successful outcome.

SUGGESTED READING

Chapter 8: Vascular access. In: *Emergency War Surgery, Third United States Revision*. Washington, DC: Department of the Army, Office of The Surgeon General, Borden Institute; 2004.

Chapter 16: Thoracic injuries. In: *Emergency War Surgery, Third United States Revision*. Washington, DC: Department of the Army, Office of The Surgeon General, Borden Institute; 2004.

Bellamy RF, Zajtchuk R, eds. *Conventional Warfare: Ballistic, Blast, and Burn Injuries*. In: *Textbook of Military Medicine*. Washington, DC: Department of the Army, Office of The Surgeon General, Borden Institute; 1991.

Approaches to the Chest Cavity

by MAJ Charles R. Mulligan, MD

The key to managing chest trauma is knowing when, and when not, to operate. An incorrect decision can lead to increased morbidity and/or mortality. Unlike civilian chest trauma, military chest trauma tends to involve more penetrating injuries. The principles of management are quite similar. A properly placed chest tube is sufficient to treat the majority of chest wounds encountered (70%–80%). Indications for early thoracotomy include chest tube output greater than 1,500 cc at initial placement, or more than 200 cc/hr for four consecutive hours, open sucking chest wound, and retained hemothorax. Other indications for thoracotomy include postcontusion infection, empyema, and bronchopleural fistula. Indications for emergency room thoracotomy include penetrating chest injuries with hemodynamic instability or collapse and nonthoracic penetrating trauma with witnessed cardiovascular collapse (resuscitative thoracotomy).

The military surgeon should be familiar with a variety of approaches to the chest cavity. The key to success is using the incision that best gets you quickly to the problem. Adequate exposure is critical, and wider tends to be better ("high, wide, and handsome"). A thorough knowledge of thoracic anatomy is critical to success.

The quickest access into the chest is through an anterolateral thoracotomy. This can be accomplished in seconds with just a scalpel. The left anterior approach provides access to the pericardium, descending aorta, proximal left subclavian artery, and the left pulmonary hilum. The right anterior approach provides access to the right pulmonary hilum and the pericardium (not as well as the left-side approach). The pitfall of this method is that it provides a less-than-ideal approach to medial-posterior parenchyma lung injuries.

A clamshell incision (bilateral anterior lateral thoracotomies with a transverse sternotomy) improves exposure to the entire pericardium and heart, as well as the thoracic inlet. It also provides quick access to the right atrial appendage following pericardiotomy for vascular access if needed during emergency resuscitations. It can be used for transmediastinal wounds that require bilateral chest cavity exploration. The disadvantage is poor access to the esophagus and posterior trachea.

Median sternotomy also provides access to the pericardium, heart, thoracic inlet, and both lungs. In skilled hands, using a sternal saw, it can be done rapidly. However, most Forward Surgical Teams (FSTs) do not have power saws, and median sternotomy using a Lebsche knife is slower. Sternotomy provides limited access to the left lower lobe, which is obscured by the heart. Left lower lobe exposure can be improved if the sternotomy is extended into the left anterior lateral chest along the submammary crease (hemiclamshell or sternothoracotomy). This also improves access to the proximal left subclavian artery and the descending aorta. Additional versatility of the incision can be obtained by extending the incision along the anterior border of the sternocleidomastoid or via a supraclavicular extension, thus providing more exposure to the subclavian and carotid vessels. The trapdoor incision (sternothoracotomy with supraclavicular extension) provides excellent exposure to the thoracic inlet. However, it limits simultaneous access to the axillary artery.

The posterolateral thoracotomy is the standard access recommended for unilateral isolated chest trauma requiring surgery. It provides the best view of the entire lung and chest wall, as well as the intrathoracic esophagus and the carina from the right. The patient is placed in the lateral decubitus position with the down leg flexed and the upper leg extended with pillows between the legs. For maximum exposure, one lung ventilation (lung isolation) is preferred, but it is not always practical in trauma. Lung isolation gives the surgeon a quiescent lung to work on; but, more importantly, it protects the uninjured lung from soilage. The incision should be as large as required to see the injuries. Entering the chest through the fifth intercostal space centers the surgeon on the major fissure, but entry can and should be tailored to the wounds/injuries expected. Widely open the interspace to provide optimum exposure. If parenchyma bleeding is the major issue or if there is a large contusion, isolate the hilum as quickly as possible to prevent soilage and air embolus and to provide hemorrhage control so that the injury can be completely evaluated and addressed. This can be done easily by placing a hand around the hilum and guiding an aortic cross-clamp or large DeBakey vascular clamp around all the structures. A hilar twist is an alternative method of control. The pulmonary vasculature is a low-pressure system and can be easily controlled with direct pressure, which is done ideally with a broad-based sponge stick with just enough pressure to stop the bleeding.

In managing parenchyma lung injury, the goal is to limit removal of viable lung and control bleeding. The injury is either bleeding or not. Within the lung parenchyma, expanding hematomas do not occur because the pleura prevents expansion with a resultant contusion. Pulmonary contusions are not acutely managed operatively.

Most penetrating lung parenchymal injuries can be managed by tractotomy or wedge resection of a peripheral tract. However, if the tract traverses the fissure, the surgeon should suspect a pulmonary artery injury, and a lobar or greater resection may be required to control the hemorrhage.

Once bleeding is controlled, the surgeon must next control the postoperative pleural space. Placement of both apical straight anterior and posterior tubes is recommended. This provides more pleural coverage than a single apical and basilar right-angle tube. It also provides better pneumostasis. A poorly controlled pleural space leads to increased morbidity.

Thoracoabdominal wounds provide a greater quandary to the military surgeon. Projectile tract and potential organs injured should dictate operative incisions. Midline laparotomy incision is usually satisfactory for most of these wounds; but, if primary liver and upper abdominal injuries are suspected, a chevron incision may be considered. The chest component of most of these wounds can be generally attended with well-placed tubes. However, if necessary, either of these incisions can be extended with a sternotomy or an anterolateral thoracotomy, which provides optimum exposure. Do not fear going across the costochondral junction or extending it down through the diaphragm. The military surgeon should be familiar with the location of the phrenic nerve and what are safe incisions to prevent its injury. The costochondral juncture is easily repaired with no. 2 VICRYL in U-stitch fashion after diaphragm closure.

The proper approach to thoracic injury varies, depending on the structure injured. Under the best of circumstances, preoperative determination of thoracic injuries is difficult. In the combat environment, the surgeon will be required often to enter the chest using clinical judgment alone. The usual indication for entering the chest will be massive hemorrhage. There is no cookbook answer to what is the right incision in this circumstance, and the surgeon should not hesitate to make a second or even third incision if required to expose the damaged structure quickly, allowing control of hemorrhage. Knowledge of three-dimensional anatomy of the thorax will serve the combat surgeon well under these circumstances.

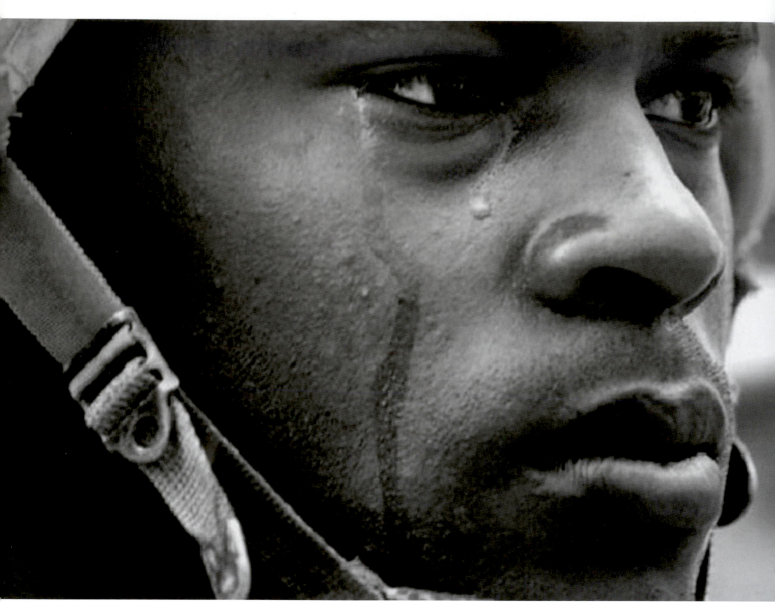

Courtesy David Leeson, *The Dallas Morning News*

Chapter V
ABDOMINOPELVIC TRAUMA

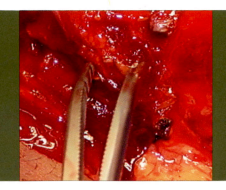

V.1
Indirect Effects of Wounding

CASE PRESENTATION

This 15-year-old host nation male presented after reportedly having been shot once with an M-16. Three wounds were apparent. A left lateral abdominal wound was the suspected entrance wound (Fig. 1). Two exit wounds were created secondary to fragmentation (Figs. 1 and 2). The patient underwent exploratory laparotomy. In surgery, there was no evidence of penetration of the peritoneum (Fig. 3). Nevertheless, there was a 3-cm, full-thickness injury of the transverse colon (Fig. 4). This wound was likely caused by cavitation commonly associated with high-velocity gunshot wounds. Because of the patient's apparent good nutritional status and the isolated extent of injury, he was treated with extended right hemicolectomy and ileocolostomy. Host nation patients do not enter the Army evacuation system and instead necessarily receive their definitive care at a combat support hospital (CSH). This patient's wounds were left open and treated with dressing changes. He recovered without complications.

TEACHING POINTS

1. This is an example of nonuniform energy transfer of a high-velocity round. The width of tissue disturbance is an indication of the magnitude of energy transfer, which may increase along the trajectory of a projectile.

2. The specific effect involved is cavitation. The physical properties of the target tissue determine the dimensions of the temporary cavity. For example, the cavity may be small in the lung, but large in the liver. Cavity size can be impressive—as much as 20-fold greater than the diameter of the bullet that caused it.

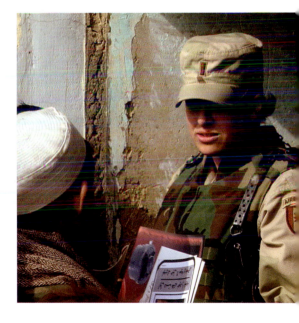

3. This gunshot wound of the extraperitoneal abdominal wall, which caused an injury of the underlying bowel, is also an example of indirect effects of wounding. Presumed by its nature to be rare, the Wound Data and Munitions Effectiveness Team (WDMET)—a database of American casualties in the Vietnam War—records only five documented examples of similar injury of 299 surviving casualties with intraabdominal trauma.

4. This case also recognizes the not uncommon scenario in which, if local medical facilities are not available or a field hospital is not established for that sole purpose, the CSH becomes the highest level of medical care available for many allied military and civilians.

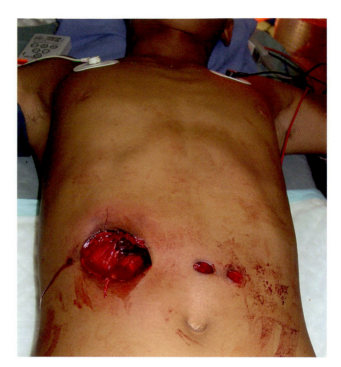

FIGURE 1. (Top) *M-16 entry and exit wounds.*

FIGURE 2. (Bottom) *Close-up of M-16 entry and exit wounds.*

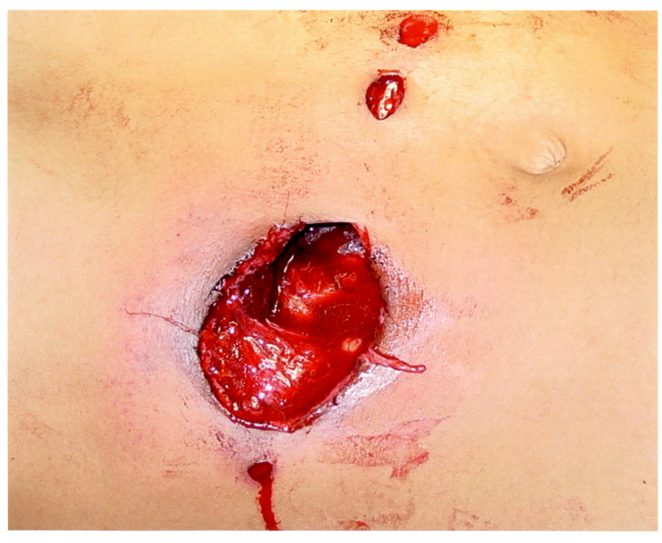

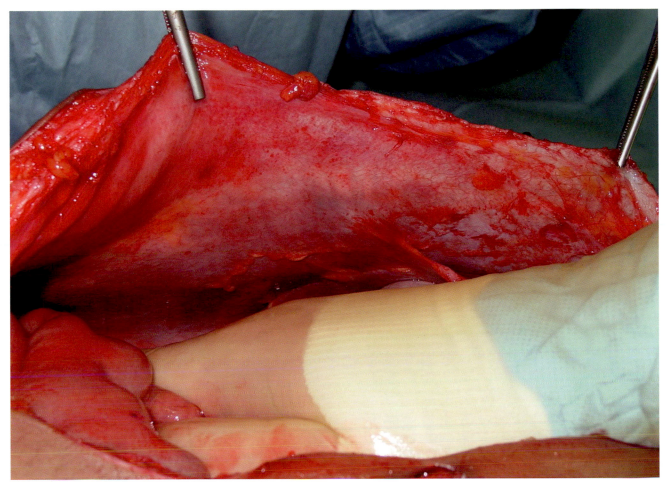

FIGURE 3. *Exploratory laparotomy. Note: There is no penetration of the reflected peritoneal wall.*

CLINICAL IMPLICATIONS

Simple, isolated colon injuries are uncommon. In host nation casualties and enemy combatants, poor nutritional status of these populations may preclude primary repair. Diversion with colostomy should be strongly considered in all patients in the presence of any of the complicating factors listed below:

1. Massive blood transfusion requirement.
2. Ongoing hypotension.
3. Hypoxia (secondary to a pulmonary injury).
4. Reperfusion (vascular) injury.
5. Multiple other injuries.
6. High-velocity injuries.
7. Extensive local tissue damage.

High-energy tangential wounds are prone to progressive soft-tissue devitalization and may evolve into necrotizing fasciitis. These wounds should be serially debrided and allowed to heal by either delayed primary closure or secondary intention.

DAMAGE CONTROL

1. In the unstable patient, control contamination with ligation/stapling of the bowel. Establishing intestinal continuity is not imperative.
2. Delay creation of the stoma until the patient is stable.
3. Document treatment for optimal follow-up through all levels of care.

SUMMARY

This is an uncommon case in which tangential injury by a high-velocity projectile presented with a relatively benign appearance. An understanding of the indirect effect of temporary cavitation in high-velocity wounds prompted formal laparotomy. Right hemicolectomy with ileocolostomy was performed. In this case,

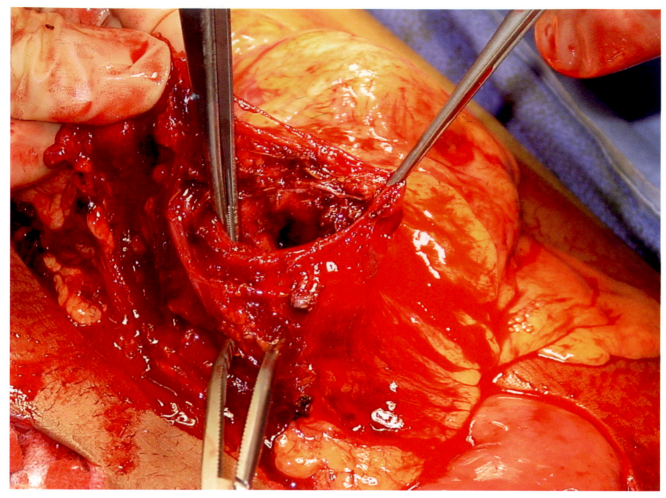

FIGURE 4. *The transverse colon has a large wound resulting from the indirect effects of the gunshot wound.*

prolonged care was necessary because the patient was a host national and could not be evacuated.

Note: See discussion of these cases on page 201.

SUGGESTED READING
Chapter 17: Abdominal injuries. In: *Emergency War Surgery, Third United States Revision*. Washington, DC: Department of the Army, Office of The Surgeon General, Borden Institute; 2004.

Bellamy RF, Zajtchuk R, eds. *Conventional Warfare: Ballistic, Blast, and Burn Injuries*. In: *Textbook of Military Medicine*. Washington, DC: Department of the Army, Office of The Surgeon General, Borden Institute; 1991.

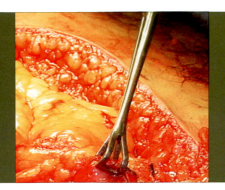

V.2
Penetrating Trauma to the Stomach and Pancreas

CASE PRESENTATION

A car bombing occurred near a combat support hospital (CSH). All staff prepared immediately for a mass casualty event. Initially, only patients with minor injuries came to the hospital. However, several hours later, a host nation policeman presented with facial, abdominal, and extremity injuries. He was awake and alert, with a mildly tender abdomen and multiple fragment wounds to the face overlying the parotid gland, the thoracoabdominal region, and the left leg (Fig. 1). His chest X-ray was significant for free air under the diaphragm (Fig. 2). During surgery, a single fragment was found that had entered the left abdomen, passed through the anterior and posterior walls of the stomach, and embedded in the pancreas. The anterior and posterior stomach wounds were closed in two layers (Figs. 3–5), and a distal pancreatectomy and splenectomy were also performed (Fig. 6). The parotid injury was minor, and the face laceration was closed. The leg wound required only washout, packing, and dressing changes.

TEACHING POINTS

1. This case is an excellent example of a patient who presented several hours after injury because of the confusion frequently encountered following an attack. At times, the CSH was notified of large-scale attacks and was informed to expect casualties. Surprisingly, these patients may not arrive for many hours.

2. In this case, enough time elapsed from the time of injury until presentation of the patient to allow free air to accumulate under the diaphragm and be visible on the chest X-ray. Patients with penetrating abdominal injury and free air under the diaphragm should undergo immediate laparotomy.

3. Penetrating injuries below the nipples, above the symphysis pubis, and between the posterior axillary lines must be treated as injuries to the abdomen and mandate exploratory laparotomy.

4. Stomach wounds require minimal debridement and are closed in two layers. The fragment that caused the injuries was found embedded in the distal pancreas. It caused significant tissue damage and therefore required distal pancreatectomy and splenectomy.

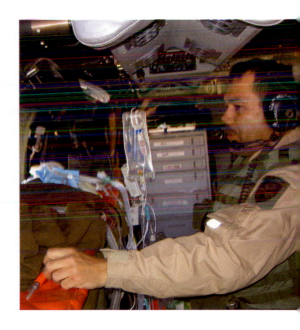

CLINICAL IMPLICATIONS

The stomach is well vascularized and usually heals well with primary closure. Arteries supplying the stomach are not end arteries and can be ligated. The following points should be emphasized:

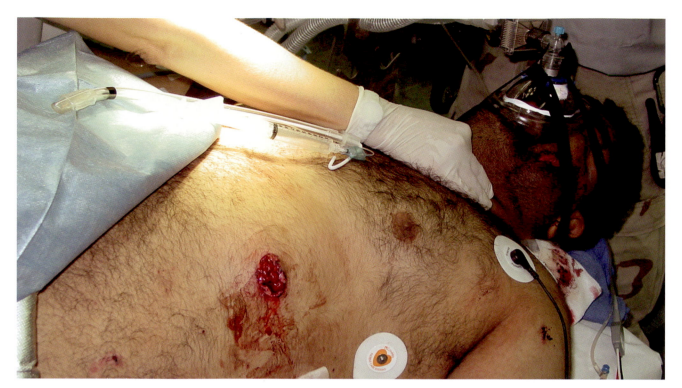

FIGURE 1. *Abdominal entrance wound before surgery. The facial wound overlying the left parotid gland is also apparent.*

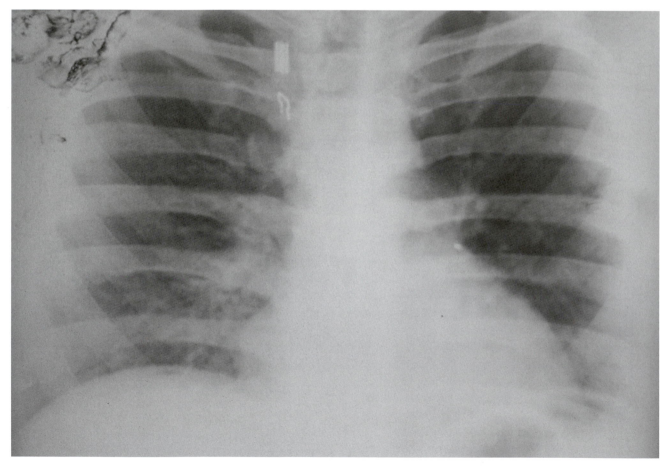

FIGURE 2. *Chest radiograph (AP) of free air under the diaphragm. (Objects are visible outside the body.)*

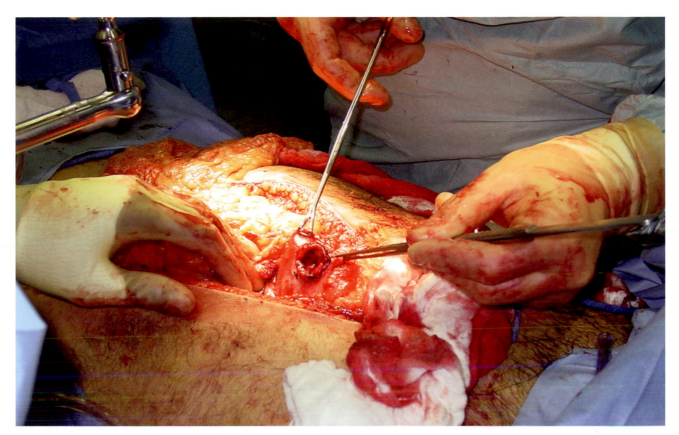

Figure 3. *Anterior stomach wound before closure.*

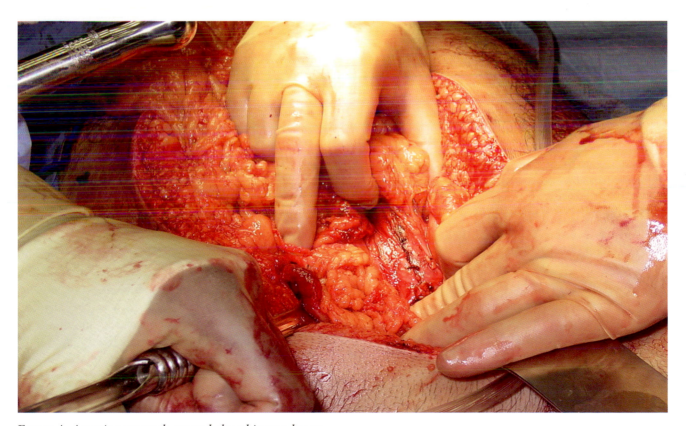

Figure 4. *Anterior stomach wound closed in two layers.*

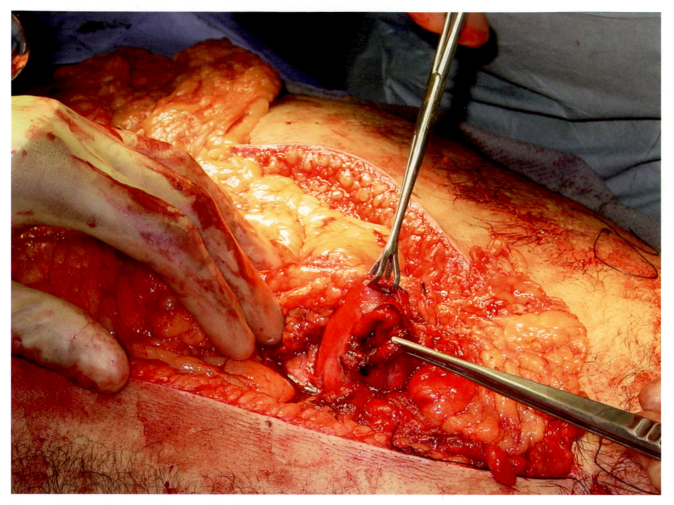

FIGURE 5. *Posterior stomach wound before repair.*

1. Enter the lesser sac to identify posterior stomach and pancreatic body and tail injuries. A Kocher maneuver should be performed to thoroughly evaluate the duodenum and head of the pancreas. Always examine the pancreas in cases involving penetrating trauma to the upper abdomen.

2. Drain all pancreatic injuries.

3. Treat transection or injury of the pancreatic duct by the following:

   a. Resection (distal pancreatectomy, as in this case).

   b. Oversewing or stapling the proximal pancreas segment.

   c. Roux-en-Y drainage of the injury.

4. The somatostatin analog, octreotide acetate (Sandostatin), administered subcutaneously (starting dose, 50 μg t.i.d.) can be initiated if a pancreatic leak occurs and may decrease output.

DAMAGE CONTROL

In an austere environment, once hemorrhage is controlled, pancreatic injury can be managed by drainage alone. If the clinical situation dictates, controlling bleeding with packing and limiting contamination by stapling off bowel injuries may be used.

SUMMARY

This case is an example of a single fragment passing through the anterior and posterior walls of the stomach and embedding in the pancreas. Management of this case was relatively straightforward, because the patient presented with a significant abdominal wall injury, tenderness, and free air under the diaphragm. This case also demonstrates that a significant delay can occur between time of actual attack and arrival of patients at a CSH, even if that hospital is within close proximity of the attack. Medical staff should

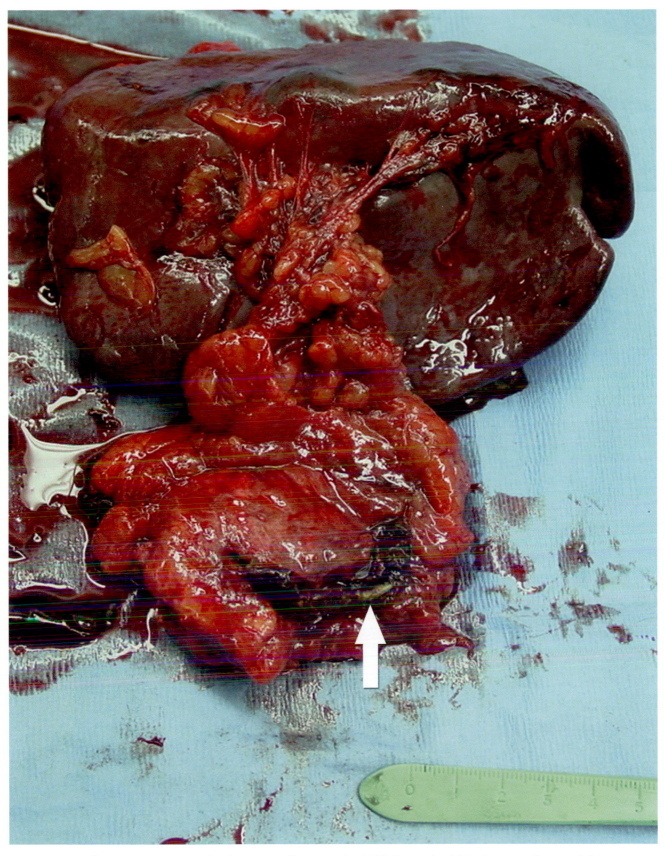

FIGURE 6. *Distal pancreatectomy and splenectomy. Fragment is visible* (arrow) *within the parenchyma of the pancreas.*

consider this when anticipating a mass casualty event. A trauma system should be in place to ensure that rest cycles are maintained and that personnel do not exhaust themselves waiting for patients to arrive.

Note: See discussion of this case on page 201.

SUGGESTED READING

Chapter 13: Face and neck injuries. In: *Emergency War Surgery, Third United States Revision*. Washington, DC: Department of the Army, Office of The Surgeon General, Borden Institute; 2004.

Chapter 16: Thoracic injuries. In: *Emergency War Surgery, Third United States Revision*. Washington, DC: Department of the Army, Office of The Surgeon General, Borden Institute; 2004.

Chapter 17: Abdominal injuries. In: *Emergency War Surgery, Third United States Revision*. Washington, DC: Department of the Surgeon General, Borden Institute; 2004.

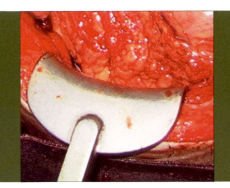

V.3
Blunt Abdominal Trauma

CASE PRESENTATION

This male patient was involved in a motor vehicle crash. He was transferred to a combat support hospital (CSH) after an initial evaluation at a host nation medical facility. Typical of these types of accidents, details were not available when the patient arrived at the hospital. On admission, he was hemodynamically and neurologically uncompromised. He had a tender abdomen. Imaging capability was limited to a cervical spine series, a portable chest X-ray, and a pelvis radiograph (all normal). A decision was made to explore the patient's abdomen. On entering the abdomen, vegetable matter was noted throughout the peritoneal cavity, as well as 500 mL of blood. The abdomen was thoroughly explored, and all injuries were limited to the upper abdomen. The most apparent injuries were to the stomach and duodenum. The stomach was almost completely transected between the body and antrum, and only 1 cm of stomach remained intact along the lesser curvature (Fig. 1). The duodenum was completely disrupted between the second and third portions. The superior mesenteric vein (SMV) was also injured just caudal to the pancreas, and the tributary veins had been torn flush with the SMV. Bleeding from the SMV was managed with fine Prolene sutures at the sites of the avulsed branches. The bleeding ends of the tributaries were managed with ligation, and the SMV remained patent after the repair. On visual inspection, the pancreas was injury-free. No other abdominal injuries were identified. Damage control laparotomy was performed. No effort was made for primary repair of the gastrointestinal tract. The open end of the proximal stomach was stapled closed. The open end of the distal stomach was also stapled. In addition, the two transected ends of the duodenum were stapled. This anatomical configuration left the patient with a blind pouch consisting of the distal stomach and the proximal duodenum. Temporary abdominal closure was performed, and the patient was resuscitated in the intensive care unit. After resuscitation, he was taken back to the operating room. Immediate restoration of his gastrointestinal anatomy was not performed. The proximal stomach was managed with tube gastrostomy, and the distal stomach and proximal duodenal pouch were managed with tube drainage. A 24-French Malecot catheter was placed through a purse-string stitch in the anterior wall of the distal stomach, and the catheter advanced through the pylorus into the duodenum. The distal stomach was brought up to the right upper quadrant of the abdominal wall and secured to the

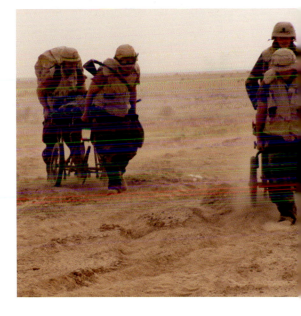

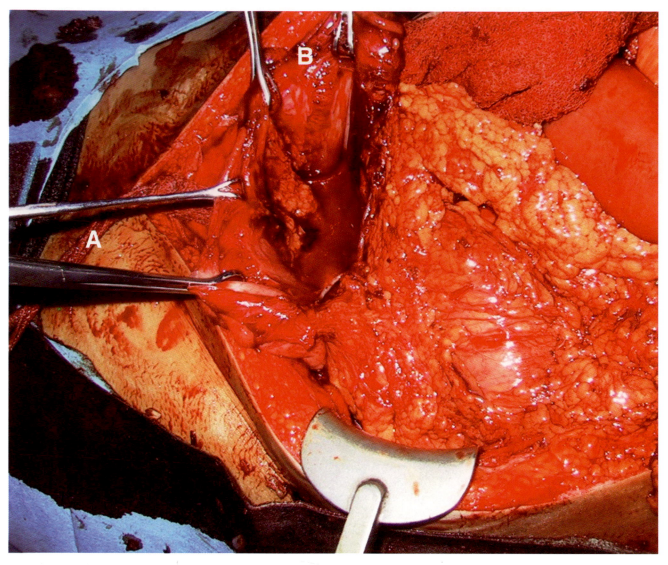

FIGURE 1. *With the patient's head to the left, the Babcock on the patient's right* (A) *is on the distal stomach remnant. The two Babcock clamps on the left side of the patient are on the proximal gastric remnant* (B). *The duodenal injury is not shown.*

parietal peritoneum. Although the pancreas had not been injured, two drains were placed adjacent to the pancreas, and the abdominal wall fascia was left open. After two more days, the patient underwent a third operation. The SMV remained patent. Nonetheless, bowel edema prevented abdominal wall closure. Abdominal integrity was restored with VICRYL mesh. Vacuum dressing was applied to promote granulation. Two days later, a tracheostomy was performed to assist in weaning the patient from the ventilator. The patient was transferred to a host nation medical facility. He had good respiratory function, jejunostomy feedings at goal, and no evidence of sepsis at the time of transfer.

TEACHING POINTS

1. Blunt injuries to the duodenum may be associated with massive upper abdominal trauma, as in this case. Early during the initial operation, consideration should be given for staged damage control surgery.
2. When produced by blunt force, gastric ruptures are often large with copious intraperitoneal soiling.
3. With massive proximal intestinal injury at initial operation, only bowel that is unquestionably devascularized or necrotic should be resected. Although bowel of questionable viability can be assessed intraoperatively (Doppler flow, fluorescein), a second-look operation in 24 hours is recommended.

CLINICAL IMPLICATIONS

1. Even though Army medical assets can be geared toward combat trauma in a combat zone, noncombat trauma still occurs. Approximately 40% of surgeries performed by one CSH during combat deployment were noncombat related.[1]

2. Army medical personnel deployed in the combat zone are resourced to provide care for combat casualties. However, many trauma patients will be host nationals depending on the medical rules of engagement and resources available. When resources are available and security measures in place, providing care to the local population may be possible.

DAMAGE CONTROL

1. This case is typical of the type of damage control surgery that is required in combat hospitals.

2. Clinical practice guidelines suggesting damage control laparotomy include the following:

    a. Multiple life-threatening injuries.
    b. Acidosis (pH < 7.2).
    c. Hypothermia (temperature < 36°C).
    d. Hypotension and shock.
    e. Combined hollow viscus and vascular injury.
    f. Coagulopathy.

SUMMARY

This patient had a combined hollow viscus and a major vascular injury. He required 8 units of packed red blood cells. His perioperative status included hypotension, and he presented a triad of hypothermia (34.6°C), acidosis (pH 7.27), and coagulopathy (partial thromboplastin time, 54 seconds). The patient's Injury Severity Score (ISS) was 16. He was treated with damage control laparotomy, and damage control techniques used early in his treatment resulted in a successful outcome. Teams preparing for deployment need to anticipate providing care to the local population and to noncombat trauma patients.

Note: See discussion of this case on pages 201–202.

REFERENCE

1. 86th Combat Support Hospital. Experience of the 86th Combat Support Hospital. Operation Iraqi Freedom-1. January 2003 through June 2003. Unpublished data.

SUGGESTED READING

Chapter 1: Weapons effects and parachute injuries. In: *Emergency War Surgery, Third United States Revision*. Washington, DC: Department of the Army, Office of The Surgeon General, Borden Institute; 2004.

Chapter 11: Critical care. In: *Emergency War Surgery, Third United States Revision*. Washington, DC: Department of the Army, Office of The Surgeon General, Borden Institute; 2004.

Chapter 17: Abdominal injuries. In: *Emergency War Surgery, Third United States Revision*. Washington, DC: Department of the Army, Office of The Surgeon General, Borden Institute; 2004.

Chapter 34: Care of enemy prisoners of war/internees. In: *Emergency War Surgery, Third United States Revision*. Washington, DC: Department of the Army, Office of The Surgeon General, Borden Institute; 2004.

US Army Center for Health Promotion and Preventive Medicine. *Clinical Practice Guidelines*. Aberdeen Proving Ground, MD: USACHPPM; March 2005. 44th Medical Command.

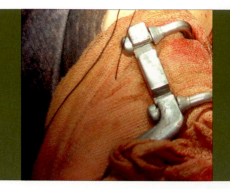

V.4
Missed Duodenal Injury

CASE PRESENTATION

This 20-year-old marine was transferred—after laparotomy and repair of penetrating gastric injury—from a level II Forward Surgical Team (FST) to a level III combat support hospital (CSH) medical treatment facility. While awaiting aeromedical evacuation, he exhibited tachycardia and hypotension, with a small amount of bilious drainage from the posterior exit wound (lower back). The patient's abdomen was reexplored prior to aeromedical evacuation. At laparotomy, bile staining was noted at the site of gastric repair. A Kocher maneuver was performed. A missed through-and-through duodenal injury was also discovered (Fig. 1). In addition, a superior pole laceration of the right kidney was found (Fig. 2). The duodenal injury was repaired with a two-layer closure anteriorly and posteriorly (Figs. 3 and 4). The renal injury was debrided, and bleeding was controlled with electrocautery. Both injuries were externally drained. The patient improved clinically and was later evacuated.

TEACHING POINTS

1. Level II surgery units (eg, FSTs) operate in austere and resource-constrained environments. Often, they perform lifesaving operations in very difficult conditions. It is critically important that medical personnel perform a thorough exploration (if time permits) when operating on penetrating abdominal trauma.

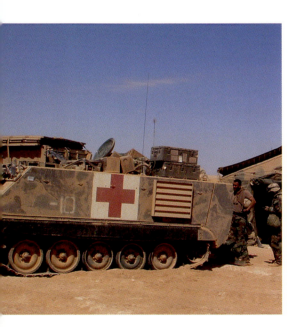

2. If the clinical situation or condition of the patient does not permit this examination, it is essential that the level II medical treatment facility communicate in some way (even if it involves writing on the abdominal dressing; Fig. 5) with the receiving level III facility to make sure that the next level of care personnel understand that reexploration prior to further evacuation is mandatory.

3. It is critical that level III medical treatment facilities carefully reevaluate patients received and consider early reoperation when patients remain unstable or deteriorate after arrival. Serial examinations and attentive observation of postoperative patients are mandatory throughout the MEDEVAC system.

CLINICAL IMPLICATIONS

Injuries to the duodenum are often associated with massive upper abdominal trauma. Damage control techniques should be considered early.

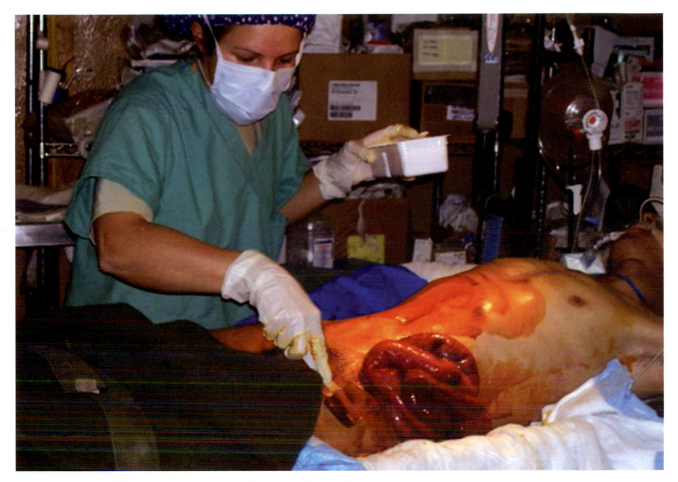

FIGURE 1. *Wound showing evisceration of the small intestine.*

CLINICAL IMPLICATIONS

Once the decision is made to take the patient to the operating room, management of a simple evisceration is straightforward.

1. The patient can be prepped widely, and the eviscerated bowel can be prepped with betadine after thorough irrigation.
2. Any other immediately life-threatening abdominal injuries should be addressed first—then reduce the bowel and assess viability.
3. The procedure should begin with a midline incision.
4. The eviscerated bowel can be examined outside of the abdominal cavity. If there are enterotomies, control contamination by closing the defects with a simple suture before reducing the bowel back into the abdomen.
5. Remember, as in an incarcerated hernia, simple reduction of the intestines may be all that is needed to return blood flow to ischemic areas.
6. All frankly necrotic bowel is removed, and a primary anastomosis or an ostomy may be performed. Choice of primary anastomosis versus ostomy and delayed primary repair depends on many factors (eg, the presence of associated injuries, hypotension, and degree of intraabdominal contamination). Primary repair in young, healthy patients who are hemodynamically stable is acceptable. An ostomy and delayed repair are reserved for unstable patients or severe, gross fecal contamination, as in a left colon or rectal injury.

DAMAGE CONTROL

1. Control airway and hemorrhage first in hemodynamically unstable patients.
2. Control gross contamination by closing enterotomies with simple sutures or staples.
3. Resect dead and ischemic bowel and delay anastomosis or creation of an ostomy until patients are hemodynamically stable.

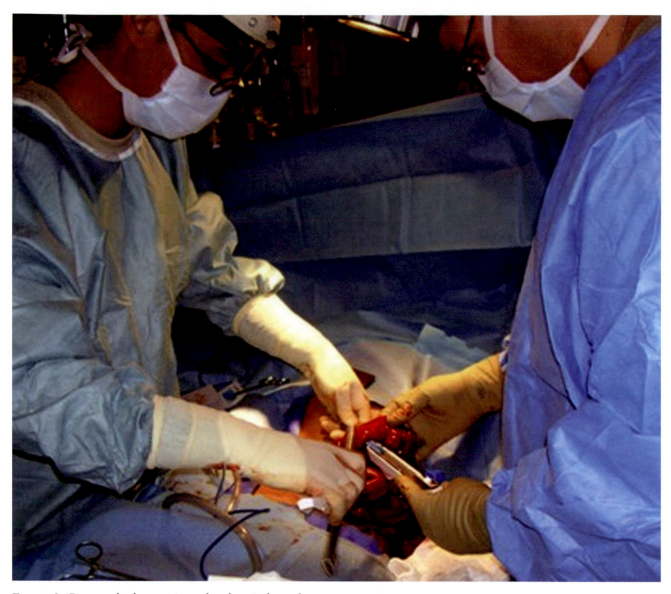

FIGURE 2. *Removal of necrotic and ischemic bowel.*

SUMMARY

In the combat setting, the management of eviscerated abdominal contents is stratified into two categories: (1) early mandatory laparotomy and (2) nonurgent laparotomy. Unlike in the civilian setting, nonoperative treatment of these patients is not appropriate.

Note: See discussion of this case on page 202.

SUGGESTED READING

Arikan S, Kocakusak A, et al. A prospective comparison of the selective observation and routine exploration methods for penetrating abdominal stab wounds with organ or omentum evisceration. *J Trauma.* 2005;58(3):526–532.

Benissa N, Zoubidi M, et al. Abdominal stab wound injury with omentum evisceration. *Ann Chir.* 2003;128(10): 710–713.

Chapter 3: Triage. In: *Emergency War Surgery, Third United States Revision.* Washington, DC: Department of the Army, Office of The Surgeon General, Borden Institute; 2004.

Chapter 17: Abdominal injuries. In: *Emergency War Surgery, Third United States Revision.* Washington, DC: Department of the Army, Office of The Surgeon General, Borden Institute; 2004.

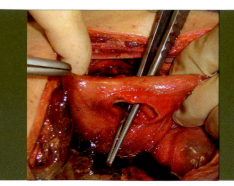

V.6
Penetrating Rectal Injury

CASE PRESENTATION

This 35-year-old male patient was riding in a military vehicle when an improvised explosive device (IED) was detonated. He was treated by medics in the field and then brought to the combat support hospital (CSH) by MEDEVAC helicopter. He arrived awake and complaining of pain in his left leg. A thorough examination revealed an obvious left femur fracture with a lateral entrance wound and a medial exit wound. The patient's pulses were normal, with no evidence of arterial injury. Further examination revealed a second penetrating wound that entered the left buttock, created a large subcutaneous tract with palpable crepitus, and exited through a larger wound in the right buttock. Examination of the perineum showed no bruising, and no other injuries were noted. The patient required external fixation of the femur fracture and exploration of the sacral wound. It was clear that the procedure would take some time to perform. A blood drive was initiated for 8 units of whole blood. Because there was minimal bleeding from the sacral wound, external fixation of the femur fracture was performed to minimize blood loss from that wound. Then the patient was placed in the prone position. The sacral wound was addressed by opening the wound tract between the entrance and exit wounds. The projectiles (rocks) had passed through the sacrum at the S2 level and completely divided the bony sacrum (Fig. 1). The muscular bleeding was packed. A full-thickness, 50% circumferential posterior rectal injury—with gross fecal contamination—was identified. There was bleeding from the patient's left side between the rectum and left lateral pelvic wall. The severed ends of the hypogastric artery were identified with difficulty and ligated. The presacral venous plexus of the upper and lower sacral fragments was compressed with packs. With hemorrhage controlled, the patient's physiological status was assessed. His temperature was 34°C, and he was clinically coagulopathic and acidotic. The decision was made therefore to proceed with damage control by rapidly closing the rectal wound with VICRYL suture, applying QuikClot hemostatic agent, and packing the wound. The skin was closed over the packs to apply pressure (Fig. 2), and the patient was then taken to the intensive care unit (ICU) for resuscitation and warming (Fig. 3). At that time, the CSH did not have active warming devices (eg, Bair Huggers), so intravenous catheter bags heated in a microwave oven and activated MRE (Meal, Ready-to-Eat) heaters wrapped in towels were used to warm

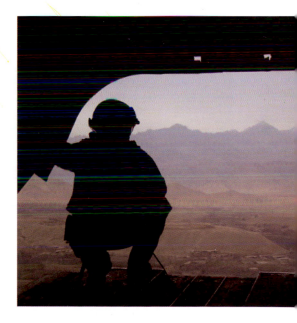

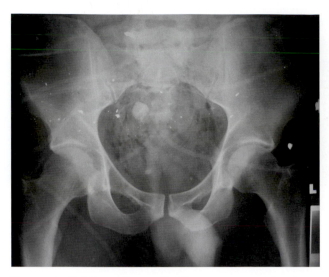

FIGURE 1. *Pelvic radiograph. Note numerous foreign bodies. The sacrum is transected at S2.*

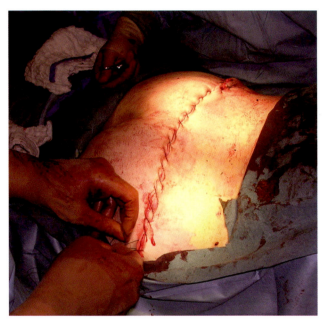

FIGURE 2. *Damage control. Skin temporarily closed over packing.*

the patient. He was given whole blood transfusions until his platelet level was above 50,000 plts/mL. With resuscitation, the patient's temperature and vital signs normalized and acidosis improved. However, the patient's abdomen became increasingly distended, and serial ultrasound examinations revealed increasing amounts of intraperitoneal fluid. Once stabilized, the patient was returned to the operating room (OR) for laparotomy to rule out intraabdominal hemorrhage and to perform a diverting colostomy to treat the rectosacral wound.

No intraabdominal wound was identified, and an end descending colostomy was performed (Fig. 4). The distal colon was closed, followed by closure of the abdomen. The following morning, 24 hours after initial injury, the patient was hemostatic. Evacuation was planned, but the timing of theater evacuation is unpredictable; therefore, the patient was taken back to the OR for washout and debridement of the rectal wound. The sacral packs were removed (Fig. 5). The raw surfaces were hemostatic, with the sandlike remnants of the QuikClot in place. Copious irrigation was used to remove the particles and necrotic tissue. Manipulation of the upper sacral body revealed a cerebrospinal fluid leak, and intraoperative consultation with a neurosurgeon was obtained. Definitive treatment of that injury was deferred to level V. Therefore, the wound was closed over closed-suction drains. Later that evening, the patient was evacuated to a level IV medical treatment facility with his surgeon attending and with CCATT (Critical Care Air Transport Team) assistance.

TEACHING POINTS

1. Combat-injured patients often present with multiple complex wounds. All variables must be considered when caring for these patients. It can be argued that the sacral injury should have been addressed first. However, it was clear that, when this patient presented, he would require staged procedures and damage control techniques.

2. The need for whole blood and other blood product transfusions must be identified early.

3. The need for damage control surgery must be made before irreversible acidosis and coagulopathy develop. Use all of your resources—physicians, nurses, and anesthetists—to resuscitate and stabilize the patient.

4. Ligation of internal iliac arteries may be effective in managing otherwise uncontrollable pelvic hemorrhage. It can be performed through the posterior wound in some situations. Bilateral ligation of the internal iliac arteries is to be avoided, if possible.

5. In the combat setting, perform the least amount of surgery possible. In this case, the cerebrospinal fluid leak was controlled, and definitive repair was deferred to a level V medical treatment facility. If possible, attempt primary closure of the thecal sac. In many cases, this cannot be done because direct access may be difficult, or because the dura tends to be diaphanous and attempts at stitching can enlarge the tear. Instead, consider a dural substitute (eg, DuraGen). Follow with a fibrin sealant.

6. CSHs are designed to treat combat trauma. Pre-deployment and peacetime training must include patient care within the field treatment facilities. In this case, equipment as fundamental as patient warmers were not included in this hospital's inventory. Army surgeons must discipline themselves to participate in predeployment training and the process that develops field hospitals and the equipment set.

CLINICAL IMPLICATIONS

When caring for patients with multiple complex wounds, remember the basics:

1. Control the airway, obtain adequate intravenous access, and resuscitate the patient with warm fluids, including whole blood when appropriate.
2. Identify sources of hemorrhage and control hemorrhage by the simplest means available. This may include stabilizing extremity and pelvic fractures. Hemostatic agents (eg, chitosan) may be useful. Fresh frozen plasma and recombinant factor VII may be available. Trauma surgeons need to understand the preparation and use of all available blood products.
3. Control gross contamination and liberally defer definitive repair of bowel injuries until the patient is stable. A temporary closure with packs and drains in place is often helpful. When the patient is stable, planned reoperation is useful.
4. Rectal wounds can be difficult to diagnose. Injury should be suspected if trauma has occurred in proximity to the rectum, if there is an abnormal rectal examination, or if a radiograph suggests injury. The following principles apply:
   a. All rectal injuries should have proximal diversion. Sigmoid end colostomy is usually adequate. If the injury has not violated the peritoneum, exploration of the extraperitoneal rectum should not be done at laparotomy unless indicated for an associated nonbowel injury. This avoids contaminating the peritoneal cavity with stool.
   b. All rectal wounds should be drained. Presacral drains should be used for extraperitoneal rectal injuries. Fecal contamination of the perirectal space mandates presacral drainage.
   c. Distal washout of the rectum is usually necessary to assess the injury. Gentle pressure when irrigating will minimize contamination of the perirectal space.

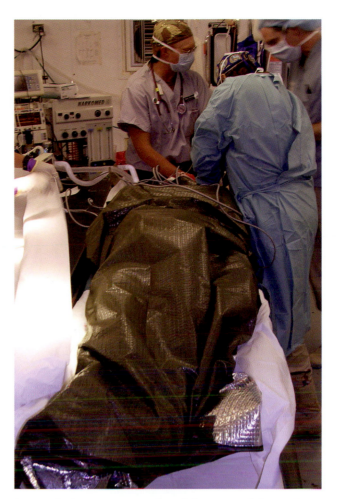

FIGURE 3. *Rewarming and stabilization of the patient in ICU.*

   d. Debridement and closure are not necessary in small- or medium-sized wounds that have been diverted and drained.
   e. Hematoma in the perirectal space should be drained either transluminally by leaving the injured rectum open or by placing drains trans-abdominally or through presacral drains.
   f. Peritonealized rectal injuries are easily accessed transabdominally and should be repaired and protected with diversion.

DAMAGE CONTROL

This case aptly illustrates the principles of damage control. Damage control is defined as the rapid initial control of hemorrhage and contamination, temporary closure, resuscitation to normal physiology in the ICU, and subsequent reexploration and definitive repair. Concerning the cerebrospinal fluid leak: sew in a patch graft or lay one down and separate it with fascia and fat.

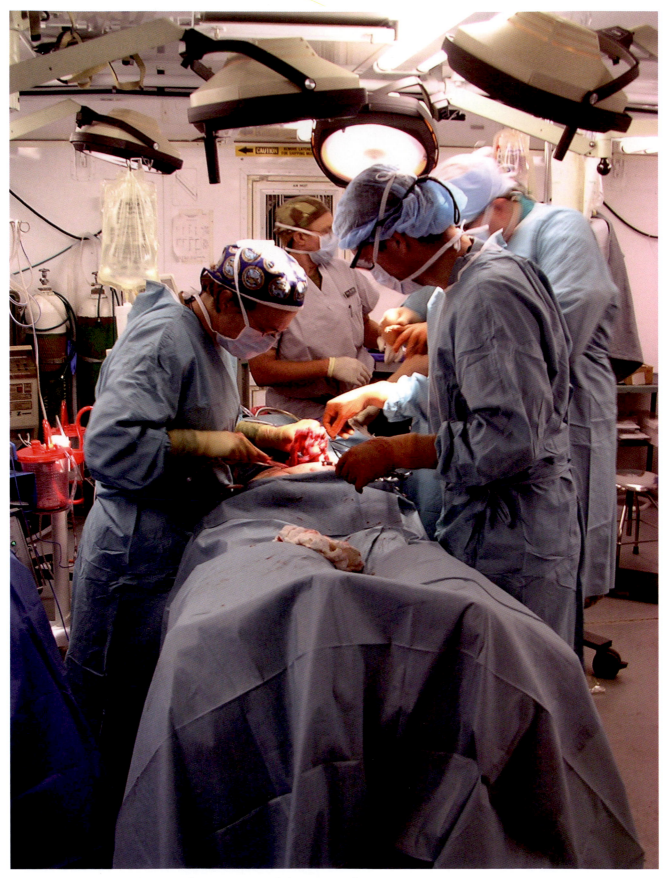

FIGURE 4. *Surgery; exploratory laparotomy and diverting colostomy.*

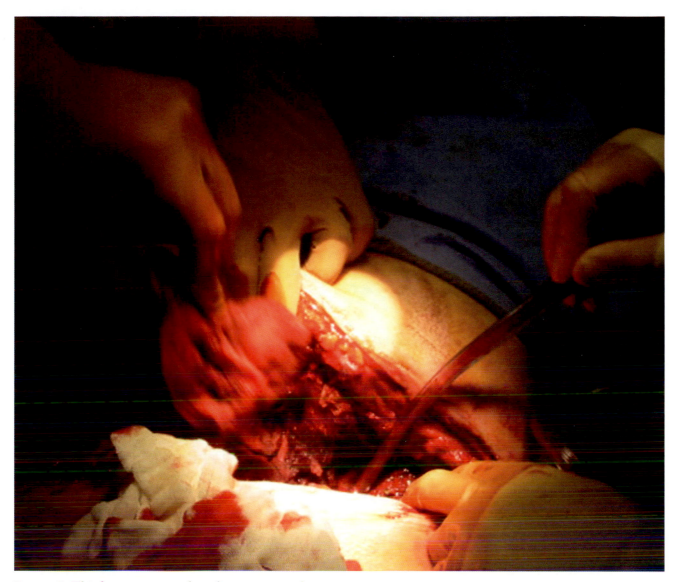

FIGURE 5. *Third surgery; sacral packs are removed.*

Divert cerebrospinal fluid with a lumbar drain. Pack the wound. Keep the patient flat.

SUMMARY

In this case, a patient with severe injuries survived those wounds by effective use of damage control techniques, including early aggressive resuscitation with whole blood and control of hemorrhage and gross contamination. When stable, the patient was returned to the OR for further required surgery and then evacuated. Perform CT/myelography at level V to rule out pseudomeningocoele.

Note: See discussion of this case on pages 202–203.

SUGGESTED READING

Chapter 4: Aeromedical evacuation. In: *Emergency War Surgery, Third United States Revision*. Washington, DC: Department of the Army, Office of The Surgeon General, Borden Institute; 2004.

Chapter 6: Hemorrhage control. In: *Emergency War Surgery, Third United States Revision*. Washington, DC: Department of the Army, Office of The Surgeon General, Borden Institute; 2004.

Chapter 12: Damage control surgery. In: *Emergency War Surgery, Third United States Revision*. Washington, DC: Department of the Army, Office of The Surgeon General, Borden Institute; 2004.

THREE PHASES OF DAMAGE CONTROL

The goal of damage control is to restore normal physiology rather than normal anatomy. It is used for the multiply injured patient, with combinations of abdominal, vascular, genitourinary, neurological, orthopaedic, and/or thoracic injury in three separate and distinct phases.

1. Primary Operation and Hemorrhage Control—surgical control of hemorrhage and removal of contamination; laparotomy terminated, abdomen packed, and temporary closure; definitive repair is deferred.
   a. Control of hemorrhage.
   b. Exploration to determine extent of injury.
   c. Control of contamination.
   d. Therapeutic packing.
   e. Abdominal closure.
2. Critical Care Considerations—normal physiology restored in the ICU by core rewarming, correction of coagulopathy, and hemodynamic normalization.
   a. Core rewarming.
   b. Reversal of acidosis.
   c. Reversal of coagulopathy.
3. Planned Reoperation—reexploration to complete the definitive surgical management or evacuation.

Chapter 17: Abdominal injuries. In: *Emergency War Surgery, Third United States Revision*. Washington, DC: Department of the Army, Office of The Surgeon General, Borden Institute; 2004.

Chapter 22: Soft-tissue injuries. In: *Emergency War Surgery, Third United States Revision*. Washington, DC: Department of the Army, Office of The Surgeon General, Borden Institute; 2004.

Chapter 23: Extremity fractures. In: *Emergency War Surgery, Third United States Revision*. Washington, DC: Department of the Army, Office of The Surgeon General, Borden Institute; 2004.

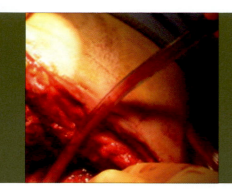

V.7
Renal Trauma

CASE PRESENTATION

A 23-year-old host nation male presented with a single gunshot wound following a sniper incident. The patient was alert and responding appropriately to questions. Initial vital signs revealed the following: blood pressure, 90/60 mm Hg; heart rate, 115 beats per minute; and temperature, 36°C. Primary and secondary surveys revealed diffuse abdominal tenderness and rebound, and a single entrance wound in the posterior axillary line on the left just below the 12th rib. The patient went directly to surgery, without imaging, based on the clinical examination. Exploratory laparotomy was negative, to include no obvious retroperitoneal hematoma. The patient received 2 units of packed red blood cells intraoperatively. Postoperatively, his vital signs stabilized. Approximately 10 hours postoperatively, the patient's vital signs became unstable, with blood pressure of 80/60 mm Hg and a heart rate of 130 beats per minute. Repeat laboratory evaluation revealed the following: hemoglobin, 7.5 g/dL; international normalized ratio (INR), 3.1; and partial thromboplastin time (PTT), 68 seconds. A CT scan was obtained (Fig. 1) and revealed a grade III right renal injury (Table 1) with no urinary extravasation and intact vessels. The bullet is shown. Because of the recent onset of hemodynamic instability and coagulopathy, a trial of nonoperative management was elected. The patient was given 2 additional units of packed red blood cells, 4 units of fresh frozen plasma, and 7,500 μg of activated Factor VII. Fluid resuscitation continued. Over the next several hours, urine output increased and vital signs stabilized. The coagulation parameters also normalized. The patient was discharged home on postoperative day 5.

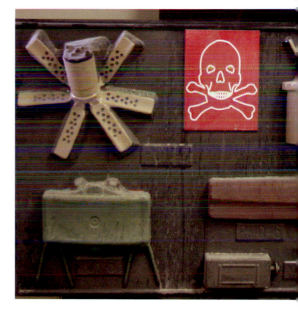

TEACHING POINTS

1. Significant retroperitoneal injuries can be missed at exploratory laparotomy. Consider early imaging with negative findings at exploration.
2. The majority of grade III renal injuries do not require operation. Coagulopathy was a complicating factor in this case.
3. In patients with grade III or IV renal injuries—with no other indication for operative exploration—a trial of aggressive resuscitation with crystalloid and blood products is the first line of intervention. Operative exploration of the retroperitoneum is reserved for nonresponders.

TABLE 1. *Renal Injury Scale*

GRADE	TYPE OF INJURY	DESCRIPTION
MINOR		
I	Contusion	Microscopic or gross hematuria; urological studies normal
	Hematoma	Subcapsular, nonexpanding without parenchymal laceration
II	Hematoma	Nonexpanding perirenal hematoma confined to renal retroperitoneum
	Laceration	<1.0-cm parenchymal depth of renal cortex without urinary extravasation
MAJOR		
III	Laceration	>1.0-cm parenchymal depth of renal cortex without collecting system rupture or urinary extravasation
IV	Laceration	Parenchymal laceration extending through renal cortex, medulla, and collecting system
	Vascular	Main renal artery or vein injury with contained hemorrhage
V	Laceration	Completely shattered kidney
	Vascular	Avulsion of renal hilum that devascularizes kidney

4. The use of activated Factor VII is controversial; in this case, it may have been organ-sparing.

CLINICAL IMPLICATIONS

1. Management of blunt and penetrating renal trauma is directed by the grade of injury. Grades I to III involve varying degrees of laceration and hematoma with no disruption of the major vessels or collecting system. Grade V represents avulsion of the pedicle and is almost always managed operatively. Grade IV involves varying degrees of collecting system and/or vascular injury. Management of grade IV injuries can involve either immediate operative exploration or a trial of aggressive resuscitation with crystalloid and blood products, depending on the availability of resources and the level of expertise of available surgeons.

2. Renal trauma patients should have a Foley catheter in place and should remain on bed rest until gross hematuria clears.

DAMAGE CONTROL

In the absence of a CT scanner, a FAST examination of the retroperitoneum may detect a retroperitoneal hematoma. If no imaging is available, a high index of suspicion for retroperitoneal injury must be maintained based on the location of entrance and exit wounds. If the patient responds to fluid and blood product resuscitation, immediate evacuation to the next level of care should be initiated. If hemodynamics remains unstable, emergent operative intervention is required, with careful attention to assessment of the retroperitoneum. Nephrectomy may be the best solution for major renal injuries when other life-threatening injuries are present. Determining the function of the contralateral kidney (confirmed by contrast study) is desirable prior to nephrectomy.

SUMMARY

The kidneys and other retroperitoneal structures are at risk with blunt and penetrating abdominal, back, and flank trauma. If operative management is not immediately indicated, the imaging modality of choice is a three-phase CT scan of the abdomen and pelvis. Based on CT scan findings, renal trauma can be graded on a scale of I to V. Grades I to III and many grade IV

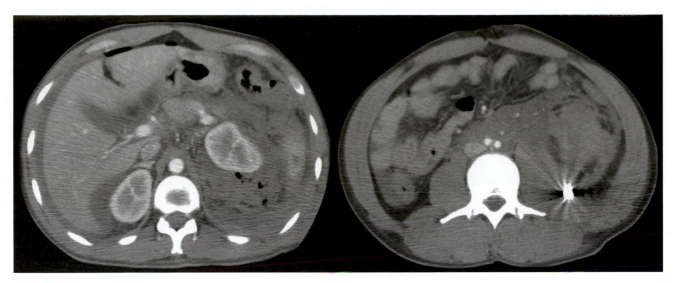

FIGURE 1. *Abdominal CT images obtained postoperatively. A large perinephric fluid collection and air lucencies* (Left), *as well as bullet fragment* (Right) *are evident.*

injuries can be managed nonoperatively with aggressive fluid and blood product resuscitation.

SUGGESTED READING

Chapter 17: Abdominal injuries. In: *Emergency War Surgery, Third United States Revision.* Washington, DC: Department of the Army, Office of The Surgeon General, Borden Institute; 2004.

Chapter 18: Genitourinary tract injuries. In: *Emergency War Surgery, Third United States Revision.* Washington, DC: Department of the Army, Office of The Surgeon General, Borden Institute; 2004.

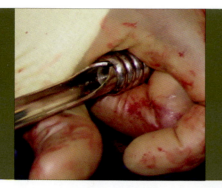

V.8
Penetrating Pelvic Trauma

CASE PRESENTATION

A 27-year-old male sustained injuries after exposure to a blast from an improvised explosive device (IED). He was the front-seat passenger in a vehicle, and the blast occurred at the right front tire. On arrival, he was alert and answering questions appropriately. Vital signs were stable. Primary and secondary surveys revealed a right ankle blast injury and penetrating wounds to the upper posterior right thigh (Figs. 1 and 2) and medial left thigh. Abdomen, genitourinary, and rectal examinations, as well as the remainder of the physical examination, were normal. A plain film was obtained of the right foot and ankle and the right thigh. An anteroposterior pelvis radiograph was ordered. Two large shrapnel fragments were identified overlying the pelvis (Fig. 3). With this information, a CT scan was then obtained of the abdomen and pelvis. The CT scan showed two fragments: one fragment was adjacent to the base of the bladder on the right, and the other fragment was adjacent to the inferior pubic ramus and posterior aspect of the right corpus cavernosum (Fig. 4). The location of the fragments raised concern for the integrity of both the urinary tract and lower gastrointestinal (GI) tract. He was brought to the operating room for washout of the right ankle and further investigation of the lower urinary and GI tracts. Proctoscopy was negative. Cystoscopy and retrograde contrast studies revealed no injury in the urethra, bladder, or distal right ureter. He was observed overnight and evacuated in 24 hours to the next higher level of care.

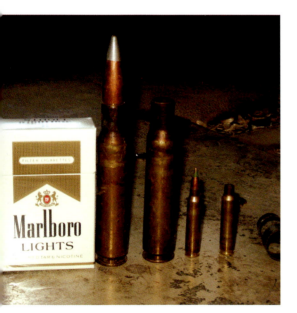

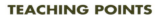

TEACHING POINTS

1. IED fragments may have a significant distance of excursion from the entrance wound. Consequently, plain films should be obtained liberally in the trauma bay.
2. When pelvic fragments are identified, the integrity of the urinary and lower GI tracts must be considered. Further diagnostic testing should be planned based on radiographic and physical examination findings.

CLINICAL IMPLICATIONS

Penetrating injuries to the pelvis are often associated with abdomino-pelvic organ injury. Diagnosis of associated injuries may require

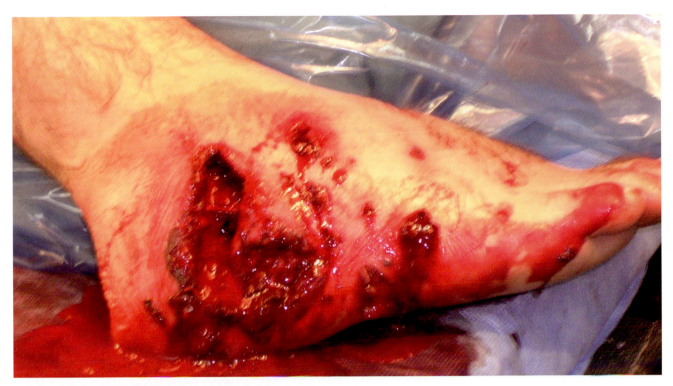

FIGURE 1. *Penetrating blast injury, right ankle.*

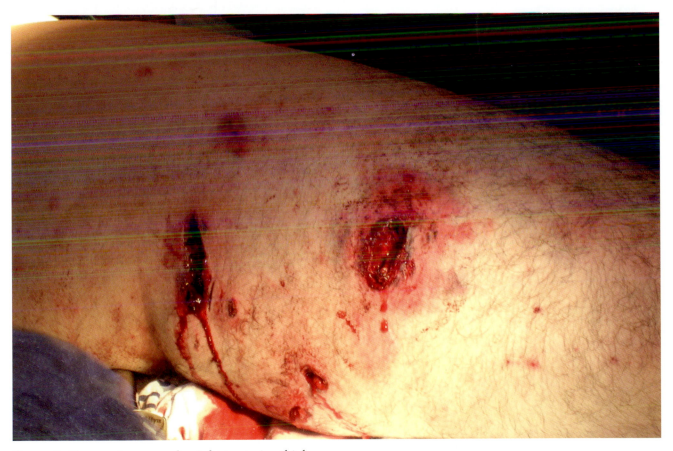

FIGURE 2. *Penetrating wounds, right posterior thigh.*

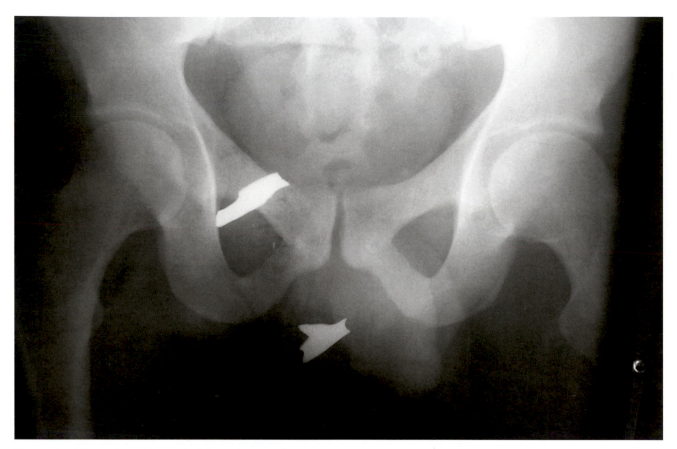

FIGURE 3. *AP pelvis radiograph. Note the two fragments.*

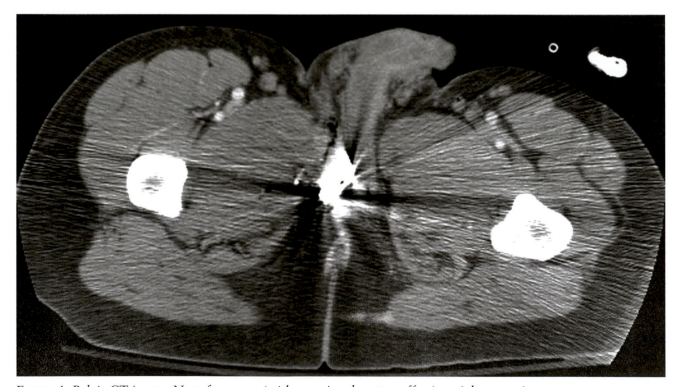

FIGURE 4. *Pelvic CT image. Note fragment (with associated scatter effect) at right posterior corpus cavernosum.*

exploratory laparotomy. Catheterization is contraindicated until urethral integrity is confirmed by retrograde urethrography.

DAMAGE CONTROL

For cases of suspected urethral trauma (blood at the meatus, scrotal hematoma, high-riding prostate), a retrograde urethrogram should be performed prior to insertion of a Foley catheter. If a urethral injury is discovered, a suprapubic catheter is recommended.

SUMMARY

IED blasts are the most common mechanism of injury in Operation Iraqi Freedom. They may result in multiple sites of trauma for a given patient. The location of the entrance wound prompts varying levels of concern for adjacent structures based on location. It must be emphasized that fragments may come to rest a significant distance from their entrance wounds. Liberal use of plain radiography and cross-sectional imaging should be utilized with this mechanism of injury.

SUGGESTED READING

Chapter 18: Genitourinary tract injuries. In: *Emergency War Surgery, Third United States Revision*. Washington, DC: Department of the Army, Office of The Surgeon General, Borden Institute; 2004.

Chapter 21: Pelvic injuries. In: *Emergency War Surgery, Third United States Revision*. Washington, DC: Department of the Army, Office of The Surgeon General, Borden Institute; 2004.

Chapter 22: Soft-tissue injuries. In: *Emergency War Surgery, Third United States Revision*. Washington, DC: Department of the Army, Office of The Surgeon General, Borden Institute; 2004.

Chapter 26: Injuries to the hands and feet. In: *Emergency War Surgery, Third United States Revision*. Washington, DC: Department of the Army, Office of The Surgeon General, Borden Institute; 2004.

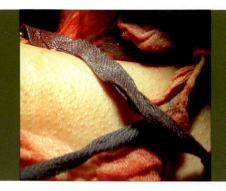

V.9
Penetrating Scrotal Trauma

CASE PRESENTATION

A 23-year-old host nation male presented as part of a mass casualty event after a suicide bomb attack. The patient was alert and complained of right hand, right groin, and right thigh pain. His injuries included a right-hand fracture and an avulsion of skin and subcutaneous tissue in the proximal/medial right thigh with a foreign body evident on examination (Fig. 1). The penile and scrotal examinations revealed diffuse edema and ecchymosis. The left testicle was palpable and unremarkable. The right testicle was nonpalpable. A radiograph of the pelvis/lower extremities revealed a foreign body superimposed on the inferior pubic ramus on the right (Fig. 2). A CT scan of the abdomen and pelvis revealed an abnormal appearance of the right testicle, air in the scrotum, and the foreign body posterior to the scrotum (Fig. 3). The patient was brought to the operating room for stabilization of the right hand, washout of the right thigh wound, and—based on radiographic findings and physical examination—scrotal exploration. On exploration, the foreign body was removed and was consistent with a human rib fragment with attached intercostal musculature (Fig. 4). The scrotum was explored through a midline incision at the median raphe. The patient had a ruptured right testicle. An orchiectomy was performed. He recovered well and was discharged on postoperative day 2.

TEACHING POINTS

1. Patients injured in suicide bomb attacks are at risk for both mechanical injury from blast effects and fragments. They are also at biological risk from "missile-ized" body parts.
2. The absence of a palpable testicle after blunt penetrating trauma should prompt scrotal exploration.

CLINICAL IMPLICATIONS

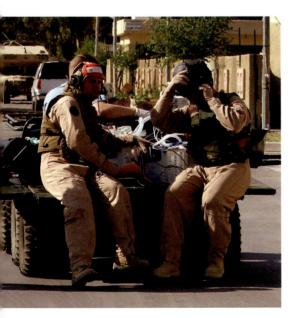

1. In many cases of scrotal trauma, as in this case, there are associated injuries prompting CT scan. CT scan and ultrasound of the scrotum are insensitive for testicular rupture and other scrotal pathology. A high index of suspicion based on mechanism of injury and physical examination findings should prompt scrotal exploration.
2. Testicular salvage after rupture is possible. Determining factors are the degree of remaining vascular supply to the tubule mass and

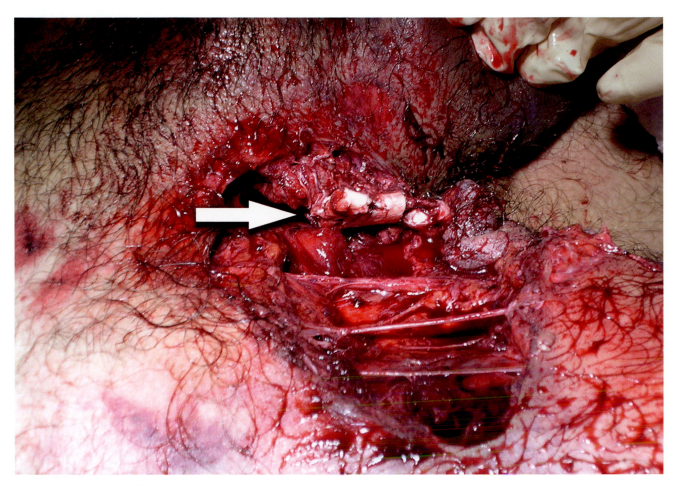

FIGURE 1. *Scrotum reflected to show proximal medial thigh wound. Note foreign body in wound* (arrow).

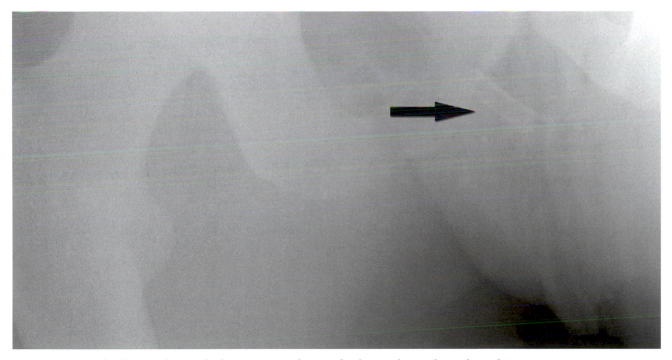

FIGURE 2. *Coned pelvic radiograph demonstrates foreign body overlying the right pubic ramus* (arrow).

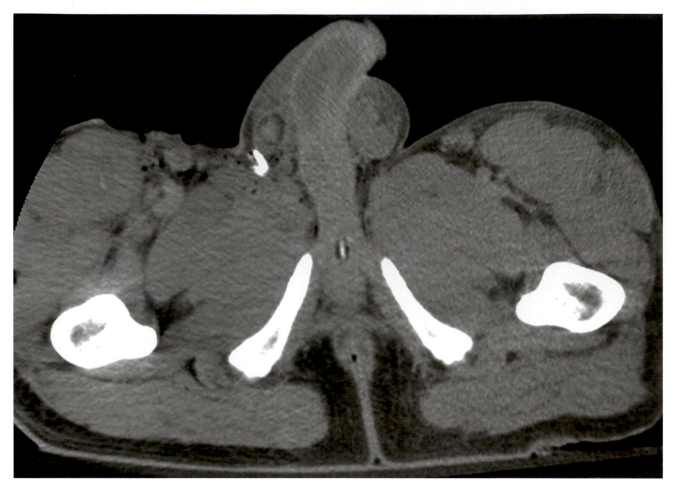

FIGURE 3. *Pelvic CT image demonstrates air in right scrotum with the foreign body located posteriorly. Right testicle is abnormal.*

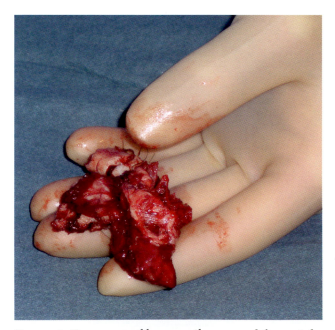

FIGURE 4. *Fragment of human rib removed from right scrotum.*

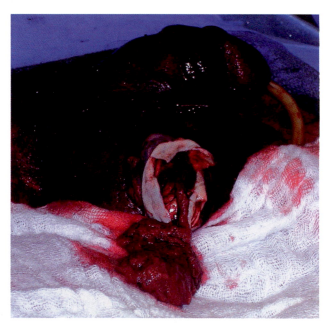

FIGURE 5. *Avulsed right testicle.*

the availability of remaining tunica albuginea to reconstruct the testicle. In this case, there was almost complete avulsion of the tubule mass (Fig. 5); therefore, orchiectomy was performed. However, as soon as the tunica albuginea (or epididymis or vas deferens) is violated, there is a breach of the blood–testis barrier, and there exists potential for the formation of antisperm antibodies regardless of the disposition of the testicle (salvage or removal). This does not guarantee infertility, but creates the risk of subfertility. If fertility becomes a clinical problem for these patients in the future, early referral to an infertility specialist is indicated.

3. In terms of testicular function, the remaining normal testicle produces enough testosterone for normal male physiological function.

DAMAGE CONTROL

In austere conditions, scrotal injuries are not emergent as long as hemostasis is achieved. If testicular salvage is to be entertained, the patient should be seen by a surgeon within 3 to 4 hours of injury. If the mission precludes immediate referral to a surgeon, it could be managed conservatively indefinitely until urological evaluation is possible.

SUMMARY

Patients injured in suicide bomb attacks are at risk for both mechanical and biological injuries. The examining provider must develop an index of suspicion for testicular injury based on mechanism and physical examination findings. CT scan and ultrasound are often unsatisfying in diagnosing testicular injury. Testicular salvage should be the goal, if mission allows, and the patient should be evacuated to the nearest urologist within 3 to 4 hours of injury. If immediate referral is not possible, and operative facilities are not immediately available, scrotal injuries can be managed conservatively indefinitely until referral is possible.

SUGGESTED READING

Chapter 17: Abdominal injuries. In: *Emergency War Surgery, Third United States Revision*. Washington, DC: Department of the Army, Office of The Surgeon General, Borden Institute; 2004.

Chapter 18: Genitourinary tract injuries. In: *Emergency War Surgery, Third United States Revision*. Washington, DC: Department of the Army, Office of The Surgeon General, Borden Institute; 2004.

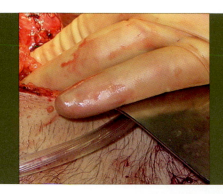

V.10
Genital Soft-Tissue Trauma

CASE PRESENTATION

While on patrol, a 29-year-old male soldier sustained multiple blast injuries when his vehicle was struck by an improvised explosive device (IED). He was resuscitated at the Forward Surgical Team (FST) facility and transferred to a level IV medical facility. In addition to dramatic soft-tissue injuries to the penis and scrotum, he suffered head, face, right hand, and bilateral lower extremity injuries. The patient underwent wound debridement and genital reconstruction that included a left orchiectomy, repair of the ruptured right testicle, urethral reconstruction over a 12-gauge French urethral catheter, penile glans reconstruction, and skin closure (Fig. 1). He was evacuated to the United States on the fifth day following his injury. The penile and urethral reconstructions failed with progression of nonviable tissue, and the repairs were taken down for additional debridement (Fig. 2). Delayed reconstruction was started 2 weeks after the injury by placement of a split-thickness skin graft to the wound bed (Fig. 3).

TEACHING POINTS

1. High-energy injury to the soft tissue of the genitalia can cause delayed tissue necrosis.
2. Early reconstruction has a greater risk of failure.
3. Closure of the corpus cavernosum is advisable for small injuries.
4. Tension-free approximation of the urethra and corpus spongiosum with absorbable suture is recommended.
5. Genital skin should be reapproximated loosely at its anatomical site.
6. Generous use of drains is recommended.

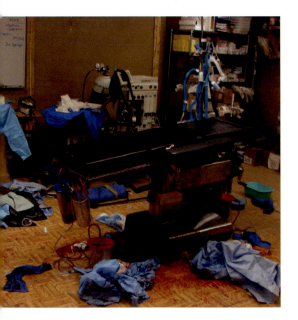

CLINICAL IMPLICATIONS

1. Genital wound debridement can be done quickly during damage control surgery. This is accomplished through judicious removal of nonviable tissue with copious irrigation or pressure lavage of the wound. Tissue devitalization from high-velocity projectiles is not always apparent at initial evaluation. Delayed necrosis can jeopardize early reconstructive efforts. Definitive wound closure should, therefore, not be attempted in this early period. Final cosmetic and functional results, however, are enhanced if loose approximation of the tissue is accomplished with several widely separated nylon sutures that can be removed at the next surgery for further debridement. The

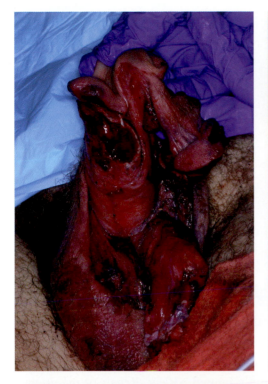
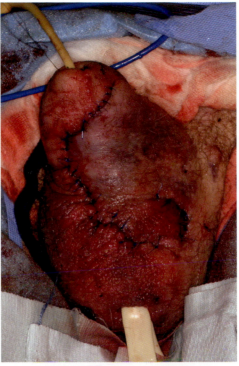

FIGURE 1. (Top Left) *Intraoperative appearance of genital trauma from blast. The left testicle has been removed and the right one repaired. The glans penis is traumatically divided with half partially attached by a skin bridge. The transected corpus cavernosum is visible below a small intact segment of glans. The proximal urethral opening is visible at the base of the shaft near the penoscrotal junction. (Top Right) An aggressive, early attempt at reconstruction. Little of the reconstructed tissue would survive.*

FIGURE 2. (Bottom) *Subsequent intraoperative appearance of the injury after all nonviable removed. The scrotum is nearly reapproximated in this image.*

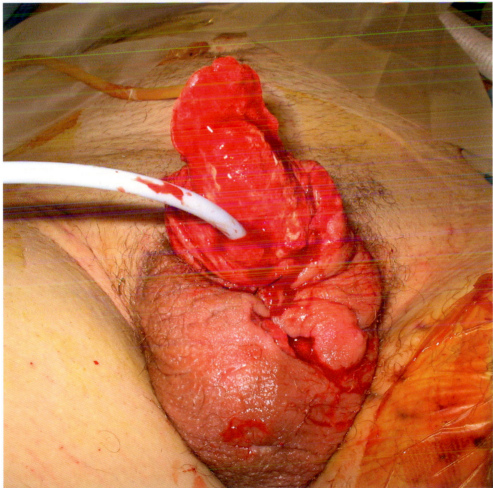

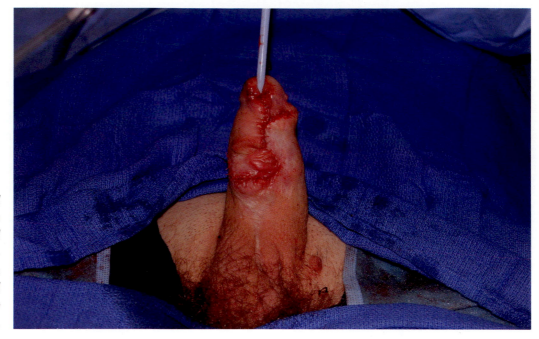

FIGURE 3. *Final reconstruction after staged buccal and split-thickness skin grafts are formed into a new urethra.*

loosely approximated wound should be drained completely with Penrose drains, small suction drains, or a wound vacuum.

2. Injury to the corpus cavernosum and urethra requires more detailed attention at the time of injury. The integrity of the urethra can be determined by retrograde urethrography or urethroscopy. Cavernosal injuries should be suspected when a large penile hematoma is present. Exploration and repair of the tunica albuginea can improve final function. This repair can be completed through the penile wound, by penile skin degloving, or by a vertical incision in the penis at the site of corporal injury. It is important to remember that the neurovascular bundle to the glans runs along the dorsum of the penis. A ventral approach to the tunica albuginea can reduce injury to these structures.

3. Small fragment injuries to the penis may not require extensive debridement. Experience shows that aggressive exploration for these small fragments is not warranted in the acute setting and can be accomplished later if symptomatic.

DAMAGE CONTROL

Genital wounds are seen frequently with concurrent wounds to the abdomen and lower extremities. Initial treatment often requires damage control principles. Rapid removal of obvious devitalized tissue, copious irrigation of the wound, loose approximation of penile skin with maximal wound drainage, and Foley catheter placement—when feasible—can be accomplished swiftly in the seriously injured patient. Repair of the urethra and corpus cavernosum with absorbable sutures may reduce bleeding and aid in damage control. Delaying closure, however, is sometimes necessary when tissue loss is severe, tissue viability is uncertain, or the patient is hemodynamically unstable.

SUMMARY

Soft-tissue injuries to the genitalia are devastating. Early surgical intervention should entail judicious wound debridement that favors observation of tissue of uncertain viability rather than aggressive removal. Delayed reconstruction appears superior to premature attempts at penile and scrotal skin closures. Loose approximation of tissue with liberal use of drains aids future reconstruction. Early approximation of urethral and corpus cavernosal injuries may assist in hemorrhage control and improve future function.

SUGGESTED READING

Chapter 18: Genitourinary tract injuries. In: *Emergency War Surgery, Third United States Revision.* Washington, DC: Department of the Army, Office of The Surgeon General, Borden Institute; 2004.

Chapter 22: Soft-tissue injuries. In: *Emergency War Surgery, Third United States Revision.* Washington, DC: Department of the Army, Office of The Surgeon General, Borden Institute; 2004.

Damage Control Surgery

by COL George E. Peoples, MD

A theme of this chapter is damage control surgery as it pertains to the injured abdomen. Usually applied to the unstable patient, and revisited throughout this book, this approach is a well-accepted concept among civilian and military trauma surgeons. Its basic requirement is a staged approach to the severely injured patient at risk for the lethal triad of hypothermia, acidosis, and coagulopathy. In general, there are three phases to damage control surgery: (1) primary surgery that assesses the extent of injury and controls hemorrhage and gross contamination; (2) intensive care unit resuscitation to address warming, to reverse acidosis, and to correct coagulopathies; and (3) planned reoperation for more definitive management of injuries. The latter steps may need to be repeated as often as necessary to correct the injuries without unduly stressing the patient.

There are, however, some notable differences in the civilian and military applications of the damage control concept. The most prominent among these is overall management of the patient. In the civilian realm, a single surgeon usually manages the entire damage control sequence. He knows firsthand the extent of the injuries, what was and was not done at the first surgery, and when best to take the patient back to the operating room, based on carefully observed and measured physiology. Contrast that to the combat-wounded soldier who may have his first procedure performed in a tent at the Forward Surgical Team (FST) facility, is then evacuated immediately to a Combat Support Hospital (CSH) for aggressive resuscitation, then flown to a level IV medical treatment facility where the next procedure is performed, and finally receives definitive repair at a level V hospital in the United States. Further compound this sequence by compressing it into 4 to 5 days. For optimal care, the military sequence requires precise communication and coordination. Unfortunately, this chain of communication is not always feasible, given the constrictions of the tactical situation, the necessity of establishing intermediary levels of care, and the uncertainty of uncontested aeromedical evacuation. In the absence of seamless transfers, military trauma surgery is dependent at its core on the understanding, practice, and flexible application of damage control surgery by all participating military surgeons.

Even with this doctrine firmly established in the military realm, deployed military surgeons must still be extra conservative in their surgical decisions. Patients must be thoroughly reassessed at each level of evacuation. Most importantly, military surgeons must be flexible and innovative in their management of injured soldiers.

Many of the concepts that have been advanced in civilian trauma centers leading to nonoperative management of certain injuries (splenic laceration), reliance on specialized services like interventional radiology (embolization), and earlier definitive repair (colon repair vs colostomy) may be impossible in combat-wounded personnel because of the unavailable imaging or intervention technologies, and/or ill-advised because of the inability to conduct continuous close follow-up, as outlined in the sequence above. Combat wounds are also different from those seen in civilian trauma centers where these advances in technology have been implemented. Combat trauma is often a result of high-energy projectiles. Multiple complex injuries are the norm. Initial management often occurs in an austere environment with limited resources and prolonged evacuation times. The patient's condition on arrival to the military surgeon is often not comparable with the civilian emergency department.

One of the greatest challenges of any evacuation system is the requirement to maintain the flow of relevant medical information through each level of care in pace with the patient's movement. The disruption of this information flow results in missed injuries, compartment syndromes, delayed treatments, and potentially unnecessary procedures. The evacuation system must strive to improve the conveyance of real-time treatment information from level to level. Follow-up information sent backwards, so that surgeons and medical units can assess and adjust their overall quality of care, is also an essential requirement.

A military-relevant algorithm of how best to care for any specific injury, including the intraabdominal injuries cited in this chapter, is virtually impossible because there are too many variables that are uncontrollable. Many of the treatment decisions for a specific injury will be necessarily influenced by the following:

- patient's condition,
- resources available (most often determined by which level of care the surgeon finds himself),
- availability of the next higher level of care (often dictated by the phase of the conflict), and
- time to evacuation (determined by the tactical situation and weather).

A surgeon at a FST who is faced with the same injury as a colleague at a CSH, may—by necessity—treat it completely differently. In the absence of pertinent and useful treatment algorithms, we rely on principles.

The military version of damage control surgery, as well as the overall surgical management of the injured soldier, relies on the premise that the patient should have only that surgery necessary to stabilize him for safe evacuation to the next level of care. This may mean *no* surgery at an FST facility if the patient is stable. The principle guiding which injuries should be addressed and when is that of escalating intervention. For a vascular injury, escalation may mean ligation if necessary, repair if circumstances permit, or bypass if not reparable (shunt if expedience is required). For a colon injury, escalation might be simple repair, exterioration, formal colostomy, repair with protective ostomy, resection with ostomy, or resection with anastomosis. This general concept is applicable to most injured organs and pairs the increasing complexity of the procedure with the sophistication of resources available, and the time required to complete it. The decision of what procedure to perform for any given injury will be dictated not only by the usual parameters of the patient's condition, severity of the specific injury, and associated injuries; but also by the level of care, resources available, tactical situation, and availability of evacuation. Military surgeons must have a working knowledge of escalating interventions for the wide array of specific intraabdominal injuries. They must embrace the concept of damage control surgery, understand the levels of care and the evacuation system, and appreciate and anticipate the constantly changing environments in which they may find themselves when caring for the combat wounded.

Abdominopelvic Trauma, Cases Review

by LTC Brennan J. Carmody, MD

The cases in this chapter highlight the vast differences between abdominal trauma encountered in military and civilian settings. High-velocity projectiles and combinations of blast and penetrating injuries can result in extensive tissue destruction that may not be immediately apparent. An understanding of these injury patterns and the application of damage control principles are crucial in minimizing morbidity and mortality.

CASE V.1 (Indirect Effects of Wounding) is an excellent example of the effects of combined blast-penetrating injuries. Despite the absence of peritoneal entry, the cavitation produced by this high-velocity abdominal wall injury led to a full-thickness colon injury. The need to rule out intraperitoneal entry led to abdominal exploration and management of the colon injury. A high level of suspicion must be maintained with these mechanisms of injury, because military bullets travel in excess of 3,000 f/s. Despite a relatively benign-appearing wound and the absence of objective evidence of intraabdominal penetration, one should have a low threshold for laparotomy. These high-energy tangential wounds are prone to progressive soft-tissue devitalization and may evolve into necrotizing fasciitis. These wounds should be serially debrided and allowed to heal by either delayed primary closure or secondary intention.

Another important teaching point involves the differences in management of colon injuries, depending on whether the patient will remain in theater or enter the evacuation chain. Most surgeons would consider it reasonable to perform a segmental colectomy with ileocolostomy in the absence of hypotension, significant fecal soilage, and significant associated injuries in any patient who would remain in theater under close supervision. In patients who will be evacuated to higher echelons of care, end colostomy should strongly be considered, given the potential for prolonged evacuation times, the break in continuity of care, and the high-injury mechanisms of energy frequently encountered.

CASE V.2 (Penetrating Trauma to the Stomach and Pancreas) illustrates the high likelihood of associated injuries in upper abdominal penetrating trauma. It is critical to explore all areas of the abdomen, including the lesser sac. Routes to access this space include the gastrocolic and gastrohepatic ligaments. Additionally, a Kocher maneuver should be performed routinely to assess the posterior aspects of the duodenum and pancreas. In damage control settings, drainage of pancreatic fluid is all that should be done. More definitive interventions can be performed when the patient has been appropriately resuscitated. Given the propensity for pancreatic anastomoses to leak, distal pancreatectomy should be considered before using pancreaticojejunostomy to the distal pancreatic remnant. The somatostatin analogue octreotide acetate (sandostatin), administered subcutaneously (starting dose: 50 µg t.i.d.), can be initiated if pancreatic leak occurs and may decrease outputs; the dose can be titrated to the point of cholestasis.

CASE V.3 (Blunt Abdominal Trauma) eloquently describes staged management of a complex duodenal injury. Combined gastrointestinal and vascular injuries are common, and patients who have sustained such trauma often present in shock with elevated Injury Severity Scores, hypotension, coagulopathy, acidosis, and hypothermia. Surgeons managing this case took the appropriate initial actions to control hemorrhage and gastrointestinal soilage, and made no efforts to reestablish gastrointestinal continuity. Following resuscitation and return to the operating room, drainage of the isolated portions of the foregut was established, along with placement of a jejunostomy for enteral feeds. Visceral edema precluded definitive abdominal wall closure, and an absorbable mesh was placed with plans for subsequent skin graft and planned ventral hernia. The patient was then transferred to a host nation medical facility.

This case illustrates several teaching points. First, definitive gastrointestinal reconstructions should only be performed after adequate resuscitation, resolution of visceral edema, and restoration of protein stores. This patient's status resulted in transfer to a local hospital prior to meeting these criteria. In patients entering the evacuation chain, temporary abdominal closure should be established in theater with definitive reconstruction performed at higher levels of care (where the patient will be more likely physiologically ready for such complex surgery). Definitive reconstruction options would include Roux-en-Y gastrojejunostomy with duodenojejunostomy to allow for drainage of biliopancreatic fluids.

Second, proper management of the open abdomen continues to evolve. Whereas placement of absorbable mesh with skin grafting and planned ventral hernia remain an option, other techniques that avoid the morbidity of the planned ventral hernia are becoming more widely used. Vertrees and colleagues[1] reported their experience with serial abdominal closure using polytetrafluoroethylene mesh as a temporary closure. In this technique, the mesh allows abdominal domain to be reestablished, and the mesh is tightened at intervals leading to early definitive abdominal closure. Such closures involved either primary closure or an onlay interposition using polypropylene mesh. No fistulae developed, although the average time from initiation of serial abdominal closure to definitive closure was 45 days (range: 15–160). A more novel approach involves the use of bioprotheses, such as AlloDerm (an acellular dermal matrix that can be used to reconstruct abdominal wall defects). This prosthetic supports vascular and collagen ingrowth. It is relatively resistant to infection and can be used for definitive abdominal closure. Advantages include a potential shorter interval between injury and definitive abdominal closure, and use in previously contaminated fields. More long-term data regarding its durability are needed. Regardless of the technique used for abdominal closure, key principles include early use of a vacuum-assisted, nonadherent covering for the abdomen (ie, the VAC Abdominal Dressing System) or a Bogota bag that protects the viscera and allows full access to the entire abdomen. Vacuum and suction dressings also improve visceral edema and allow quantification of fluid losses.

Such early management will allow a full range of options for abdominal closure.

CASE V.4 (Missed Duodenal Injury) reiterates the need for thorough exploration following penetrating upper abdominal injury. The close proximity of gastrointestinal, vascular, and urological structures makes concomitant injury likely. Delay in diagnosis of duodenal injuries is associated with substantial morbidity and mortality. Occasionally, inflammatory changes will preclude primary repair of an otherwise minor injury. In such cases, placement of an appropriately sized Malecot drain can convert the injury to a tube duodenostomy that allows control of secretions. This option should be combined with a gastrostomy tube and wide drainage. Alternatives include repair with duodenal diverticularization or pyloric exclusion. This case also highlights the need for prompt communication between surgeons and facilities in cases in which full exploration was not feasible. Regardless of the thoroughness of prior procedures, a low threshold to reexplore unstable or deteriorating patients should be maintained, given the potential for missed or evolving injuries, recurrent or persistent hemorrhage, or undrained collections. This is especially critical in patients who will enter the evacuation system where continuity of care can be compromised.

In **CASE V.5** (Traumatic Evisceration), surgeons encounter and manage traumatic evisceration following blast injury. Key points include prehospital management (saline gauze, no efforts to reduce the viscera), control of enterotomies prior to reduction, full abdominal exploration, and resection of frankly nonviable intestine. When viability is questionable, the abdomen can be temporarily closed with reassessment in 24 to 48 hours. Occasionally, edema of the eviscerated bowel may require enlargement of the fascial defect (analogous incarcerated ventral hernias). Management of the fascial defect at the evisceration site can be problematic, especially in the setting of blast injury or high-velocity projectiles. Prostheses such as VICRYL or AlloDerm reestablish abdominal wall integrity and decrease the likelihood of postoperative evisceration through the entrance wound. Progressive devitalization of soft tissue is common, and the wound should be serially washed out and debrided as necessary.

CASE V.6 (Penetrating Rectal Injury) includes many of the war surgery tenets previously described: damage control techniques for combined visceral and vascular injuries, early resuscitation and rewarming, and return to the operating theater for further required surgery. Prompt initiation of a whole-blood drive was a key decision. As similar devastating injuries have become more common, deployed laboratories and blood banks have become incredibly efficient in acquiring and preparing whole blood. Activated Factor VII is also now widely available and has a role in similar situations. Ligation of the internal iliac arteries is effective in managing otherwise uncontrollable pelvic hemorrhage and can be performed through the posterior wound in some situations. It is more commonly performed transabdominally. Rectal injury should be suspected in nearly all settings of penetrating buttock wounds and ruled out with rigid proctoscopy. Small extraperitoneal rectal wounds do not need to be repaired; proximal diversion, presacral drainage, and gentle distal rectal washout should suffice.

This case illustrates the creativity displayed by hospital personnel to actively rewarm their patient using MRE (Meal, Ready-to-Eat) warmers. I have also personally seen space heaters and hair dryers used in similar scenarios. It is such innovation that we must constantly use as we care for the wounded, with increasingly severe injuries, in austere environments.

REFERENCE

1. Vertrees A, Kellicut D, et al. Early definitive abdominal closure using serial closure technique on injured soldiers returning from Afghanistan and Iraq. *J Am Coll Surg.* 2006;202: 762–772.

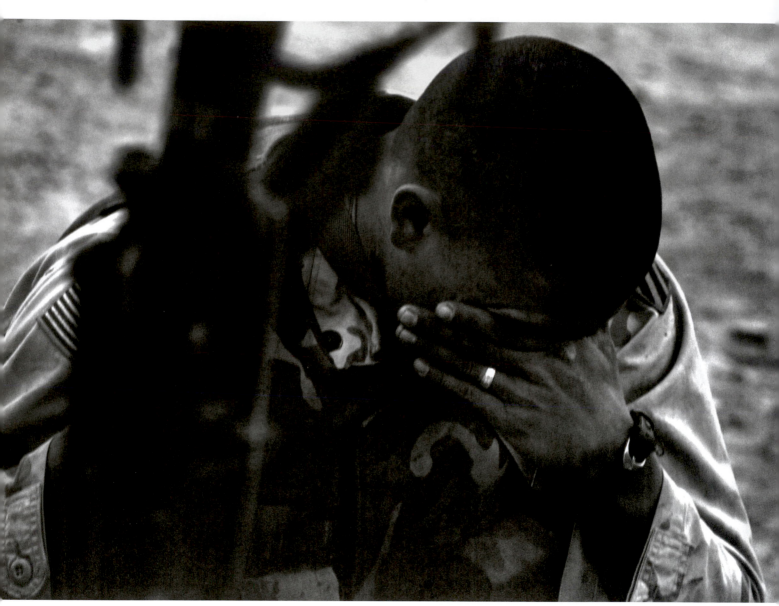

Courtesy David Leeson, *The Dallas Morning News*

Chapter VI
SOFT-TISSUE TRAUMA AND BURNS

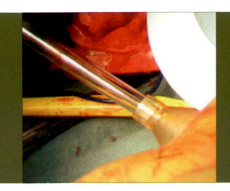

VI.1
Lower Extremity Compartment Syndrome

CASE PRESENTATION

This male patient sustained a blast injury that resulted in multiple fragment wounds to his left leg. He presented shortly after wounding and complained of severe, unrelenting pain in his left leg. The wounds were not considered severe (Fig. 1). Plain radiographs revealed no fractures, but did reveal multiple fragments (Fig. 2). The extremity was neurologically intact, and there was no evidence of vascular injury. During physical examination, the compartments were tense, with severe pain on palpation. Pain was also noted during passive range of motion of the toes. A clinical diagnosis of compartment syndrome was made. The patient was taken to the operating room for irrigation and debridement of his wounds and a four-compartment fasciotomy (Figs. 3 and 4). Intraoperatively, all compartments were tense, and the muscles of all four compartments were very swollen when released. No necrotic muscle was noted. Dressings soaked with Dakin's solution were placed on the affected areas. Postoperatively, symptoms were relieved completely, and the patient remained neurologically intact with a normal vascular examination.

TEACHING POINTS

1. Compartment syndrome is a common result of wounding. It can occur even in the absence of fractures or impressive soft-tissue wounds. It is important to note that compartment syndrome can be caused by one small fragment that makes a very small entry wound.

2. Do not be misled by a small wound or unimpressive radiograph. The diagnosis is made on clinical grounds and demands an urgent fasciotomy to avoid severe disability.

3. If no Stryker pressure monitors are available in theater and a pressure measurement is required, an arterial line setup can be used in the intensive care unit or operating room to measure the pressure of involved compartments. Compartment pressure measurements, however, are fraught with confounders. Pressures vary with the patient's hydration, blood pressure, nature and age of injury, and altitude, among other factors. Pressures higher than 25 to 30 mm Hg are cause for concern, but no specific value, per se, mandates surgical release. If the diagnosis of compartment syndrome is suspected on clinical grounds, obtaining a measurement should not delay surgical treatment or postpone compartment release (see Chapter VII Commentary by Ficke).

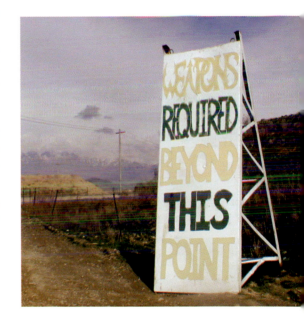

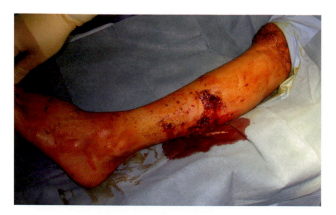

FIGURE 1. *Wound prior to surgery.*

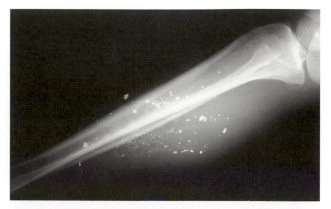

FIGURE 2. *Radiograph of multiple fragments in soft tissue, but no fracture.*

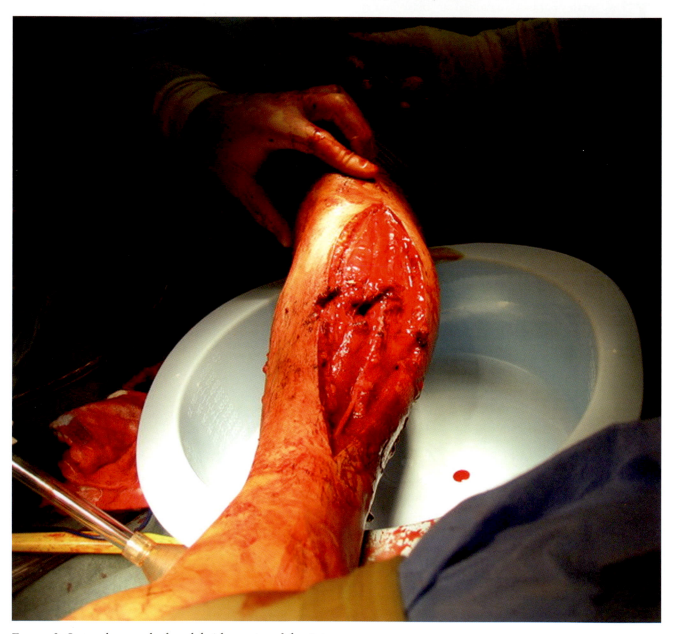

FIGURE 3. *Lateral wound after debridement and fasciotomy.*

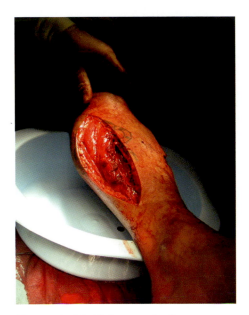

FIGURE 4. *Medial wound after debridement and fasciotomy.*

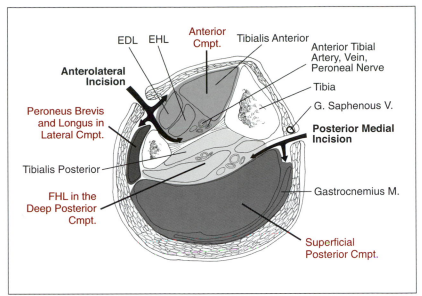

FIGURE 5. *Calf compartments. Cmpt.: compartment; EDL: extensor digitorum longus; EHL: extensor hallucis longus; FHL: flexor hallucis longus; G.: greater; M.: muscle; V.: vein.*

4. Postoperative care: Consider low-dose heparin for deep vein thrombosis prophylaxis. Postoperative deep vein thrombosis in trauma is common. Use caution if patient is multiply injured or has head/eye injuries.

5. Slight elevation of the injured extremity improves postoperative edema.

6. If available, a wound VAC may be used in lieu of Dakin's soaked dressings.

CLINICAL IMPLICATIONS

1. Any wounded soldier can present with compartment syndrome at any point along the evacuation chain. To avoid long-term patient disability, the possibility of this condition appearing in any medical treatment facility must be anticipated and looked for. Head-injured patients and patients with a depressed level of consciousness obviously will require closer monitoring for compartment syndrome.

2. Early clinical signs: pain out of proportion with physical findings, pain with passive stretching, and a tense swollen compartment. Loss of pulses is a late finding.

3. Late clinical signs: paresthesia, pulselessness, pallor, and paralysis.

4. Recheck for compartment syndrome all along the evacuation route.

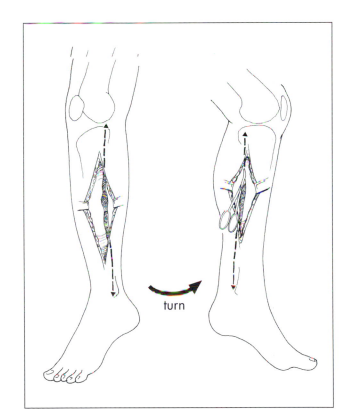

FIGURE 6. *Anteromedial incision of the calf.*

DAKIN'S SOLUTION

Developed during World War I, this solution was the result of a collaboration between Americans Henry Drysdale Dakin (1880–1952) and Alexis Carrel (1873–1944). It is also known as Carrel-Dakin solution, Carrel-Dakin fluid, and Dakin's fluid. It is a highly diluted, neutral antiseptic solution for cleaning wounds. The solution is made of sodium hypochlorite (0.45%–0.5%) and boric acid (4%). However, it is unstable and cannot be stored for more than a few days. It must be prepared fresh as needed.

Note: Century Pharmaceuticals, Inc (Indianapolis, Indiana), modified Dr Dakin's original formula and made it stable for more than 12 months. **Full strength** contains the highest concentration of sodium hypochlorite (0.50%) tolerable to the skin. **Half strength** contains 0.25% sodium hypochlorite. **Quarter strength** contains 0.125% sodium hypochlorite. Diluted Dakin's solution (or Di-Dak-Sol) contains 0.0125% sodium hypochlorite.

5. Early fasciotomy is recommended in the combat zone. Incisions should be long; in this case from 5 cm below the knee joint distally to the musculotendinous junction, with assurance of release of all four compartments.

6. Consider liberal use of fasciotomies in patients facing long-distance aeromedical evacuation.

DAMAGE CONTROL

Four-compartment fasciotomy is a primary damage control technique. All general and orthopaedic surgeons working at level II and level III medical treatment facilities should be able to perform this procedure (Figs. 5 and 6; also see Commentary on Case VII.8 by Ficke on page 312).

SUMMARY

Compartment syndrome is commonly encountered in the combat zone. Combat surgeons must be extremely watchful for this condition. Surgeons must consider this diagnosis and treat patients prophylactically, especially if patients are to be evacuated during which frequent examination or surgical intervention is not possible. In this case, diagnosis was made on clinical grounds. The patient's symptoms were relieved completely by performing a four-compartment fasciotomy.

SUGGESTED READING

Chapter 22: Soft-tissue injuries. In: *Emergency War Surgery, Third United States Revision*. Washington, DC: Department of the Army, Office of The Surgeon General, Borden Institute; 2004.

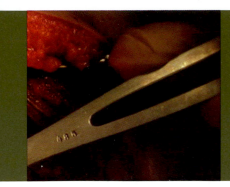

VI.2
Sciatic Nerve Laceration

CASE PRESENTATION

This 22-year-old host nation male sustained a fragment wound to the left buttock from an improvised explosive device (IED; Fig. 1). The entrance wound measured 4 cm. Communication with the patient was limited due to a language barrier. However, the patient complained of numbness to the lateral side of his left foot. Physical examination revealed an intact motor examination, but decreased pin-prick sensation at the left L5, S1, and S2 levels. Plain radiographs revealed a retained fragment at the level of the left femoral neck (Fig. 2). No fractures were identified. The patient was taken to the operating room and placed in the right lateral decubitus position. A posterolateral approach to the hip was used to explore the sciatic nerve (Fig. 3). The sciatic nerve was partially lacerated in the posteromedial portion. A 3-cm fragment was removed from the superficial surface of the quadratus femoris muscle (Fig. 4), and the wound was irrigated with pulse lavage. The surgical wound was closed, and the traumatic wound was packed with wet-to-dry dressings soaked with Dakin's solution. The patient was discharged from the hospital on postoperative day 1. Follow-up was not possible.

TEACHING POINTS

1. Gunshot and fragment wounds to the buttock frequently result in injury to underlying structures, including muscle, bone, and nerves. In this case, no fracture was noted, but a potentially more severe and less treatable injury to the sciatic nerve was noted on physical examination.
2. The language barrier limited patient interaction, even with the help of an interpreter. For this reason, it is often difficult to obtain a good, reliable, or reproducible preoperative examination and patient history.
3. Never underestimate the damage from blast injury. Usually, muscles are shredded and bones severely comminuted. The zone of injury is always larger than the obvious wound tract, and can be accompanied by thermal injury to the skin and subcutaneous tissues.

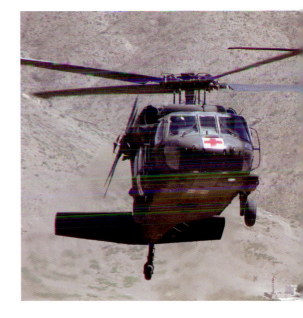

CLINICAL IMPLICATIONS

Suspected peripheral nerve injury of the extremities can be difficult to diagnose and is associated with significant morbidity. The following principles apply:

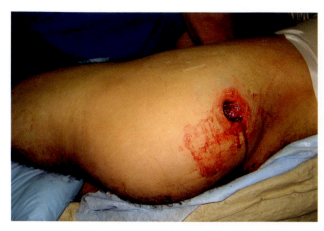

FIGURE 1. *A 4-cm fragment entrance wound from an IED.*

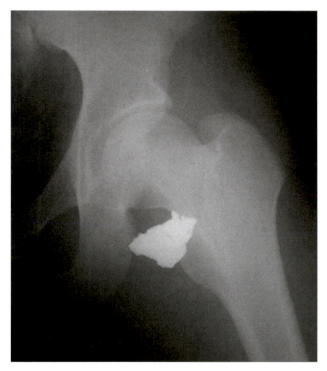

FIGURE 2. *Radiograph of fragment that injured the left sciatic nerve.*

1. When the proximal upper and lower extremities are involved, abdominal and thoracic injuries must be ruled out, because fragments can easily track into these body cavities.

2. Soft-tissue injuries with neurological deficits must be explored to decompress the nerve and document injury.

3. When appropriate, consider compartment syndrome-in-evolution as a possible explanation for patient symptoms.

4. If nerve grafting is to occur at a later date, tag severed nerves. Tagging of the ends of severed nerves is often the only option available during the initial phases of surgical care. This action may seem trivial in the face of massive tissue injury. However, it often proves valuable to our colleagues down the line as patients' wounds heal, and they are able to undergo reconstructive and restorative operations. The prognosis following peripheral nerve injury is highly variable. Nerve injury needs to be recognized immediately and the extent of impairment carefully documented. Resolution may not occur with the passage of time. Neurosurgical consultation should be requested early, because many patients will require operative intervention. Recent advances in the treatment of peripheral nerve injuries include the use of the operating microscope and intraoperative nerve action potential recordings.

DAMAGE CONTROL

Primary repair of peripheral nerves is often *not* performed and is contraindicated when damage control surgery is necessary. To prevent dessication, use soft tissue or moist dressings for coverage.

SUMMARY

This patient sustained a peripheral nerve injury accompanying the soft-tissue wound. The major concern was compression of the nerve by a fragment—a problem potentially resolved by excision of the fragment. Another possible concern was gluteal compartment syndrome (see Case VIII.10), which could adversely affect hip abductor function. Whenever an individual sustains a blast injury to exposed limbs, completed primary and secondary surveys of Advanced Trauma Life Support (ATLS)—with appropriate radiographs, CT, and general surgical consultation—are required to avoid missing potentially serious life-threatening injuries to the trunk.

SUGGESTED READING

Chapter 22: Soft-tissue injuries. In: *Emergency War Surgery, Third United States Revision*. Washington, DC: Department of the Army, Office of The Surgeon General, Borden Institute; 2004.

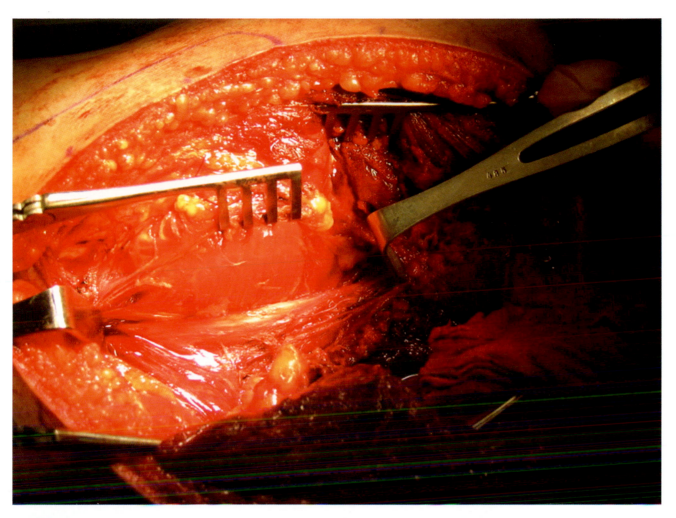

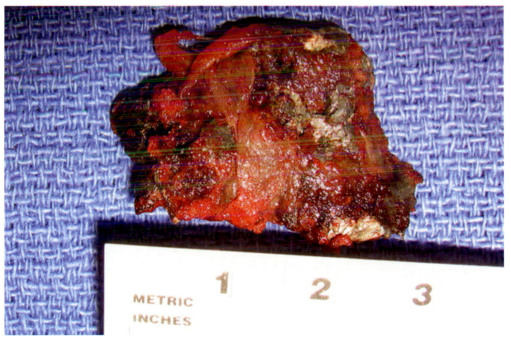

FIGURE 3. (Top) *Partial injury to the sciatic nerve and surrounding tissue.*

FIGURE 4. (Bottom) *A 3-cm fragment from the quadratus femoris muscle.*

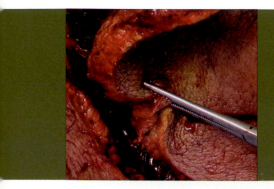

VI.3
Posttraumatic Necrotizing Fasciitis

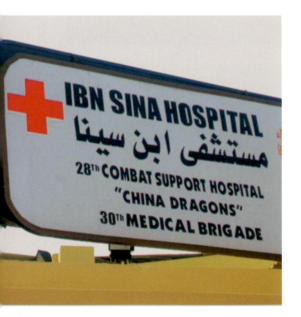

CASE PRESENTATION

This middle-aged male presented with two high-velocity (see sidebar on page 23) gunshot wounds. The first bullet penetrated the left lateral abdomen, injuring the descending colon and spleen. It traveled superior toward the left hemidiaphragm. The second bullet penetrated the left lateral thigh and also traveled superiorly, passing the posterior pelvis, the rectum, and the posterior sacrum. The patient presented in extremis and was taken immediately to the operating room for exploratory laparotomy. He required left hemicolectomy with transverse colostomy and a splenectomy. There was no intraperitoneal injury of the rectum; the rectum was left in situ, with the proximal stump stapled off at the pelvic brim. The extraperitoneal rectum sustained substantial injury, which was managed with distal washout and posterior drainage. By postoperative day 5, he developed persistent high fever and a spreading erythema on his back and right lateral abdominal wall, both suspicious for invasive infection. Open biopsy of the right lateral abdominal wall revealed viable fascia, but abundant gram-negative rods consistent with coliforms were present in the subcutaneous fat (Fig. 1). The patient was returned to the operating room. The bullet had transected the pelvis and rectum, lodged deep in his back (Fig. 2), contaminated the soft-tissue planes, and produced an aggressive necrotizing fasciitis. All dead and threatened muscle and fascia were excised. An initial incision revealed the dead (gray/black) fascia on his back (Fig. 3). This was resected back to viable tissue. Eventually, most of the fascia of the posterior thorax, the left gluteus, and the left lateral thigh were excised (Figs. 4 and 5). The patient's hospital treatment was long and complicated by bacteremic sepsis and multiple organ system failure. He eventually recovered. The large, open wound was treated as a full-thickness burn, with aggressive daily debridement, washing with chlorhexidene gluconate solution, and coverage with burn creams (silver sulfadiazine or mafenide). Once the wound no longer had a septic appearance and had begun to granulate, a large wound VAC was used to manage the open surface area (Figs. 6 and 7). This area was covered with split-thickness skin grafts in multiple stages. The patient was eventually discharged (Fig. 8).

TEACHING POINTS

1. This case demonstrates the devastating soft-tissue injury that typically accompanies high-velocity gunshot wounds. The penetrating missile is not sterile. In colon or rectal transit of the fragment(s), contamination

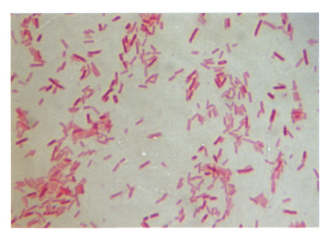

FIGURE 1. *Photomicrograph of Gram stain revealing abundant gram-negative bacilli in the subcutaneous and perifascial fat.*

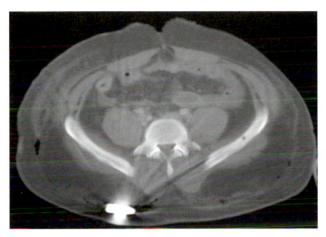

FIGURE 2. *Axial CT of a bullet that traversed the pelvis and lodged in the back. Note subcutaneous emphysema.*

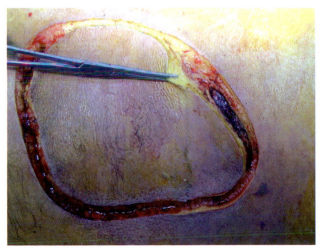

FIGURE 3. *Initial incision of the necrotic-appearing fascia of the back.*

with fecal flora potentiates infection. Aggressive debridement of the penetrating wound and blast cavity, as well as washout of the wound, can help prevent or mitigate subsequent local sepsis.

2. During the initial operation, retained bullets or fragments are generally not removed unless the missile is easily accessible, the patient is stable, and retrieval carries no risk of additional injury. Necrotizing soft-tissue infection might have been prevented or lessened in its severity and extent if planned reoperation by hospital day 2 or 3 had included washout and debridement of the cavity wound.

3. Necrotizing fasciitis is a rapidly spreading, morbid, and often fatal infection. Clinical suspicion and early detection are essential to prevent a fatal outcome. In theater, resources might not be available to support soft-tissue biopsy, Gram stain, and microscopic verification of invading organisms. Simple visual inspection of the soft tissues, fascia, and underlying musculature is all that is necessary to support the diagnosis and aggressive debridement of viable tissue. Typical findings can include the following:

    a. Hemodynamic deterioration.
    b. Tense, shiny skin, bullae, or crepitus in the region.
    c. Soft-tissue gas might be present on plain radiographs.
    d. A foul, gray, dishwater-like fluid emanating from the infected tissues (on operation).
    e. Pale-appearing necrotic fascia that is easily separated from its investing tissues.
    f. Discolored, noncontractile, nonbleeding muscle (if involved).

4. Care of a patient with necrotizing fasciitis is likely to be prolonged, and places great demands on available personnel and resources. Even in the best circumstances, survival is limited. In the case of numerous injured patients or a high critical care census, limited resources, or ongoing operations in theater, expectant management (or watchful waiting) might be the more suitable response. Obviously, this will be a difficult decision to make, and should involve the treating physicians and medical team, an ethics committee (if available), and the hospital command.

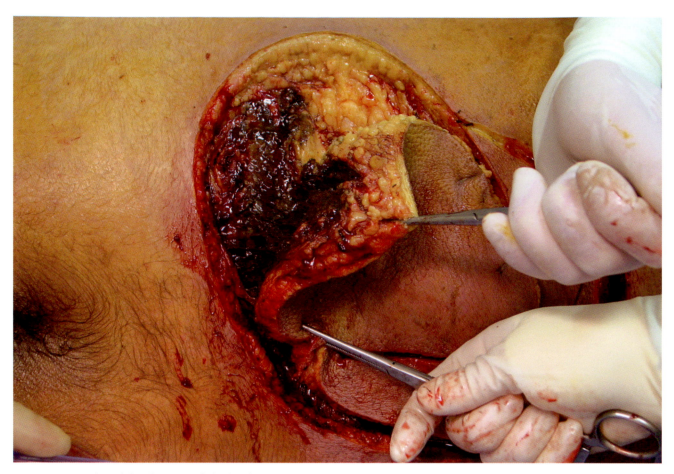

FIGURE 4. *Further debridement of the back.*

CLINICAL IMPLICATIONS

1. Necrotizing soft-tissue infection is a potentially devastating outcome of battlefield wounding.
2. Treatment is primarily surgical and involves aggressive resuscitation, broad-spectrum intravenous antibiotic coverage of all probable organisms, and emergent radical excision of all involved, nonviable tissues—including a low threshold for amputation.
3. The infection is usually caused by mixed aerobic and anaerobic bacteria and can be the result of clostridial myonecrosis or polymicrobial infection, most commonly secondary to *Streptococcus, Staphylococcus, Enterococcus, Enterobacteriaceae, Bacteroides*, or *Clostridia*. Penicillin G should be used if infection is due to streptococci or clostridia, imipenem-cilastin if polymicrobial; add vancomycin if MRSA is suspected.

DAMAGE CONTROL

Stop major hemorrhage, and stop or control major sources of contamination by performing stapled resection of the bowel and temporary colostomy formation. Drain the extraperitoneal rectal injury. Definitive reconstruction or resection may be delayed. Retrieve the fragment only if it is easy. The retrieval process should be delayed or omitted altogether if clinical circumstances do not permit this action.

SUMMARY

This case demonstrates several principles of high-velocity ballistic injury: colonic and rectal injuries predispose to septic complications; a strong clinical awareness of the patient's condition is necessary to detect complications; and early, aggressive treatment of necrotizing soft-tissue infection can lead to ultimate patient survival if appropriate resources are available.

SUGGESTED READING

Chapter 10: Infections. In: *Emergency War Surgery, Third United States Revision*. Washington, DC: Department of the Army, Office of The Surgeon General, Borden Institute; 2004.

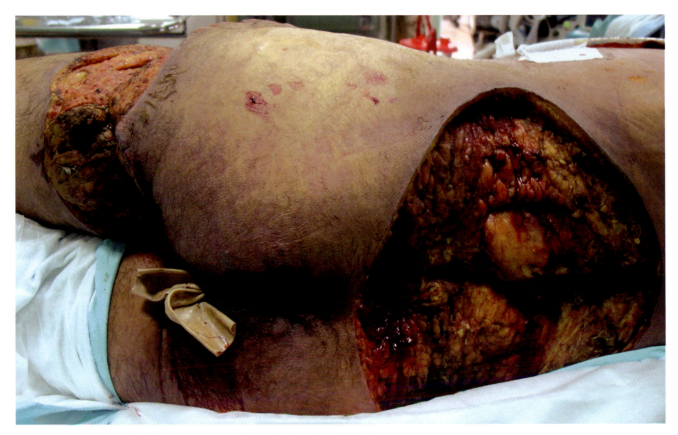

FIGURE 5. *Continued debridement involving the back and thigh.*

WOUND VAC

The Vacuum-Assisted Closure (VAC) Therapy System is used to facilitate wound healing by converting an open wound to a closed wound. VAC consists of an evacuation tube embedded in a polyurethane foam dressing (or sponge). After the dressing is placed in the wound bed and sealed by an occlusive dressing, the tube is attached to a vacuum unit. Application of this negative pressure causes the following:

- The foam to collapse—resulting in removal of excess fluids.
- Increased blood flow.
- Decreased bacterial colonization.
- Granulation formation.
- Wound closure.

Procedure

- Debride all devitalized tissue and contaminated material.
- Cut sterile polyurethane sponge to conform with the wound surface.
- Be sure that the deepest portions of the wound are in contact with the sponge.
- Ensure that the sponge makes contact with the entire wound surface.
- Place end of tube on surface of the sponge.
- Apply adhesive plastic sheet over the skin sponge and around the tubing (this seals the vacuum).
- Run tube from the sponge to the VAC pump device.
- Use a continuous setting of 125 mm Hg, which is most common (range: –50 mm Hg to –200 mm Hg).
- Change sponge every 48 to 96 hours (except for skin grafts—in which case the sponge is removed on day 4).

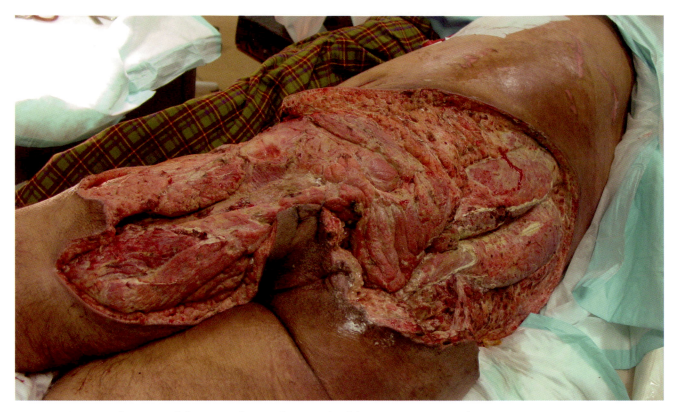

FIGURE 6. *Eventual extent of the wound now showing healthy-appearing muscle.*

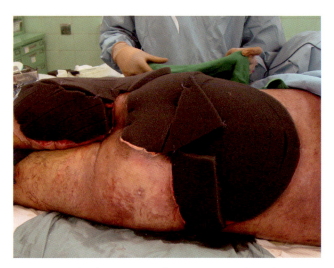

FIGURE 7. *The large wound was managed with a wound VAC device.*

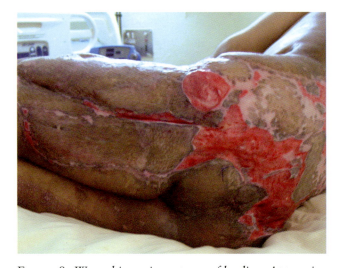

FIGURE 8. *Wound in various stages of healing. Approximately 60% of the wound surface is covered with skin grafts.*

Chapter 17: Abdominal injuries. In: *Emergency War Surgery, Third United States Revision*. Washington, DC: Department of the Army, Office of The Surgeon General, Borden Institute; 2004.

Chapter 22: Soft-tissue injuries. In: *Emergency War Surgery, Third United States Revision*. Washington, DC: Department of the Army, Office of The Surgeon General, Borden Institute; 2004.

McGrath V, Fabian TC, et al. Rectal trauma: Management based on anatomic distinctions. *Am Surg.* 1998;64:1136–1141.

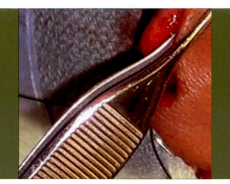

VI.4
Median Forehead Flap

CASE PRESENTATION

After a firefight, this 30-year-old host nation male presented to the combat support hospital (CSH) with a gunshot wound to the face that resulted in loss of his anterior nose (Fig. 1). After wound debridement, a median forehead flap was fashioned based on forehead vessels that were preoperatively localized using a handheld Doppler ultrasound (Fig. 2). The flap was then rotated into the defect (Fig. 3), and the flap bed was closed and the forehead flap sutured into place (Fig. 4). A stent for the right nostril was fashioned and left in place. The flap healed well and remained 100% viable with acceptable cosmetic and functional results (Fig. 5). After 6 weeks, the median forehead flap was revised to eliminate the proximal fold of skin from the original rotation (Fig. 6).

TEACHING POINTS

1. Generally, injured soldiers can be treated with wound debridement and irrigation, followed by dressing changes and evacuation. However, this approach often cannot be used for patients who cannot be evacuated.

2. Complex soft-tissue injuries are common in combat zones. Surgeons deploying to combat zones need to understand how to manage these wounds to include local and rotational flaps.

3. Closure of war wounds or coverage of complex or large wounds should be delayed until necrotic tissue is clearly demarcated and debrided, and the wound appears healthy. This can be accomplished through serial operative debridements and washout, along with either wet-to-dry dressing changes or a wound VAC, if available.

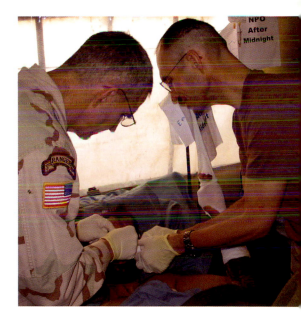

CLINICAL IMPLICATIONS

All war wounds are considered contaminated and should not be closed primarily. The goal of wound management is to preserve function, minimize morbidity, and prevent infections. The following principles apply:

1. Appropriate antibiotics should be administered for all war wounds (see *Emergency War Surgery, Third United States Revision*, page 10.5).

2. Risk of infection is decreased if debridement and washout occur within 6 hours.

3. Debridement of facial injuries should be as conservative as possible because the blood supply to the face is extensive. Allow questionably viable tissue the opportunity to demarcate. Often, tenuous-appearing tissue on second look will recover.

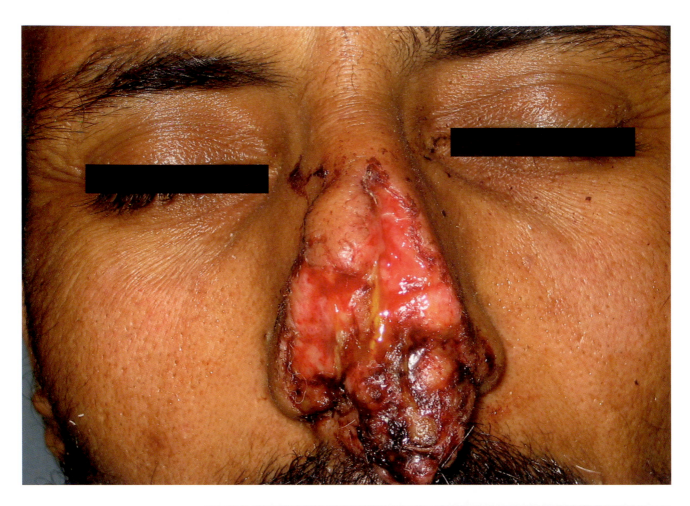

FIGURE 1. (Top) *Patient's nasal injury.*

FIGURE 2. (Bottom) (A) *Illustration of median forehead flap blood supply.* (B) *Illustration of rotated flap.*

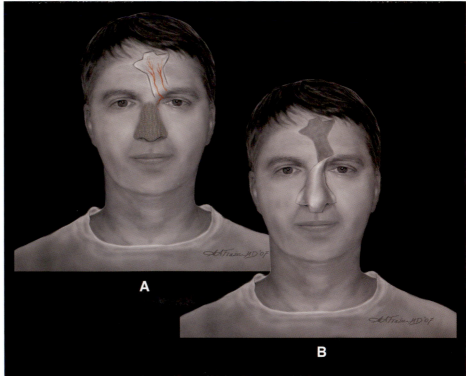

A

B

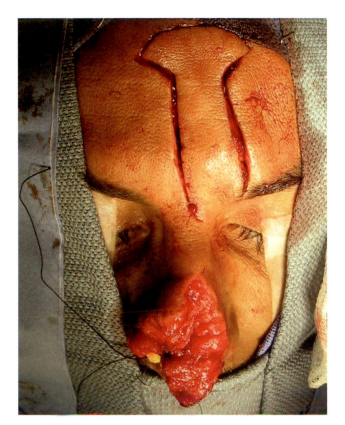 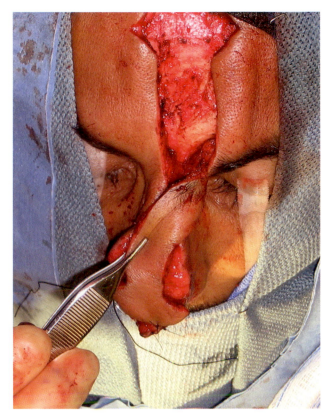

FIGURE 3. (Left) *Forehead flap prior to rotation.* (Right) *Actual flap rotated into position.*

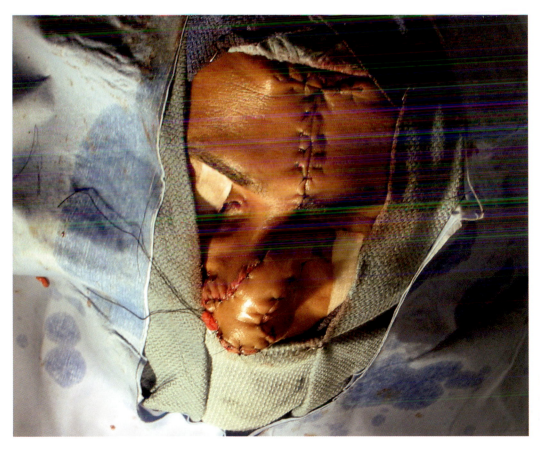

FIGURE 4. *Flap sutured into position with flap bed closed.*

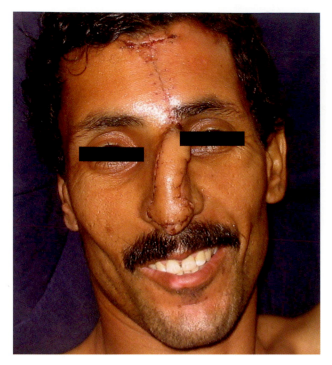

FIGURE 5. *Post-op day 7.*

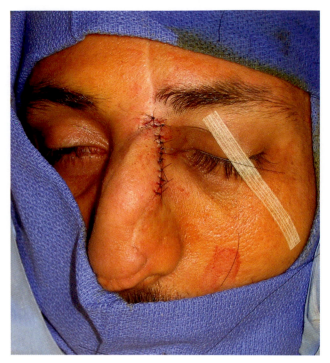

FIGURE 6. *Revision of forehead flap.*

4. Foreign material and necrotic tissue should be excised and aggressively irrigated.
5. Debridement and washout should be repeated at 24 to 72 hours.
6. Early soft-tissue coverage is desirable within 3 to 5 days—when the wound is clean—to prevent secondary infection.
7. When total or subtotal reconstruction of a nose is required, the nasal lining is required. An option for nasal lining reconstruction includes using a skin graft braced with cartilage to prevent graft contraction, resulting in a closed nostril.

SUMMARY

This case illustrates the importance of basic, soft-tissue repair skills for deployed surgeons, including local and rotational flaps.

SUGGESTED READING

Chapter 13: Face and neck injuries. In: *Emergency War Surgery, Third United States Revision.* Washington, DC: Department of the Army, Office of The Surgeon General, Borden Institute; 2004.

Chapter 22: Soft-tissue injuries. In: *Emergency War Surgery, Third United States Revision.* Washington, DC: Department of the Army, Office of The Surgeon General, Borden Institute; 2004.

Mathes SJ, Nahai F. *Reconstructive Surgery: Principles, Anatomy, & Technique.* New York: Churchill Livingstone; 1996.

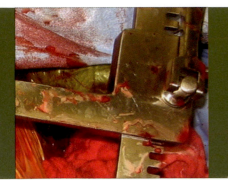

VI.5
Soft-Tissue Coverage of Combat Wounds: A Series of Cases

CASE PRESENTATIONS

Following is a collection of eight cases that presented to a combat support hospital (CSH) during a 7-month period in Iraq. All had sustained, in addition to other injuries, gunshot or penetrating blast injuries that resulted in large wounds with bone and significant skin and soft-tissue loss. These latter injuries demanded special attention because wound coverage was problematic. Either due to the size of the open wound and/or because the debrided surface included exposed bone or muscle, or synthetic material, none of these wounds would accept direct skin grafting. Alternative means of soft-tissue coverage had to be accomplished in an austere environment if amputation was to be avoided. Amputation of the involved limbs was, by far, the most likely outcome for civilians at their depleted, overstretched local hospitals. Indeed, operative decisions in deployed American facilities must necessarily factor in considerations of available resources, limited bed space (which may be occupied for weeks by the patients described in the cases included here), limited manpower, unforeseen casualty flow, and patient status before opting to undertake complex and time-consuming reparative surgery.

CASE 1 (Fig. 1)

A host nation male civilian presented to a CSH with exposed anterior tibial bone in the middle to distal third of the leg due to soft-tissue loss. The wound was debrided, and the wound VAC was applied in an attempt to obtain granulation tissue over the bone in preparation for a later skin graft. This plan of action was not successful, and the wound was finally closed with a saphenous vein fasciocutaneous flap. A skin graft was applied over the donor site defect. The patient left the hospital ambulating and without further complications.

CASE 2 (Fig. 2)

This male patient's injury, an abdominal wall defect, was repaired with synthetic mesh. The rectus abdominis muscle was not available because of the initial wound through the rectus muscle. In this case, the wound was covered over the mesh with a tensor fascia lata fasciocutaneous flap. The excess tissue (or "dog-ear" tissue) created by the 180-degree rotation of the flap will be removed in a second intervention for flap revision.

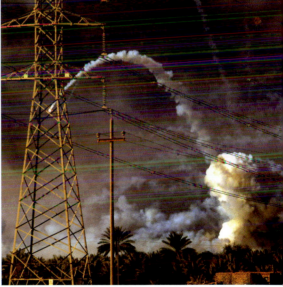

Courtesy David Leeson, *The Dallas Morning News*

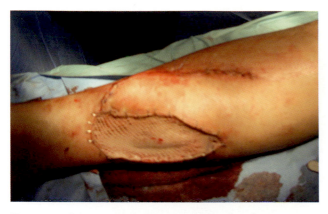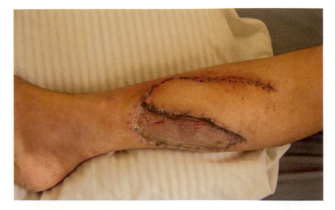

FIGURE 1. **Case 1.** (Left) *Patient immediately post-op.* (Right) *Patient on post-op day 5.*

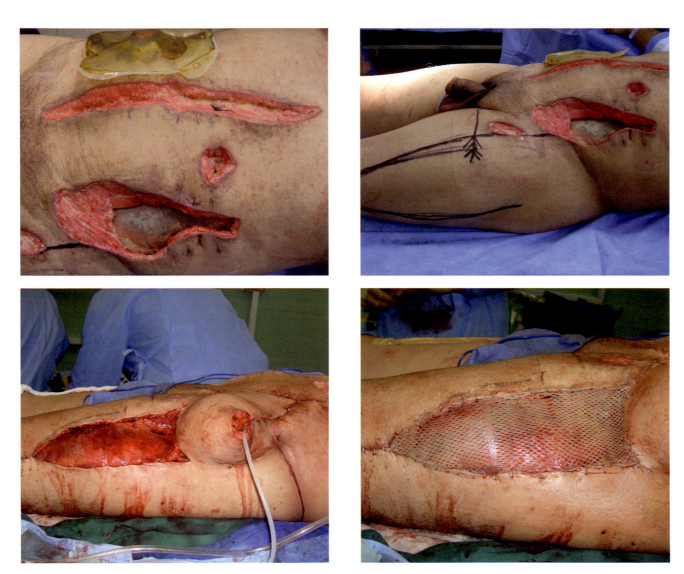

FIGURE 2. **Case 2.** (Top Left) *Exposed VICRYL mesh.* (Top Right) *Flap design.* (Bottom Left) *The tensor fascia lata fasciocutaneous flap is in place.* (Bottom Right) *Donor site with skin grafted.*

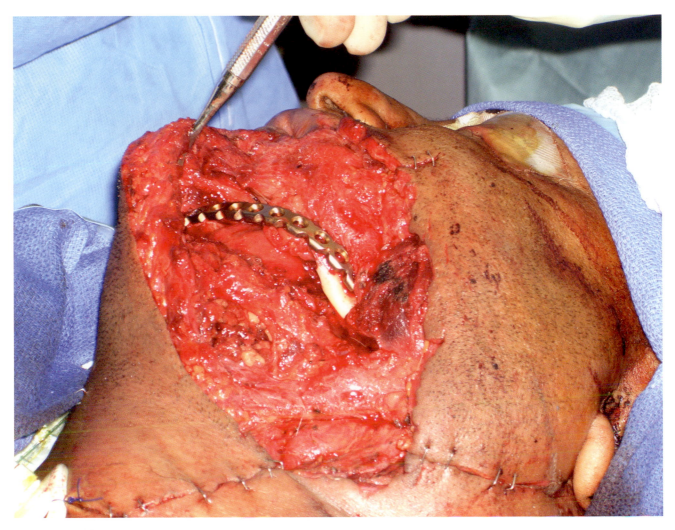

CASE 3 (Fig. 3)

This male patient had a severe blast injury to the face and neck that resulted in loss of a significant portion of the skin and a comminuted mandibular fracture with overt bone loss. The oral and maxillofacial surgeon repaired the mandibular fracture with plating (see Fig. 3, top). Closure of the skin deficiency was provided by a pedicled pectoralis major myocutaneous flap. In this case, the surgeons were forced to proceed with coverage at the initial surgery because of the nature and location of the wound.

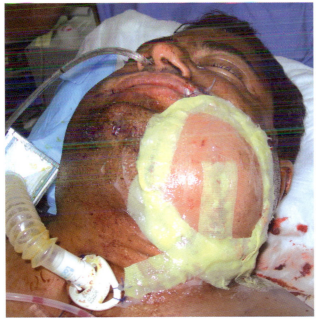

FIGURE 3. **Case 3.** (Top) *Mandibular fracture, plating will approximate mandibular fragments.* (Bottom) *Pectoralis muscle flap is in place.*

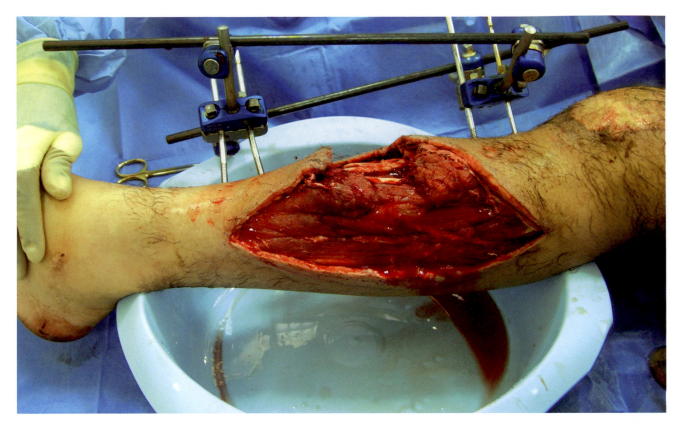

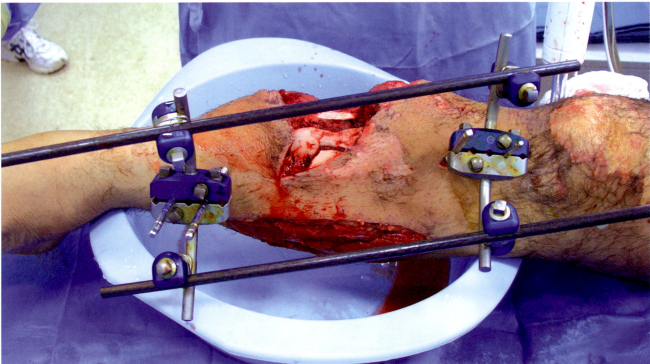

Figure 4. **Case 4.** (Top) *Lateral view of the exposed tibial fracture.* (Bottom) *Medial view of the exposed tibial fracture.*

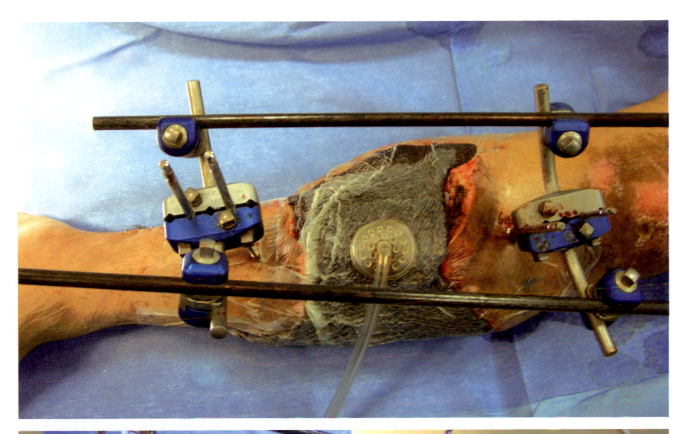

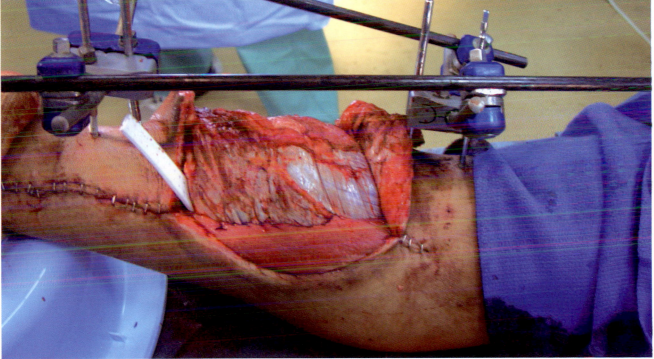

FIGURE 4. **Case 4 (cont'd).** (Top) *Wound VAC positioned over the soleus flap.* (Bottom) *Soleus flap is in place.*

FIGURE 4. Case 4 (cont'd). (Top) *Post-op day 7—the result of the wound VAC.* (Bottom) *Completed result after split thickness skin graft over the soleus muscle.*

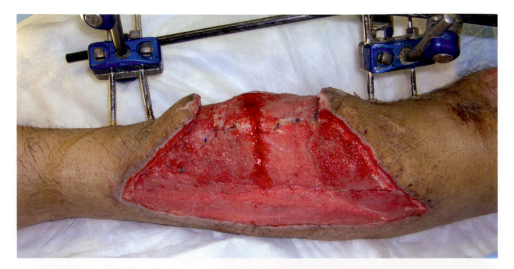

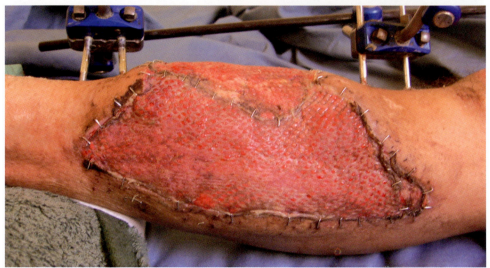

CASE 4 (Fig. 4)

This male patient sustained a complex open fracture of the left tibia from penetrating explosive injury. He underwent debridement and external fixation on the day of the injury (Fig. 4, page 226). Fasciotomies were also performed. The skin defect had exposed tibial bone in the middle third of the leg. Because of swelling and edema, and possible further muscle damage, a muscle flap was not attempted at this time. A wound VAC was applied (Fig. 4, top, page 227) and changed every other day. About 7 days later, muscle swelling had resolved, and a soleus muscle flap was applied (Fig. 4, bottom, page 227). During the procedure, the muscle was found to be bruised and contused. Therefore, the skin graft over the soleus muscle was delayed for another 6 days. Meanwhile, the wound VAC was applied to the muscle flap. The patient recovered well from his injury and subsequent surgeries (Fig. 4, page 228). Follow-up was scheduled later for the final orthopaedic repair.

CASE 5 (Figs. 5–7)

These three cases (patients A–C) were related to orthopaedic injuries resulting in loss of soft-tissue coverage over the exposed bones and/or hardware in the elbow area. Three patients required random abdominal skin flaps of the Tagliacozzi method (see accompanying box, page 232). These male patients had severe injuries to the elbow area, all received by either gunshot wound or penetrating blast. The flaps covered the bone and hardware after the orthopaedic surgeons had performed a limb salvage procedure. In the local host nation medical system, these injuries would have necessarily resulted in amputations of the involved limbs. Separation of the pedicle and insetting the flap were performed 2 to 3 weeks after the flap covered the wound, depending on development of vascularity within the flap.

CASE 5
Patient A: Exposed Elbow Joint

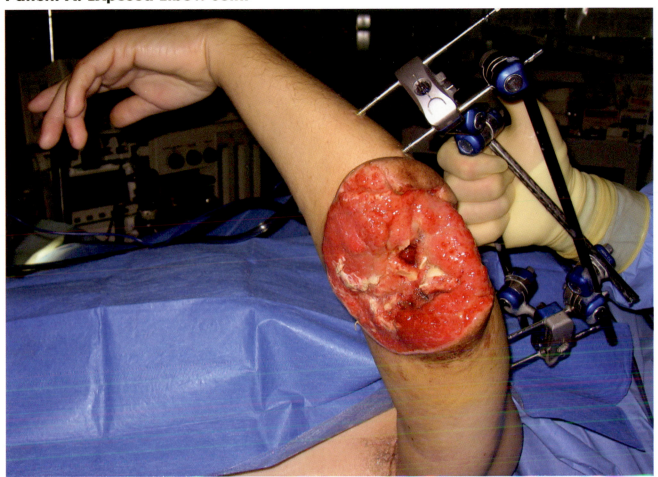

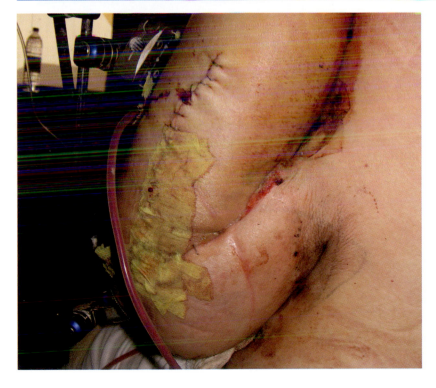

FIGURE 5. Case 5. (Top) *Preflap view of elbow wound.* (Bottom) *Random skin flap.*

CASE 5
Patient B: Elbow Injuries

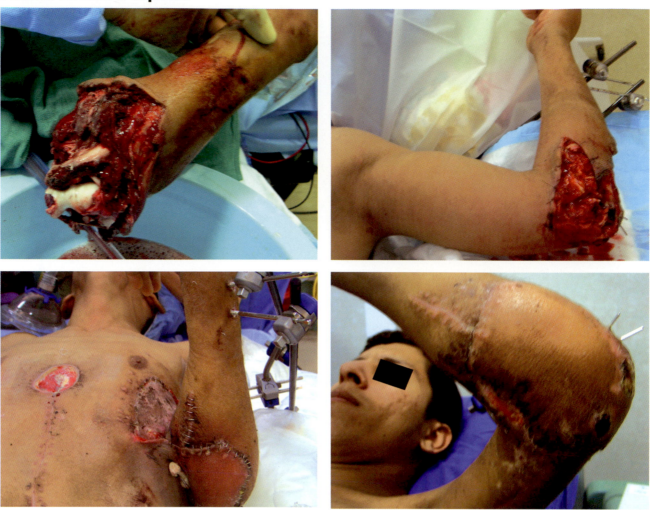

FIGURE 6. Case 5. (Top Left) *Initial injury of the elbow.* (Top Right) *Elbow injury after reduction of dislocation.* (Bottom Left) *Flap is in place.* (Bottom Right) *Two weeks after flap separation.*

CASE 5
Patient C: Elbow Injuries

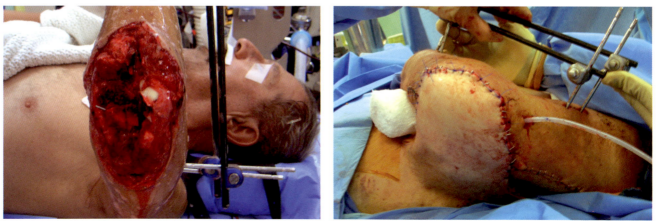

FIGURE 7. Case 5. (Left) *Elbow is missing a significant amount of soft tissue.* (Right) *Post-op flap.*

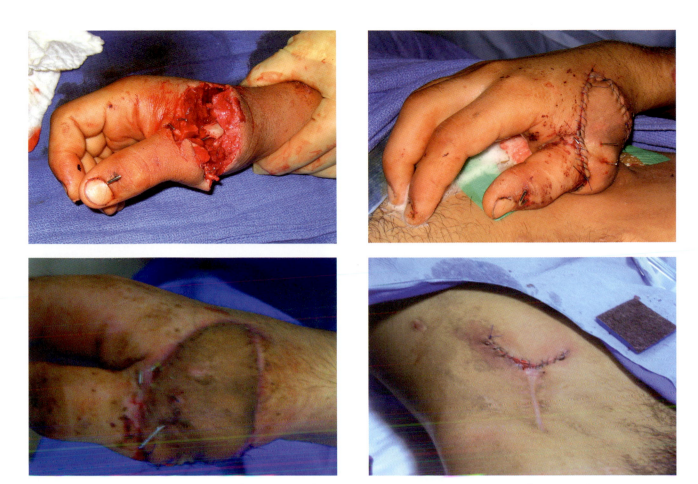

FIGURE 8. **Case 6.** (Top Left) *Exposed bone graft (note pin).* (Top Right) *Random skin flap from the groin area.* (Bottom Left) *After separation of the pedicle.* (Bottom Right) *Secondary closure of the donor site.*

CASE 6 (Fig. 8)

This host nation male sustained blast injuries to all four extremities. His hand injuries included a right thumb metacarpal fracture with bone loss and large dorsal soft-tissue loss. A random abdominal skin flap over the dorsum of his right hand was required because of missing tissue to cover the exposed bone graft (Fig. 8). The patient underwent multiple irrigation and debridement procedures of his right hand. The wound was then treated with Dakin's solution until it was granulating well (see Fig. 4, Case VII.4). When the wound was deemed surgically clean, an iliac crest bone graft was pinned in place at the thumb metacarpal bone defect site. An abdominal pedicle flap was placed on the dorsal hand soft-tissue defect. Three weeks after placement of the flap, the patient returned for separation and closure.

CASE 7 (Fig. 9)

A host nation male suffered a fragment injury to the posterior aspect of his foot with exposed bone (Fig. 9, page 232). Once the wound was managed with serial debridement and washouts, soft-tissue coverage was required. The lower third of the leg is a difficult area to cover with a local flap. One option is the sural nerve flap. This flap is based on the sural nerve blood supply and the small perforating artery that is 5 cm proximal to the lateral mallelous. This retrograde blood flow is sufficient to perfuse the distally placed flap. A paddle of skin, subcutaneous fat, and fascia are fashioned at midcalf and the sural nerve identified (Fig. 9, top and bottom, page 233). The skin between the perforator and the paddle is divided, and a strip of subcutaneous fat and fascia 2 cm wide (1 cm on each side of the nerve) is elevated—along with the paddle and the sural nerve—to the perforator (Fig. 9, top, page 234). The flap is then rotated over the defect and sutured in place (Fig. 9, bottom left, page 234). The skin defects are primarily closed or skin grafted (Fig. 9, bottom right, page 234). Some skin loss in the distal paddle is common.[1]

CASE 8 (Fig. 10)

An enemy prisoner of war suffered a fragment injury to the lower leg just below the knee. The skin defect on this

TAGLIACOZZI METHOD

Plastic surgery is believed to have begun during the Renaissance with Gasparo Tagliacozzi (1545–1599), an Italian surgeon who did pioneering work in the field of plastic surgery. He is credited as being the first practitioner of the art of plastic surgery. Tagliacozzi often repaired noses lost in duels or noses that were damaged by syphilis. He created a method of nasal reconstruction (the Tagliacozzi flap or the Italian flap) in which a flap from the upper part of the arm is gradually transferred to the nose.

Additional Information

- For many centuries, nose reconstruction using distant pedicle flaps was done.
- The Tagliacozzi flap was a popular technique in Europe in the 1600s.
- In the early 19th century, the Indian flap method was popular (using the mid-forehead for nose reconstruction).
- In the United States, V. H. Kanzanjian popularized the modern forehead flap.
- Note: The forehead flap can result in excellent cosmetic outcomes for particular kinds of nasal wounds (see Case VI.4). Optimal outcomes depend on patient selection criteria, wound selection, surgical technique, and postoperative management.

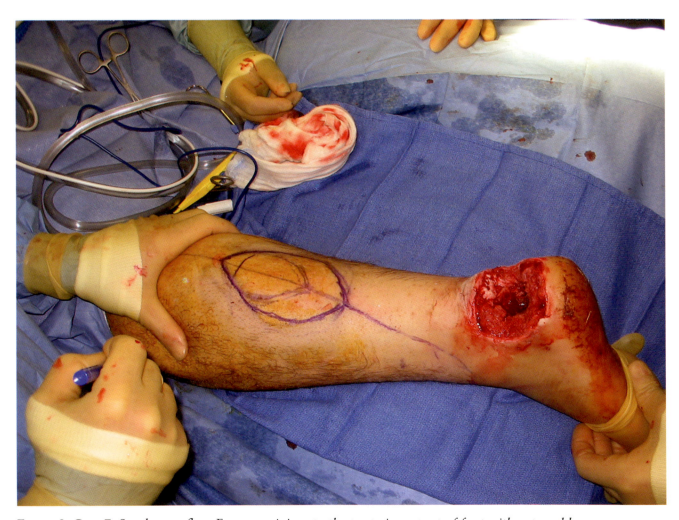

FIGURE 9. **Case 7.** *Sural nerve flap. Fragment injury to the posterior aspect of foot with exposed bone.*

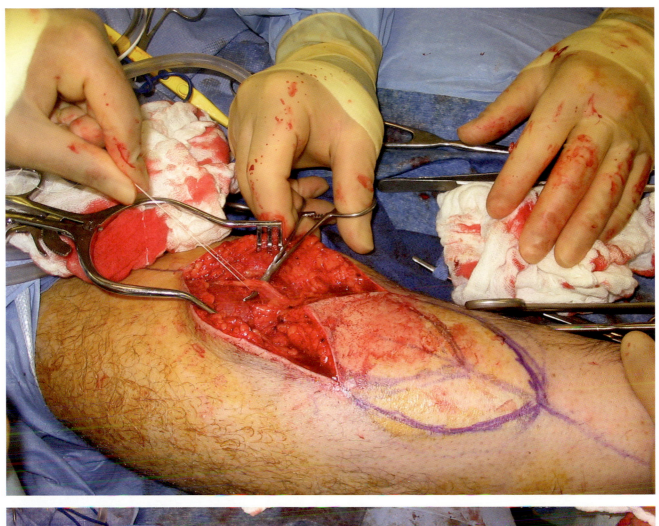

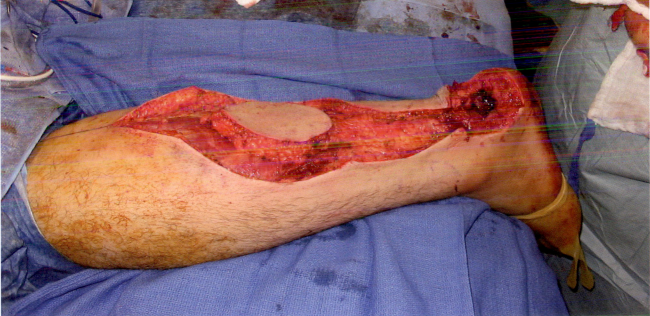

FIGURE 9. **Case 7 (cont'd).** (Top) *Sural nerve is identified.* (Bottom) *A paddle of skin, subcutaneous fat, and fascia are fashioned at midcalf.*

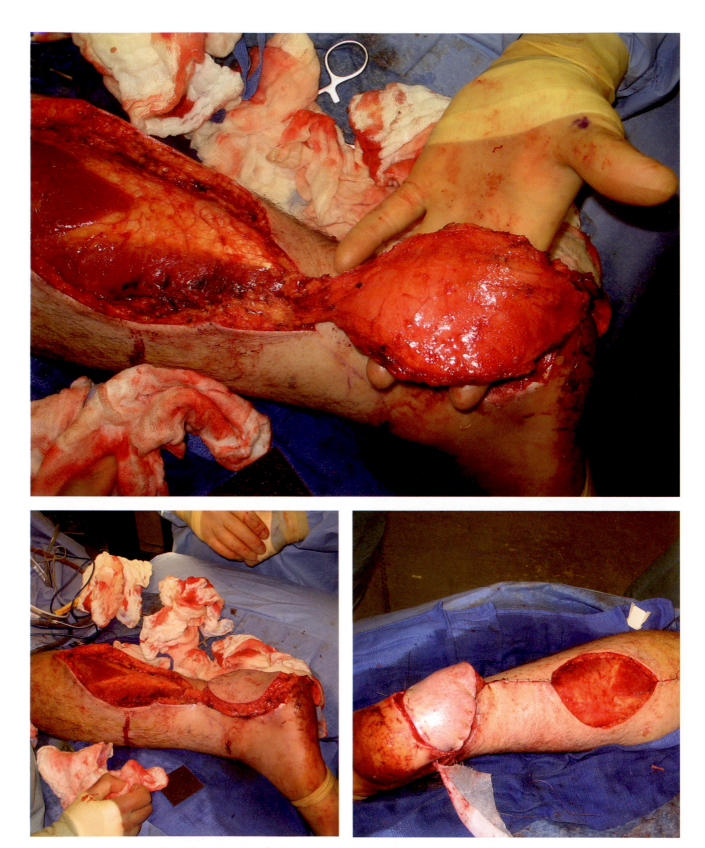

FIGURE 9. **Case 7 (cont'd).** (Top) *A strip of subcutaneous fat and fascia is elevated.* (Bottom Left) *Flap is rotated over the defect and sutured in place.* (Bottom Right) *Skin grafted.*

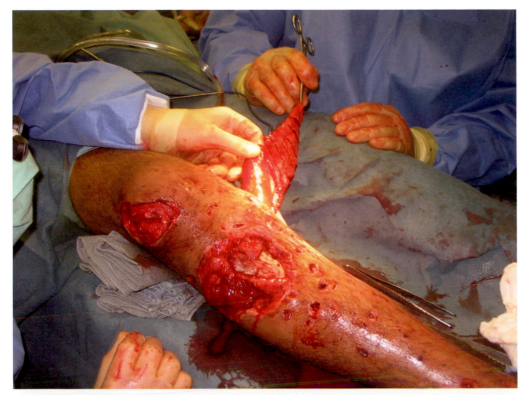

FIGURE 10. Case 8.
*Gastrocnemius muscle flap.
(Top) The skin defect on this anterior wound with tibia exposed. (Bottom) The gastrocnemius is exposed and one half divided just above the Achilles tendon. The muscle is split between the two heads and elevated superiorly.*

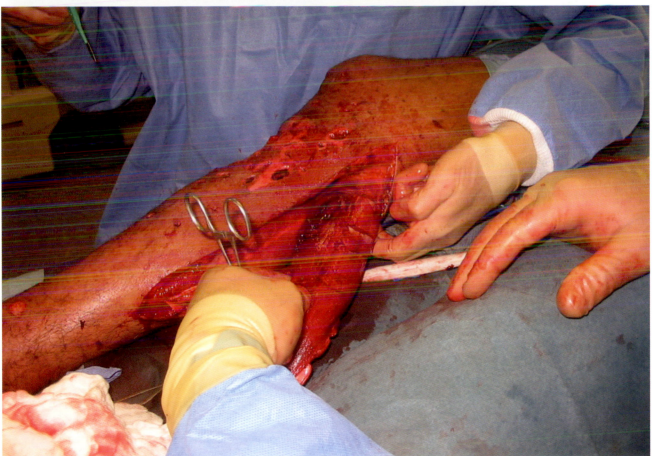

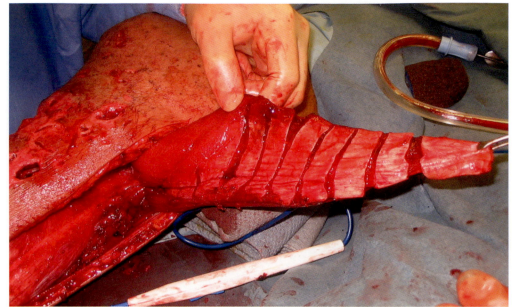

FIGURE 10.
Case 8 (cont'd).
(Top) *Scoring the fascia in a "step-ladder" fashion.*
(Bottom) *The muscle is brought through the tunnel to the defect.*

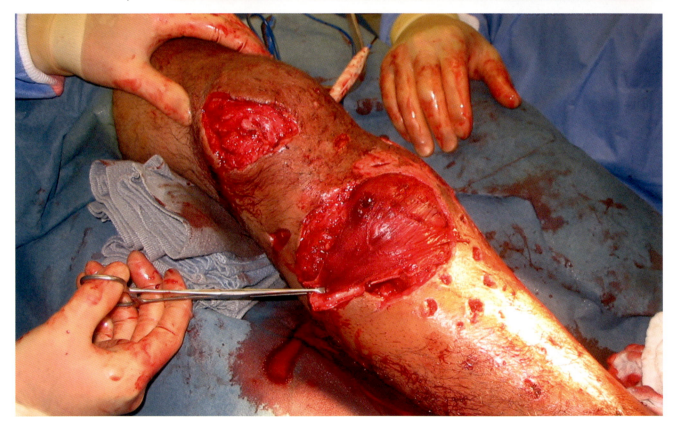

anterior wound was large, and the tibia was exposed (Fig. 10, top, page 235). Coverage for the upper part of the lower leg can be generally accomplished with a gastrocnemius muscle flap. The gastrocnemius is exposed and one half divided just above the Achilles tendon. The muscle is split between the two heads and elevated superiorly (Fig. 10, bottom, page 235). A subcutaneous tunnel is made that accommodates the muscle. Additional length may be achieved (if needed) by scoring the fascia in a "step-ladder" fashion (Fig. 10, top, page 236). The muscle is brought through the tunnel to the defect (Fig. 10, bottom, page 236). The flap is sutured in place and covered with a split-thickness skin graft.

TEACHING POINTS

1. Battlefield trauma produces difficult injuries in all areas of the body. These injuries are complex because of the high-energy damage to the tissues. The first step in managing these wounds is to perform adequate debridement. It is not appropriate to close these wounds primarily because tissue damage is extensive and often not evident initially. It is important to perform early and repeated debridement until the wound is clean and ready for closure. This may take 5 to 7 days or even longer.

2. It is best to perform delayed primary closure within 5 to 7 days after all devitalized tissue has been identified and debrided. Tissue damage is not always evident at initial surgery. Resist the temptation to close high-velocity injuries early.

3. The "Ladder of Reconstruction" principle calls for proceeding from the simplest method to obtain closure toward more complicated methods of coverage. The simplest method is to obtain primary closure if there is enough tissue/skin available.

4. If the defect is missing skin, then the next step is to proceed with skin grafting. Often, this is not possible because exposed bone or exposure of synthetic materials does not accept skin grafting. Use the wound VAC liberally to protect and prepare the wound for skin grafting, as well as to replace the tie-down bolster over the skin graft.

5. In the abdominal area, try to spare the rectus muscle whenever possible. In these cases, it was evident that the rectus could have been used more frequently for reconstruction of a variety of wounds had it been available. The most common reason for its unavailability was colostomies.

6. The soleus muscle is the best choice for reconstruction of injuries of the middle third of the leg.

DAMAGE CONTROL

Delayed primary closure (3–5 days) requires a clean wound that can be closed without undue tension. This state may be difficult to achieve in war wounds. Definitive closure with skin grafts and muscle and pedicle flaps should not be done in theater when evacuation is possible. These techniques may be required, however, for injured civilians, allied wounded, and enemy prisoners of war. In the austere environment of combat medicine, and under circumstance beyond the surgeon's control (finite resources, patient instability, "op tempo," limited expertise), amputation is a necessary consideration.

SUMMARY

When confronted with a difficult wound in theater, the plan for closure should proceed from the simplest method possible to more sophisticated methods. Most important is to remove all nonviable tissue, which may take several days and several surgical debridements. After the wound is clean, begin with delayed primary closure, if possible. Next, proceed with skin grafting. The wound VAC should be used liberally to prepare wounds for skin grafting and to use over skin grafts in lieu of the usual tie-down bolster to secure the graft. Alternative choices involve muscle flaps (with skin grafting) or fasciocutaneous flaps. The combat zone does not provide the resources for more sophisticated methods of reconstruction (eg, free flaps). For this reason, surgeons will be faced with these limitations and will be challenged to use their knowledge and imagination to obtain closure of difficult wounds.

REFERENCE

1. Hasegawa M. The distally based superficial sural artery flap. *Plast Reconstr Surg*. 1994;93(5):1012–1020.

SUGGESTED READING

Chapter 13: Face and neck injuries. In: *Emergency War Surgery, Third United States Revision*. Washington, DC: Department of the Army, Office of The Surgeon General, Borden Institute; 2004.

Chapter 17: Abdominal injuries. In: *Emergency War Surgery, Third United States Revision*. Washington, DC: Department of the Army, Office of The Surgeon General, Borden Institute; 2004.

Chapter 22: Soft-tissue injuries. In: *Emergency War Surgery, Third United States Revision*. Washington, DC: Department of the Army, Office of The Surgeon General, Borden Institute; 2004.

Chapter 23: Extremity fractures. In: *Emergency War Surgery, Third United States Revision*. Washington, DC: Department of the Army, Office of The Surgeon General, Borden Institute; 2004.

Chapter 24: Open joint injuries. In: *Emergency War Surgery, Third United States Revision*. Washington, DC: Department of the Army, Office of The Surgeon General, Borden Institute; 2004.

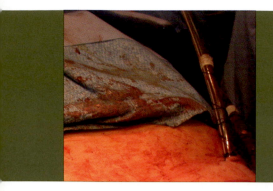

VI.6
80% Body Burn

CASE PRESENTATION

A 23-year-old male suffered severe burns during munitions disposal activities. He was found on fire after extricating himself from his burning vehicle. The fire was extinguished, and the patient was transported rapidly by helicopter MEDEVAC to the nearest level III medical treatment facility. On arrival in the Emergency Medical Treatment (EMT) area (Figs. 1 and 2), he was intubated immediately and taken to the operating room (OR) for resuscitation and initial burn wound therapy. The initial estimate of surface area burned was 80%, with extensive burns to the head, face, upper extremities, trunk (front and back), and lower extremities (Figs. 3 and 4). Escharotomies were performed on both upper extremities (Figs. 5–7), with some bleeding evident in the escharotomy sites. The burns were washed vigorously and irrigated using gauze and normal saline, with minimal sharp debridement. Once cleaned, the burns were covered with Silvadene cream, and the wounds were dressed with Kerlex rolls and burn packs (Figs. 8–10). The patient was transported to the intensive care unit (ICU; Figs. 11 and 12). Initial urine output was less than 10 cc for the first hour, with evidence of severe hemolysis (Fig. 13). After intensive volume repletion and resuscitation, his vital signs improved and his urine output exceeded 30 cc per hour. He was then transported to a level IV medical treatment facility within 12 hours of admission. The patient was met by Army burn team members from the Institute of Surgical Research (ISR; Brooke Army Medical Center, San Antonio, Texas). At the level IV medical treatment facility, he underwent bilateral upper extremity amputations above the elbows to remove his completely burned arms. After further resuscitation, he was transported to the ISR in San Antonio. The patient died there several days later.

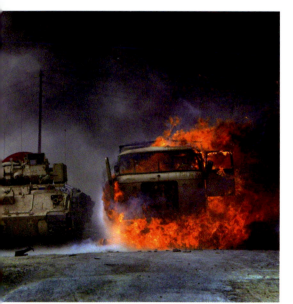

Courtesy David Leeson, *The Dallas Morning News*

TEACHING POINTS

1. Although large surface area burns are complex and difficult to manage long term, the initial management and resuscitation are usually straightforward:

    a. Secure the airway: In severe facial burns, intubation is mandatory at the time of presentation since, within hours, airway edema may make it impossible to establish the airway.

    b. An estimate of the burn surface area (Fig. 14) and time of the burn will initially guide the fluid resuscitation. For the first 24

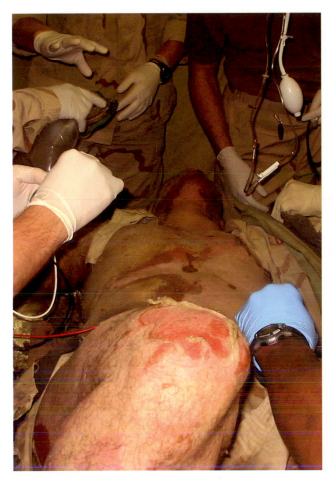

FIGURE 1. *Patient on arrival at CSH, EMT area.*

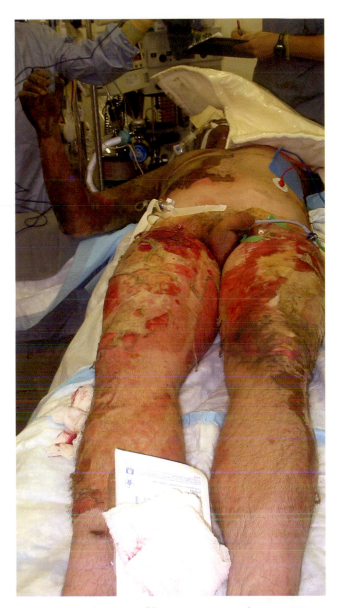

FIGURE 3. *Treatment of lower extremity burns, OR. Note protected area that was covered by boots.*

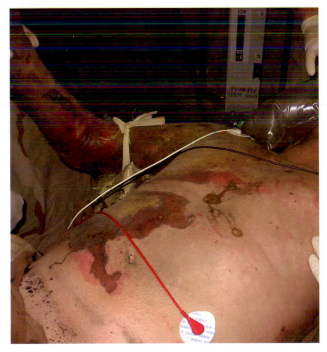

FIGURE 2. *Patient in EMT. Note extent of chest burns.*

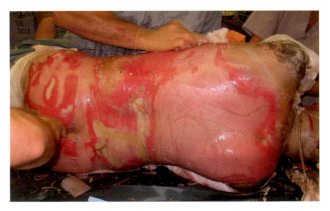

FIGURE 4. *Extent of back burns.*

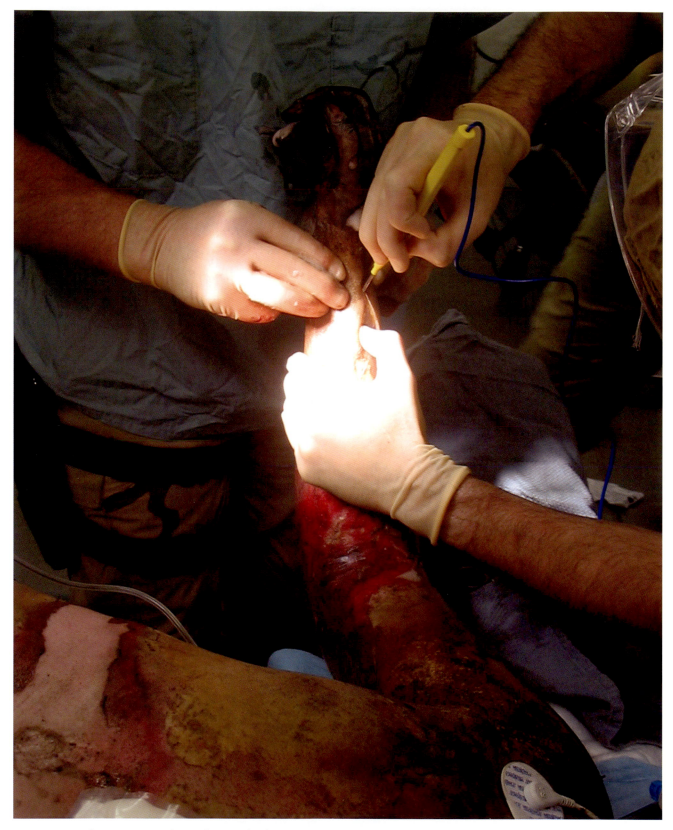

FIGURE 5. *Escharotomy performed on right forearm.*

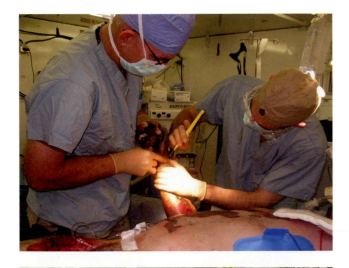

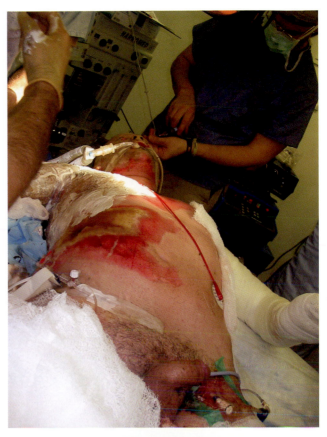

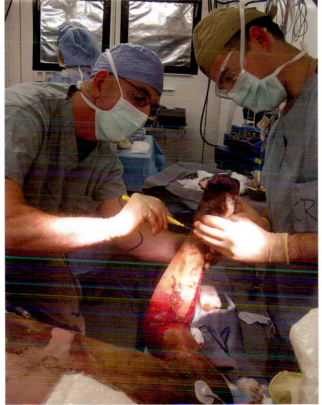

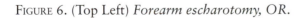

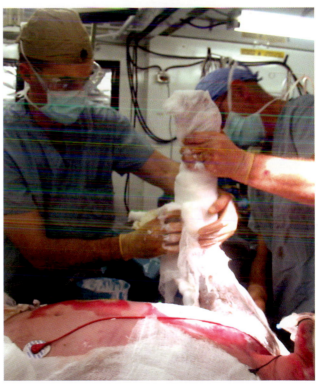

FIGURE 6. (Top Left) *Forearm escharotomy, OR.*

FIGURE 7. (Bottom Left) *Forearm escharotomy, OR.*

FIGURE 8. (Top Right) *Burns covered with Silvadene and Kerlex, OR.*

FIGURE 9. (Bottom Right) *Wound dressing, OR.*

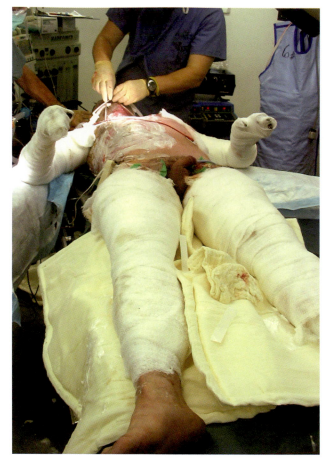

FIGURE 10. *Burns dressed, OR.*

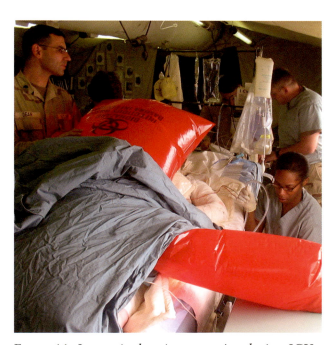

FIGURE 11. *Improvised patient-warming device, ICU.*

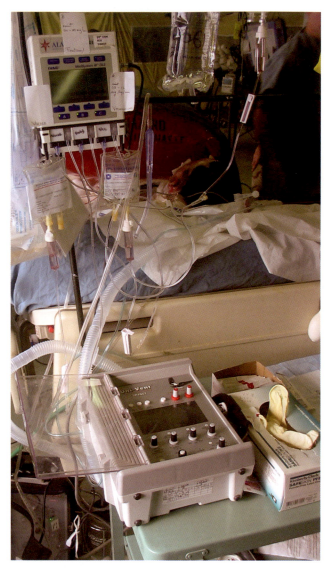

FIGURE 12. *ICU care. Note patient's ventilator at bottom of photo.*

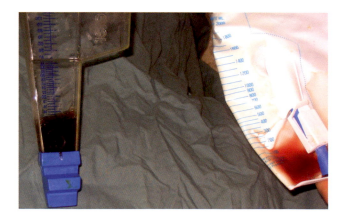

FIGURE 13. *Hemoglobinuria in urometer.*

hours, lactated Ringer's solution at 2 mL × % body burn (second- and third-degree) × the patient's weight in kilograms should be given, with one-half of the estimated fluid given within 8 hours of the burn and the remaining half of the fluid given in the next 16 hours. (This is only an estimate.) The patient's urine output and response to resuscitation must be monitored, and resuscitation must be adjusted accordingly.

   c. The OR is the best location for initial debridement and cleaning of burn wounds. With the patient under general anesthesia, scrubbing and sharp debridement—if necessary—and wound dressing are easily performed without patient discomfort.

2. For large burns, once the patient is stable enough for transport, rapid evacuation (within 48 hours) to a dedicated burn facility is imperative. It is important to deliver the patient to a burn center with appropriate staffing and logistical support to begin the complex and difficult process of minimizing burn wound sepsis (rare before 72 hours) and the arduous process of closing the open burn wounds.

CLINICAL IMPLICATIONS

Burns constitute 5% to 20% of combat casualties during conventional warfare and are particularly common on sea vessels and in closed, armored fighting vehicles. Relatively small burn wounds require aggressive and sustained care and can severely strain the logistical and manpower resources of deployed military medical units. Patients with greater than 80% surface area burns have extremely high mortality rates and if the situation warrants may be triaged expectant.

Note: See Appendix D, Clinical Practice Guidelines on Burn Care.

1. Priorities in the care of burn patient casualties is the same as for all other trauma patients. In the burn patient, special attention to exposure, removal of clothing that continues to burn the patient, and prevention of hypothermia are important. Often the depth of burn injury cannot be ascertained immediately. Burn patients may have concurrent penetrating and blunt injuries as a result of explosion or combat.

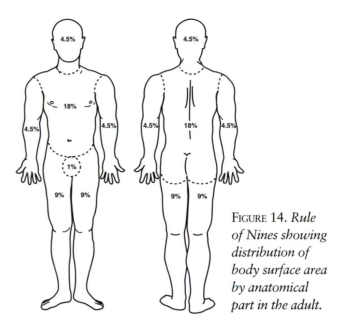

FIGURE 14. *Rule of Nines showing distribution of body surface area by anatomical part in the adult.*

2. Inhalation injury is more common with extensive cutaneous burns, a history of injury in a closed space, facial burns, and at the extremes of age. These patients require supplemental oxygen, pulse oximetry, chest X-ray, and arterial blood gas measurement.

3. Carbon monoxide poisoning results in cardiac and neurological symptoms. Patients with suspected carbon monoxide poisoning require 100% oxygen for at least 3 hours or until symptoms resolve.

4. After calculating initial fluid requirements, titrate fluid resuscitation to maintain urine output at 30 to 50 ml per hour or 1 mL/kg/h in children.

5. Children weighing less than 30 kg have a greater surface-to-weight ratio, and their fluid requirements are greater. Use lactated Ringer's solution at 3 cc/kg/% burn. Children should also receive a standard maintenance infusion of D5 1/2 normal saline concurrently.

6. After 24 hours, discontinue lactated Ringer's solution, and use 5% albumin and normal saline if available unless the wound is less than 30% body surface area.

7. Initial burn wound care includes adequate intravenous pain management, removal of foreign bodies, debridement, cleansing with surgical soap (use only saline around the face), unroofing of blisters, and application of a topical antimicrobial.

8. Burn victims must be adequately immunized against tetanus. If transport to higher level care will take more than 24 hours, they should be treated with a 5-day course of penicillin or similar antibiotics.

9. Progressive diminution of audible arterial flow by Doppler study is an indication for escharotomy. Doppler pulses must be sought in the palmar arch.

10. High-voltage electric injury requires consideration of deep muscle injury, with resultant rhabdomyolysis, hyperkalemia, acute renal failure, and compartment syndrome. Cardiac monitoring, aggressive fluid and electrolyte management, fasciotomy, and debridement are often required.

11. Chemical burns require the removal of the offending agent. Brush dry material off the skin surface before copious water lavage. If the burn is alkali, lavage may be required for several hours. Otherwise, chemical burns are managed the same as other burns.

DAMAGE CONTROL

Inhalation injury may be manifested by stridor, hoarseness, cough, carbonaceous sputum, or dyspnea. It may cause airway obstruction at any time during the first two postburn days. Prior to transport, prophylactically intubate patients with any evidence or suspicion of inhalation injury. Circumferential burns of the chest prevent effective chest motion. If this occurs, perform immediate thoracic escharotomy as a lifesaving procedure to permit adequate chest excursion.

SUMMARY

Burn injuries continue to be a common war injury that can tax the resources of field hospitals. In its 2003 deployment, injuries in 4.6% (86/1,867) of inpatients admitted to the 28th Combat Support Hospital (CSH) included burns. The mortality rate was 8%.[1] Initial treatment should focus on stabilizing the patient by appropriate airway management, fluid resuscitation, wound care, and pain control, with early evacuation to a designated burn center. Burn patients should be anticipated, and protocols should be in place to facilitate these evacuations. Infection control in the deployed setting was described by the 28th CSH as "a Herculean task" and directly impacted the care of host nationals who could not be evacuated.

REFERENCE

1. Stout LR, Jezior JR, et al. Wartime burn care in Iraq: 28th Combat Support Hospital, 2003. *Mil Med*. 2007;172(11):1148–1153.

SUGGESTED READING

Chapter 28: Burns. In: *Emergency War Surgery, Third United States Revision*. Washington, DC: Department of the Army, Office of The Surgeon General, Borden Institute; 2004.

COMMENTARY
Soft-Tissue Trauma and Burns

by LTC Evan M. Renz, MD, FACS

EXTREMITY COMPARTMENT SYNDROME

Few topics in war surgery have elicited as much discussion among combat surgeons serving in the current war as that of extremity compartment syndrome. Timely diagnosis and treatment of this problem can pose a challenge to even the most experienced field surgeon. Despite our best training and intentions, there may be great difficulty in performing an adequate fasciotomy, even by experienced surgeons. Ritenour et al[1] carefully examined the morbity and mortality associated with delayed diagnosis and treatment of combat casualties at risk for extremity compartment syndrome. Their detailed review of more than 300 combat casualties who underwent fasciotomies opens our eyes to the unmistakable importance of this pathologic process, the absolute necessity for surgeons to be skilled in the art of the fasciotomy, and the potentially devastating costs associated with failure to anticipate and treat the problem. Ritenour et al noted that 17% of patients who underwent fasciotomies in the operational theaters of Iraq and Afghanistan (2005–2006) later underwent revision of one or more fasciotomy sites on arrival at the level IV medical treatment facility in Landstuhl, Germany. Most revisions involved the lower leg and required extension of the fascial incisions. In those patients with compartments found unopened, the anterior and deep posterior compartments were most often untreated. General guidance regarding fasciotomies performed in the combat environment, or in a situation in which a prolonged transfer time is expected, remains the complete release of skin and fascia of all compartments in the extremity to be decompressed. Surgeons must maintain a high index of suspicion for delayed compartment syndrome in casualties with severe diffuse injuries, large burns, and extensive volume resuscitation.

OPEN WOUNDS AND VAC DRESSING

Negative pressure wound dressings—such as the VAC dressing—offer many benefits to the surgeon caring for the patient with extensive combat wounds, including the ability to provide a sterile wound dressing in a closed environment that protects against further contamination, while at the same time providing stability in the form of a soft splint to the affected region. Many surgeons appreciate the ability to place the conforming sponge into the cavernous spaces of a wound, which "pulls" residual irrigation fluid and potential wound contaminants from the wound. Conversely, no therapy is without its risks, and caution must be exercised when placing a negative pressure dressing over any surface that has the potential for significant bleeding, desiccation, or damage from continuous negative pressure. Placing a VAC dressing directly over muscle, fascia, or subcutaneous tissue for up to several days generally works extremely well in preparing the wound for delayed closure or skin grafting. Leaving a VAC dressing on a wound in need of further debridement can result in a foul-smelling environment, best avoided by earlier dressing change. All in all, the VAC dressing system has endeared itself with most surgeons who continue to find new and innovative ways to use it.[2]

One of the advantages of the VAC is the ability of the patient to move with the dressing in place. When using the VAC device on patients who are awake and functional, it is beneficial to route the suction line toward the torso, thereby avoiding interference from the lines during range-of-motion activities and ambulation.

BURNS

After 4 years of war in Iraq, more than 500 US soldiers and Marines sustained thermal injuries serious enough to warrant specialized care at burn centers. The range of thermal injuries is broad, involving less than 1% of the person's total body surface area to as high as 95% in survivors to date. Although the severity of injury, and mortality, generally parallels that of the size of the cutaneous burn, even a relatively small burn—such as the all-too-common isolated hand burn—can yield devastating, long-term consequences for the casualty. There are a number of key points worthy of emphasis in the case described by the authors.

Many war-related burns are a result of an explosion. The energy from an explosion is seldom limited to the thermal component. To date, more than 50% of all burn patients admitted to the US Army Institute of Surgical Research Burn Center (San Antonio, Texas) had at least one other significant injury, most commonly fractures of an extremity. It is very easy for a provider to become focused on the burned skin and overlook the underlying injury, whether it is a fracture or other penetrating injury. The key here is to treat the burn patient like any other trauma patient requiring a thorough head-to-toe assessment.

Airway protection and support of breathing are early and important steps in treatment of the burn patient, particularly if there is evidence of inhalation injury. Preemptive intubation can be lifesaving. Securing the airway cannot be stressed enough, especially when the patient is going to be evacuated by air. Standard techniques of securing the tube using tape or prefabricated adhesive devices are generally ineffective in the presence of facial burns. Securing the tube with umbilical tape, which can be adjusted as facial edema increases, is recommended.

One of the most critical aspects of care for the burn patient is that of fluid resuscitation. Both under- and overresuscitation can result in severe, unintended consequences. Overresuscitation can worsen edema in the extremities and the abdomen, leading to compartment syndromes in either or both. Monitoring urine output as an indicator of adequate resuscitation remains perhaps the single most useful tool we have, especially in a deployed environment. This process requires close attention and action when targets are not met. Guidelines and tools designed to assist the deployed military provider are available in CENTCOM's Clinical Practice Guidelines for Burn Care on the Joint Patient Tracking Application Web site. (See Appendix D.) Also included on the site is a printable Burn Resuscitation Flow Sheet designed to assist in the process of fluid resuscitation, document the process, and facilitate continuity of care for the burn casualty.[3]

Placement of an indwelling urinary catheter is essential to the process of fluid resuscitation of the burn patient. Occasionally, burn patients are transferred to level III medical treatment facilities without a catheter in place, or with a suprapubic catheter in place for the stated reason that the genitalia were burned. Even in cases of full-thickness burns involving the penis, it is extremely rare that the urethral orifice cannot be intubated. Debridement of the glans may be required, followed by careful dilation of the orifice by the physician to place the catheter. This process is associated with far less risk than placement of a suprapubic catheter.

Initial cleansing and debridement of burns should be postponed until they can be accomplished in a clean environment (eg, the operating room). Until then, the burn casualty should be covered in clean, dry material. There is no advantage to using commercially available cooling gel blankets, especially in the burn patient with large surface area involvement who is already at risk of hypothermia. Once in a proper environment, the wounds can be cleaned and dressed using a number of commonly available products (eg, Silvadene cream or 5% Sulfamyalon [mafenide] solution). Another effective option for burn care is the use of silver nylon dressings. Silver nylon materials, such as Silverlon and Silverseal, provide antimicrobial action through the release of silver ions from the fabric.

The burn patient is prone to edema formation, especially as fluid resuscitation continues. Patients sustaining full-thickness burns, especially circumferential burns involving one or more extremities, often require escharotomies to combat the effects of edema. Escharotomies, and subsequent fasciotomies, should be performed through burned skin, sparing uninjured skin for future harvesting of donor autografts. Escharotomies may be performed using either scalpel or—as depicted here—utilizing electrocautery, which offers the advantages of coagulation along the skin edge if bleeding is present. Elevating the burned extremities above the level of the heart also reduces the adverse effects of edema.

Lastly, consultation with a surgeon at the US Army Institute of Surgical Research Burn Center is available by phone 24 hours a day. Consultation using e-mail is also available. Early physician-to-physician communication regarding casualties is encouraged because it facilitates continuity of care if rapid evacuation is planned. The number of severe burn casualties will help determine whether to deploy a Burn Flight Team to transport the patients.

Our experience from this war has confirmed that even the most severely burned casualties may be safely evacuated back to the continental United States.[4] When air evacuation to a definitive care facility is available, the decision to place a burn patient in an expectant status, based on his or her clinical condition, should be carefully considered.

REFERENCES

1. Ritenour AE, Dorlac WC, Fang R. Complications after fasciotomy revision and delayed compartment release in combat patients. *J Trauma*. In press.

2. Leininger BE, Rasmussen TE, et al. Experience with wound VAC and delayed primary closure of contaminated soft tissue injuries in Iraq. *J Trauma*. 2006;61:1207–1211.

3. Ennis JL, Chung KK, et al. Joint Theater Trauma System implementation of Burn Resuscitation Guidelines improves outcomes in severely burned military casualties. *J Trauma*. In press.

4. Renz EM, Cancio LC, et al. Long-range transport of war-related casualties. *J Trauma*. In press.

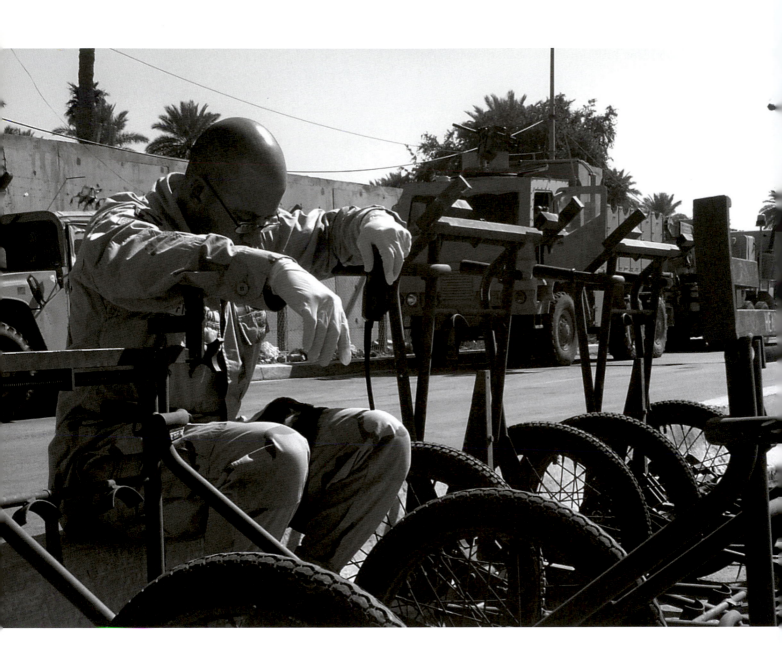

Chapter VII
ORTHOPAEDIC TRAUMA

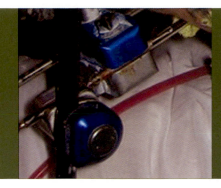

VII.1
Gunshot Wound With Loss of the Elbow

CASE PRESENTATION

This male patient, an interpreter for Special Operations Forces, sustained a gunshot wound to the left elbow. He was transported to the local host nation hospital where he was offered an above-elbow amputation, which he declined. Forty-eight hours later, he presented to the combat support hospital (CSH) with a large, dorsal elbow wound (Fig. 1). The proximal ulna was missing, but the hand appeared neurologically intact, except for decreased light-touch sensation in ulnar nerve distribution (Fig. 2). All motor function was intact. Plain radiographs revealed a distal humerus fracture and a missing proximal ulna (Figs. 3 and 4). The patient underwent irrigation, debridement, and external fixation from the humerus to the ulna (Figs. 5 and 6). The ulnar nerve was severed. All loose bone was removed, and a dressing soaked with Dakin's solution was placed in anticipation of wet-to-dry dressing changes. The wound required multiple irrigations and debridements. Intravenous antibiotics, including cefazolin and gentamicin, were administered. When the wound was surgically clean, open reduction and internal fixation of the distal humerus were performed, as well as radial head excision and elbow arthrodesis. Wound coverage was obtained with an abdominal pedicle flap. The patient was discharged on postoperative day 5 to a hospital in Jordan for continued care (Figs. 7 and 8).

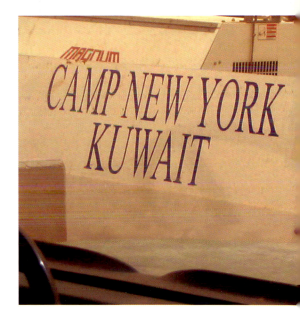

TEACHING POINTS

1. This patient was provided with full reconstructive care in a level III medical treatment facility. This specialized care posed difficult problems because instrumentation options are limited in theater. Large bone defects are also a particular problem because no bone bank is available in theater. This situation sometimes makes decisions regarding treatment options difficult for the deployed surgeon.

2. This patient presented with intact motor function and decreased light-touch sensation in the ulnar nerve distribution. This condition is most likely caused by the presence of a Martin-Gruber anastomosis that connects the median and ulnar nerves distally.

3. At the host nation hospital, he was offered an above-elbow amputation, despite the fact that his hand still worked. If the patient could obtain a prosthesis, this level of amputation could be very functional. In the host nation, however, prostheses are hard to come by. Advanced

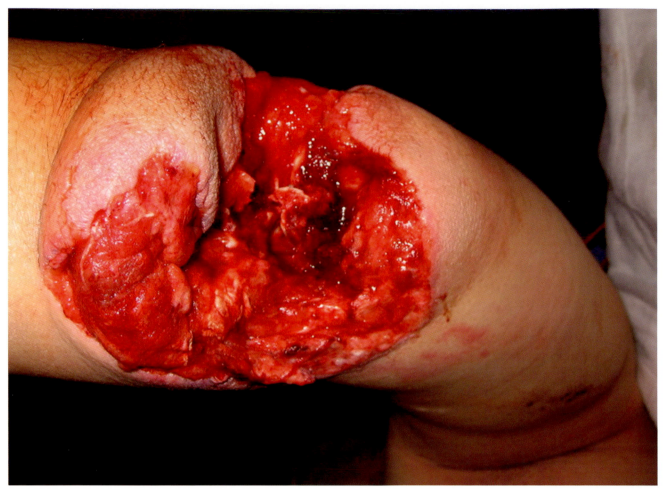

FIGURE 1. *Extensive soft-tissue and bone injuries of the elbow.*

prosthetics and expensive surgical implants (eg, an elbow arthroplasty or osteoarticular allograft) are not available. For this reason, an elbow arthrodesis was performed.

CLINICAL IMPLICATIONS

1. Wounds to soft-tissue and osseous structures around the elbow are common because the elbow is not protected by body armor. These wounds can involve fractures and arterial and nerve injuries, with the ulnar nerve frequently injured.

2. If a nerve laceration is noted and the patient has no function distally, nerve repair with an end-to-end technique or with a NeuraGen tube technique versus cable grafting can be done. These techniques are difficult to perform without a microscope and microvascular instruments. Therefore, every surgeon should bring surgical loupes to theater.

3. Wound coverage is always a problem with the elbow. Free flaps in theater are rarely performed and are fraught with significant complications. Therefore, in this patient—with the help of a plastic surgeon—an older technique of pedicle flap grafting was used.

4. Severe bone defects are difficult to address in theater. The solution to these defects is generally an amputation. In this case, reconstruction of the bone was attempted using an autograft from the iliac crest or fibula.

5. Another treatment alternative is to shorten the bone instead of reconstructing it. If bone reconstruction is successful, the procedure negates the need for a lifetime use of prosthetics in a location where they are difficult to obtain and maintain.

DAMAGE CONTROL

External fixation across the injured joint allows safe

MARTIN-GRUBER ANASTOMOSIS

Originally described by Martin in 1763 and later by Gruber in 1870, this is an anomalous innervation pattern occurring between the median and ulnar nerves in the forearm. Specifically, fibers from the median nerve cross over to the ulnar nerve in the forearm. Martin-Gruber anastomosis is the most common anomalous innervation of the hand, with an incidence of 15% to 28%.

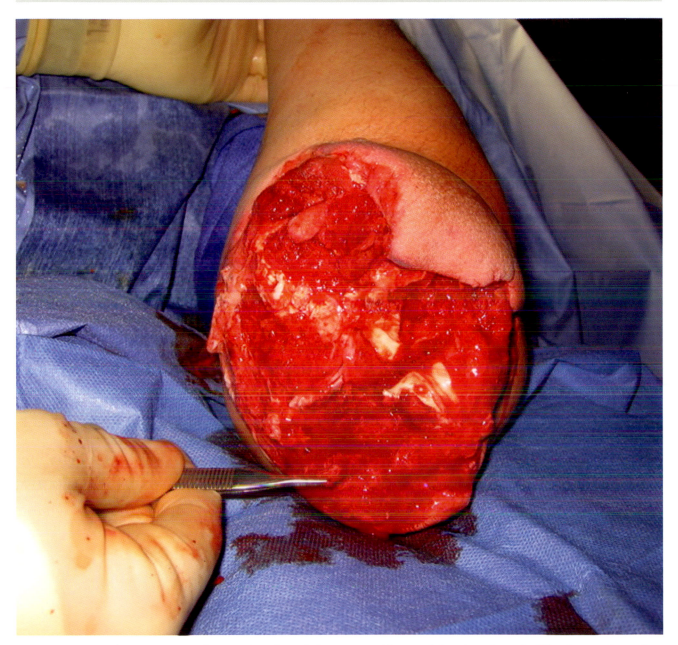

FIGURE 2. *Surgical instrument indicates the severed ulnar nerve. (Surgical draping gives the false impression of an amputation.)*

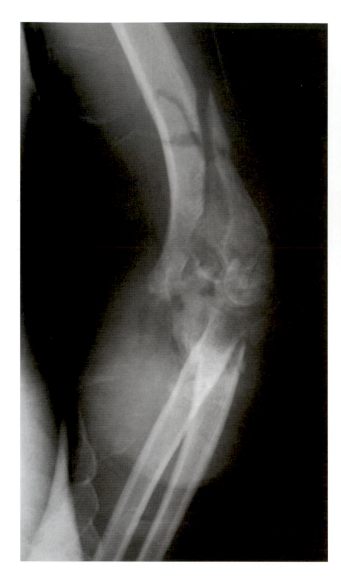

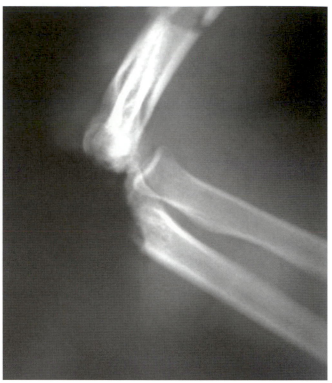

FIGURE 3. (Top Left) *Radiograph of left elbow wound. There is a fracture of the distal humerus.*

FIGURE 4. (Top Right) *Radiograph of elbow. Note loss of proximal ulna.*

FIGURE 5. (Bottom) *External fixation spanning the elbow joint. Wound care can be easily performed. If appropriate, the patient can be evacuated from the CSH.*

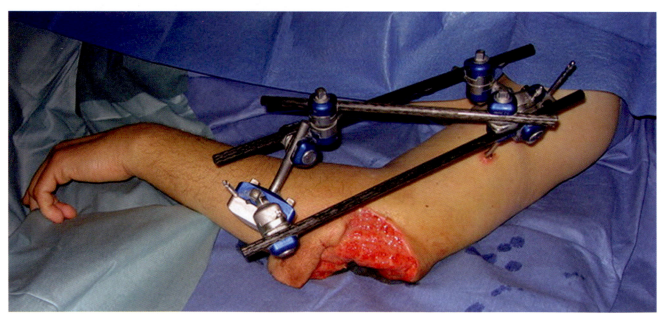

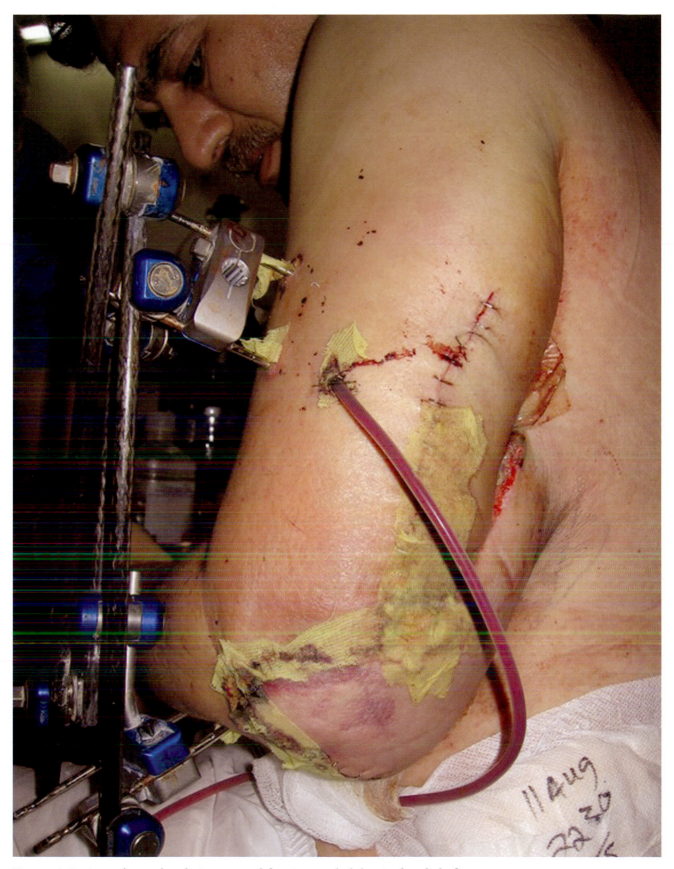

FIGURE 6. *Patient after arthrodesis, external fixation, and abdominal pedicle flap.*

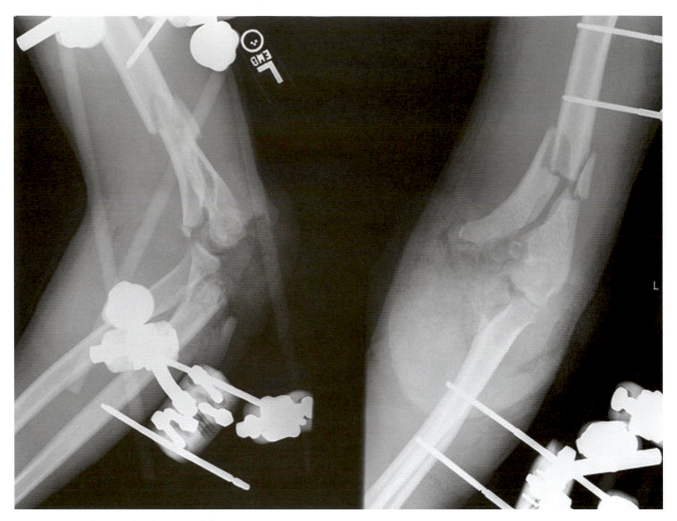

FIGURE 7. *Radiograph of external fixation.*

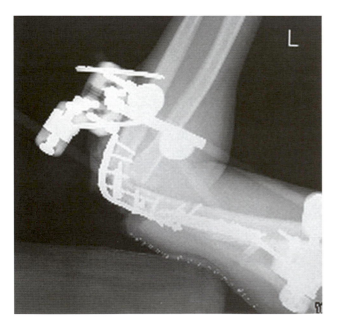

FIGURE 8. *Radiograph after arthrodesis, external fixation, and abdominal pedicle flap.*

transfer out of theater. The wound should be adequately debrided and washed out before evacuation. If possible, evacuation should be coordinated with the receiving hospital to allow timely, additional wound washouts. Nerve endings should be tagged to allow grafting at a later date.

SUMMARY

This case demonstrates a need for highly sophisticated, technically adequate, surgical capabilities in theater. CSHs are not intended to provide this type of surgery because of the rapid evacuation of American wounded. However, at times, complex surgeries are still necessary and are appropriate in the combat zone.

SUGGESTED READING

Chapter 24: Open-joint injuries. In: *Emergency War Surgery, Third United States Revision.* Washington, DC: Department of the Army, Office of The Surgeon General, Borden Institute; 2004.

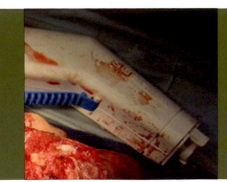

VII.2
Hand and Face Blast Injuries; Polytrauma Management

CASE PRESENTATION

This male patient was the driver of a high-mobility multipurpose wheeled vehicle (HMMWV or "Humvee") in a convoy that was hit by a blast from an improvised explosive device (IED). The patient sustained severe facial injuries (Fig. 1), as well as right forearm and hand injuries (Fig. 2). He presented to the combat support hospital (CSH) awake and attempting to talk. After resuscitation, he was taken to the operating room. His first surgery lasted 8 hours, and involved general, ophthalmic, oral and maxillofacial, plastic, and orthopaedic surgeries. Priority was given to the patient's eye and facial wounds, which were irrigated and reapproximated. A tracheostomy was performed. After his facial injuries were treated, the severe hand injuries were addressed. During intraoperative evaluation, an obvious volar forearm wound and a severe dorsal hand wound, with full-thickness tissue loss from the dorsal skin to the volar aspect of the metacarpals, were found. His fingers were blue, and his hand was folded over through the fractured metacarpals. Apropos of this injury, the question was whether or not to amputate any fingers. The surgery team elected to save the fingers. A volar forearm fasciotomy was performed (Fig. 3). The hand wound was irrigated and debrided. All dead tissue and loose bone were removed. Kirschner wire spacers were placed to recreate the anatomical cascade of the hand (Fig. 4). After placing the wire spacers and extending the hand out to length, finger perfusion improved, with good capillary refill and improved temperature. Wet-to-dry dressings soaked with Dakin's solution were placed on the affected areas. The forearm and hand were splinted. The patient was started on intravenous antibiotics and was evacuated the day of injury. The hand was reconstructed by the Hand Surgery Service at Walter Reed Army Medical Center (WRAMC). The index finger, which was completely missing the metacarpal, was used to reconstruct the other missing metacarpals and extensor mechanism. The skin of the volar index finger was rotated through the first web space to cover the skin defect of the dorsum of the hand.

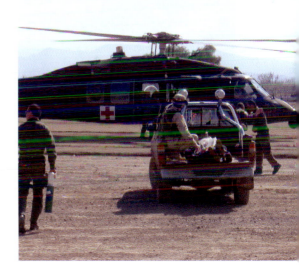

TEACHING POINTS

1. Blast injuries cause severe injuries to multiple body parts. In this case, severe facial injuries, ocular injuries, and hand injuries occurred. It is crucial that a surgeon not become fixated on any one injury. Advanced Trauma Life Support (ATLS) principles must be followed. In this patient, the airway had to be controlled.

2. The goal of the combat surgeon at the forward CSH is to give the reconstructive surgeon at the level V medical treatment facility in the United States something to work with for reconstruction. The oral and maxillofacial, plastic, and ophthalmic surgeons addressed facial injuries (Fig. 5). From an orthopaedic perspective, the goal was to retain tissue and get as many viable fingers back to WRAMC alive as possible. It appeared that the middle finger and the ring finger could be reconstructed. However, it was not clear that the index finger could be salvaged. Therefore, an attempt was made to save the index finger for reconstructive purposes.

CLINICAL IMPLICATIONS

1. Nearly every surgical service in the CSH was required to manage this multiply injured patient.
2. The most life-threatening injuries should be addressed first, followed by threats to eyesight and limbs.
3. It is vital to salvage as much tissue as possible for later reconstruction.

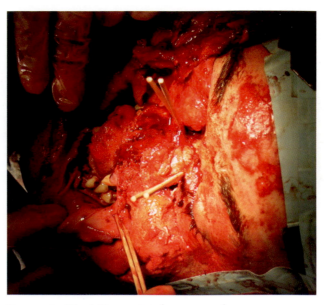

FIGURE 1. (Top) *Extensive face wounds.*

FIGURE 2. (Bottom) *Hand and forearm at presentation.*

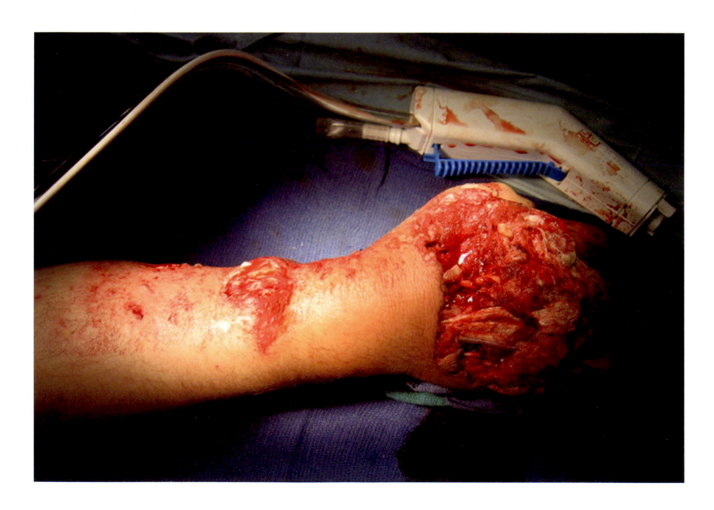

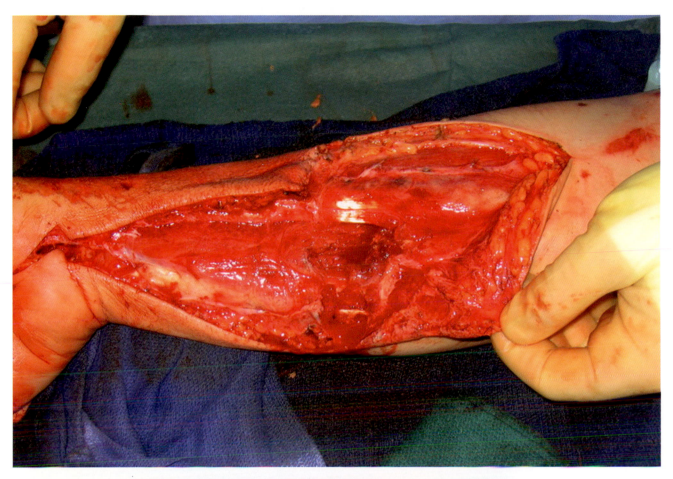

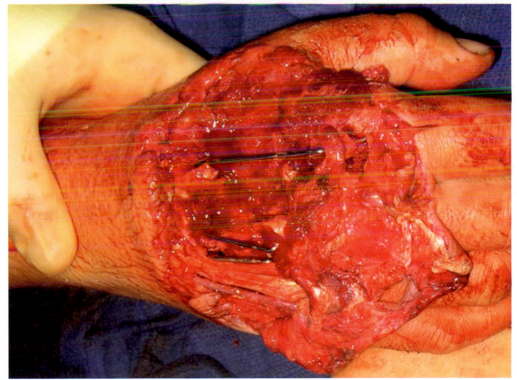

FIGURE 3. (Top)
*Volar forearm
debridement and
fasciotomy.*

FIGURE 4. (Bottom)
*Debridement
and placement of
Kirschner wires.*

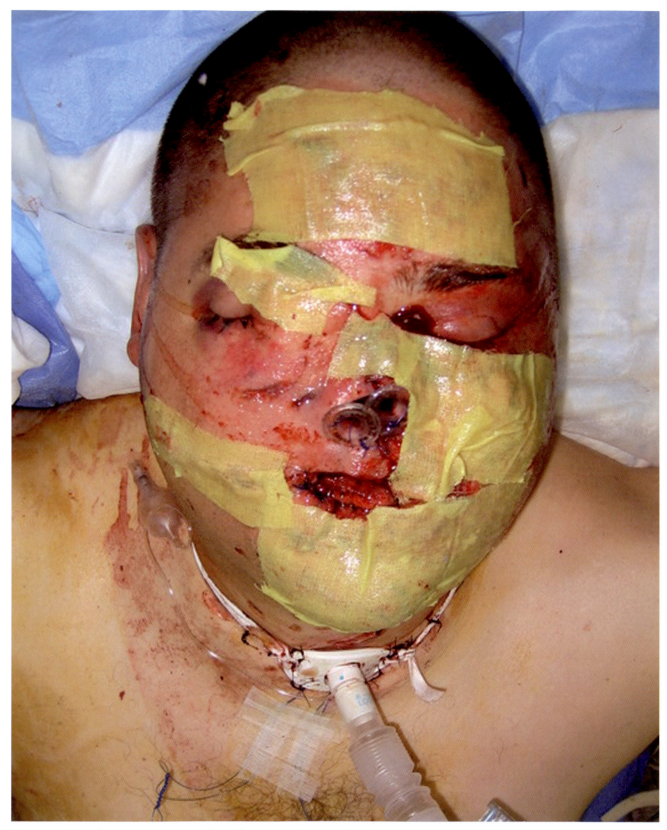

FIGURE 5. *Facial reconstruction and tracheostomy (post-op).*

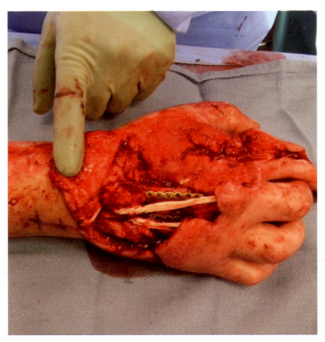

FIGURE 6. *Reconstruction performed by the Hand Surgery Service at Walter Reed Army Medical Center.*

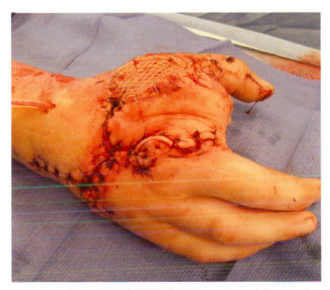

FIGURE 7. *Reconstruction after a rotational flap and skin graft have been performed.*

KIRSCHNER WIRES

Kirschner wires (or K-wires) are thin, rigid wires used to stabilize bone fragments. These wires are drilled into bone to hold the fragments in place. Kirschner wires were introduced in 1909 by Martin Kirschner (1879–1942).

DAMAGE CONTROL

The first priority is to attend to life-threatening injuries. Debride necrotic tissue and perform appropriate fasciotomies while preserving as much tissue as possible for later reconstruction. Amputation may be required for a patient in shock who is not responding to resuscitation or who needs other lifesaving procedures.

SUMMARY

There is a frequent need in the combat environment for a multispecialty team approach to the management of polytrauma. Treatment priorities must be set, and ATLS protocols must be followed. In this case, after the airway was properly secured and the admission Glasgow Coma Scale (GCS) score was > 8, facial and right arm wound management were undertaken with the intent to preserve as much tissue as possible for future reconstruction (Figs. 6 and 7).

SUGGESTED READING

Chapter 13: Face and neck injuries. In: *Emergency War Surgery, Third United States Revision*. Washington, DC: Department of the Army, Office of The Surgeon General, Borden Institute; 2004.

Chapter 25: Amputations. In: *Emergency War Surgery, Third United States Revision*. Washington, DC: Department of the Army, Office of The Surgeon General, Borden Institute; 2004.

Chapter 26: Injuries to the hands and feet. In: *Emergency War Surgery, Third United States Revision*. Washington, DC: Department of the Army, Office of The Surgeon General, Borden Institute; 2004.

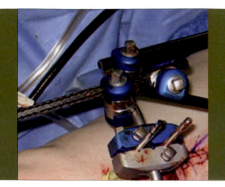

VII.3
Open Femur Fracture

CASE PRESENTATION

This male patient sustained a penetrating blast injury to his left thigh from an improvised explosive device (IED). Physical examination revealed an isolated injury to the left thigh, with a 3-cm wound at the distal third of the anterolateral thigh. Neurological and vascular examinations were normal. The thigh was moderately swollen, and a retained fragment noted radiographically was not palpable. Plain radiographs showed a long, spiral oblique fracture of the femur, with a fragment proximal to the fracture site (Fig. 1). In the operating room, he underwent irrigation and debridement of the fracture and placement of an external fixator spanning the knee joint (Figs. 2 and 3). The traumatic wound was extended to improve exposure. This extension was closed at the end of the procedure, leaving the traumatic wound open. The open wound was packed with wet-to-dry dressings soaked with Dakin's solution. Intravenous antibiotics were administered, and the patient was evacuated on the day of injury.

TEACHING POINTS

1. Fractures to long bones are very common injuries that result from either penetrating blast injuries or gunshot wounds. They must be irrigated, debrided, and stabilized before evacuation from theater.
2. Complete primary and secondary surveys must be performed because long bone fractures are sometimes accompanied by other major life-threatening injuries.
3. Significant blood loss frequently accompanies a femur fracture. This condition might necessitate transfusion before the patient is accepted into the medical evacuation system.
4. In this patient, the external fixator was placed spanning the knee joint out of concern that placing pins in the distal femur would risk intraarticular pin positioning in the suprapatellar pouch, increasing the risk of joint sepsis.
5. Retained fragments are often seen in theater. There is always a question of whether or not to remove these fragments. In general, there is no urgency to remove them. If the fragments are easily accessible in the traumatic wound, they are removed routinely. If the fragments are remote from the surgical site, they can be left in place. If fragments later become symptomatic, they can be removed electively.

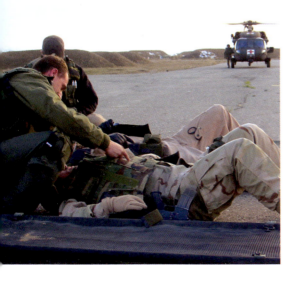

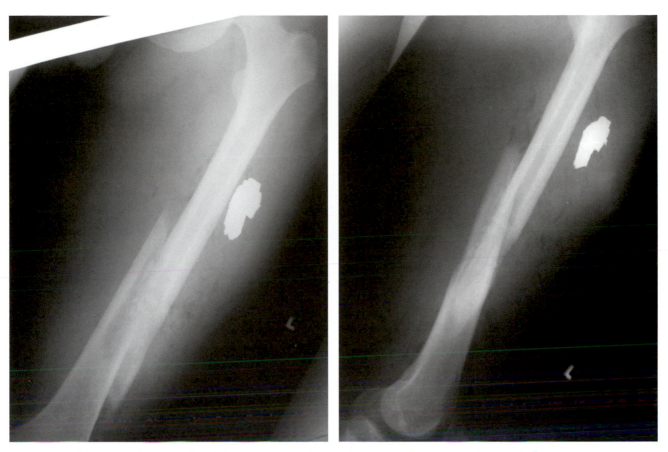

FIGURE 1. PA (Left) *and lateral* (Right) *radiographs show midfemoral fracture and metallic fragment that caused the injury. There is extensive soft-tissue air.*

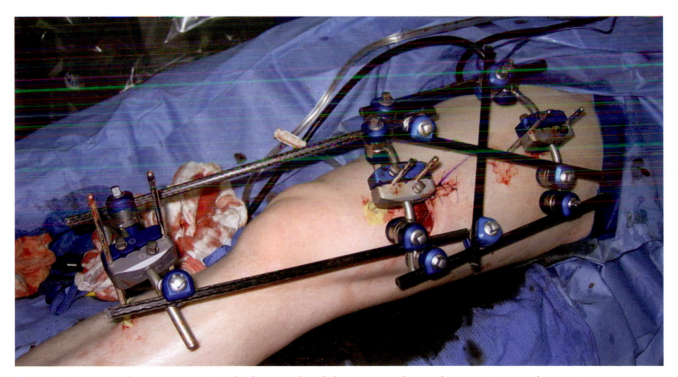

FIGURE 2. *External fixation spanning the knee and stabilizing open femur fracture in a combat environment.*

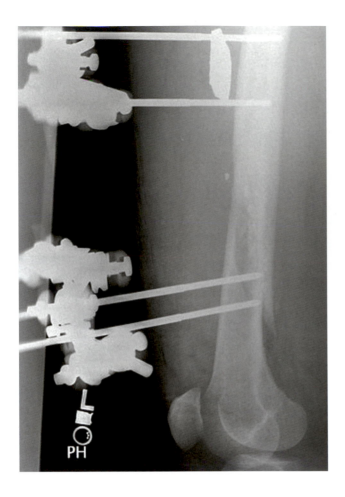

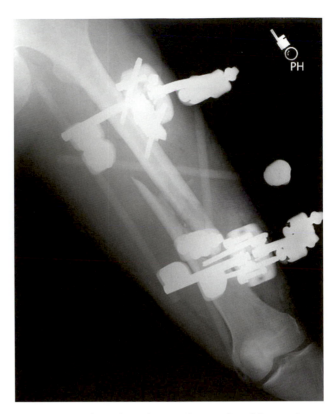

FIGURE 3. (Left and Right) *Radiographs of femoral pin placements. Fixator extension across the joint to the tibia is not shown in these films.*

CLINICAL IMPLICATIONS

Deployed surgeons will see many long bone fractures in general and many femur fractures in particular. They need to be confident stabilizing these fractures with either splints or external fixators. The following principles are important to consider:

1. In a patient with a femur fracture, blood loss might be substantial and must be addressed before entry into the medical evacuation system.
2. Open femur fractures have a historical infection rate of approximately 40%, and these fractures should be irrigated and debrided as soon as possible to minimize infection risk.
3. Initial neurovascular findings should be documented, and the examination should be repeated frequently.
4. Intravenous antibiotics should be started as soon as possible.
5. If wound debridement is performed, bone fragments attached to viable soft tissue and large bone fragments should be retained.

6. Indications for spanning the knee with external fixation include distal femur fractures, proximal tibial fractures, extensive knee injuries, and vascular repairs in the popliteal fossa.

DAMAGE CONTROL

Transportation casts are an acceptable alternative to external fixation.

SUMMARY

Open femur fractures are some of the most commonly encountered injuries in the current combat environment. All general and orthopaedic surgeons should have a thorough understanding of extremity anatomy and treatment options for these injuries. Surgeons should be familiar with the standard constructs of external fixation.

SUGGESTED READING

Chapter 23: Extremity fractures. In: *Emergency War Surgery, Third United States Revision.* Washington, DC: Department of the Army, Office of The Surgeon General, Borden Institute; 2004.

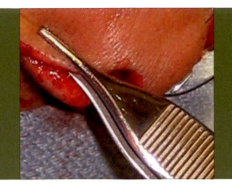

VII.4
Blast Injury of the Hand

CASE PRESENTATION

This male patient sustained blast injuries to all four extremities. His hand injuries included a right thumb metacarpal fracture with bone loss and large, dorsal soft-tissue loss. In addition, he sustained multiple fragment wounds of both lower extremities, a traumatic ankle arthrotomy with retained fragments, and a left-hand small finger fracture. He underwent irrigation and debridement of all wounds. The right thumb metacarpal head articular surface was stabilized with a longitudinal pin (Figs. 1 and 2). The left finger fracture was also pinned. Wet-to-dry dressings soaked with Dakin's solution were placed on all open wounds. Both upper extremities were splinted. Intravenous antibiotics were administered. The patient underwent multiple irrigation and debridement procedures of his right hand. The wound was then treated with Dakin's solution until it was granulating well (Fig. 3). When the wound was deemed surgically clean, an iliac crest bone graft was pinned in place at the thumb metacarpal bone defect site. An abdominal pedicle flap was placed on the dorsal hand soft-tissue defect. Three weeks after placement of the flap, the patient (a host national) returned for separation and closure.

TEACHING POINTS

1. Wounds to the hand frequently involve bone, muscle, tendon, nerve, and skin loss. It is important to obtain soft-tissue control before performing definitive treatment of a fracture. This patient required multiple procedures and formal dressing changes for weeks before the definitive procedure was performed.

2. Two major options were available for treatment of the thumb injury: amputation and reconstruction. At initial surgery, the thumb metacarpal head was stabilized with pins. This allowed for the possibility, if needed, of metacarpal bone loss reconstruction and later arthrodesis of the metacarpophalangeal joint.

3. Another major problem was dorsal hand soft-tissue loss. Ordinarily, this would be treated with a free flap. In theater, no free flaps are used. The solution to this issue was abdominal pedicle flap coverage of the dorsum of the hand (Figs. 4–6), performed with the help of a plastic surgeon.

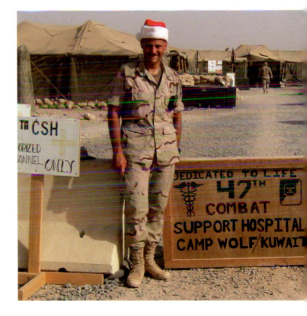

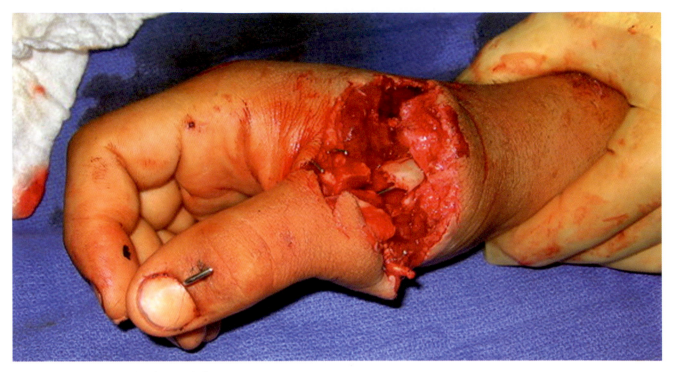

FIGURE 1. *Right thumb after stabilization.*

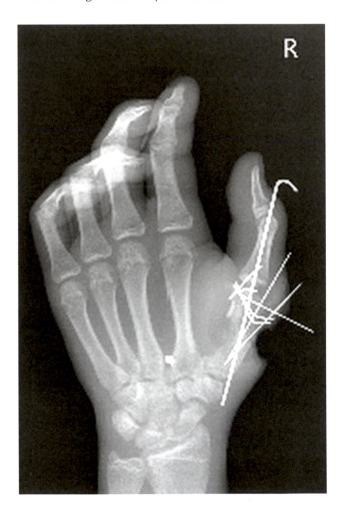

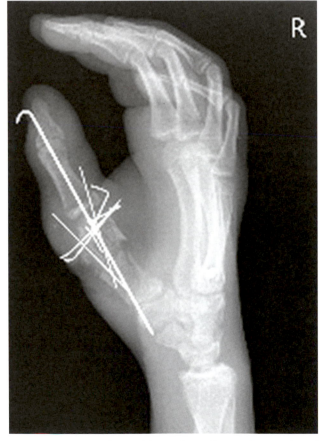

FIGURE 2. *AP* (Left) *and lateral* (Right) *radiographs of hand fracture stabilization with Kirschner wires.*

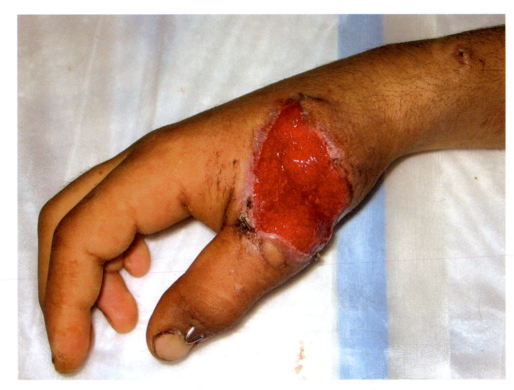

FIGURE 3. (Top)
*Excellent granulation
of wound.*

FIGURE 4. (Bottom)
*Effective use of a pedicle
flap to obtain adequate
soft-tissue coverage.*

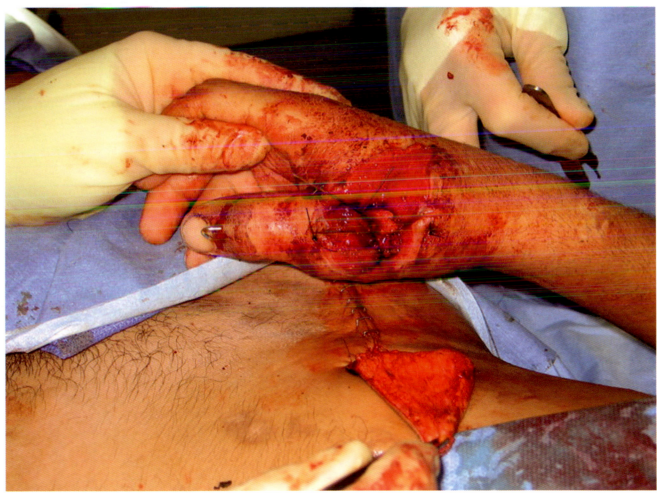

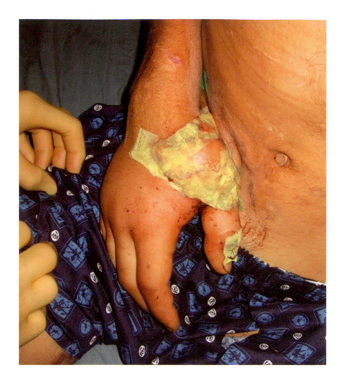

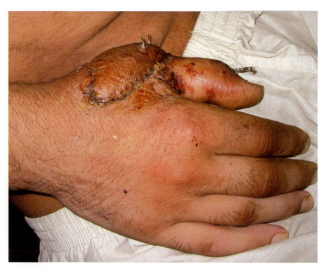

FIGURE 5. (Left) *Hand after the pedicle flap has healed.*

FIGURE 6. (Right) *Close-up of hand after the pedicle flap has healed.*

CLINICAL IMPLICATIONS

Complex reconstructive surgery is performed in theater, generally on host nationals, with the following cautions:

1. It is important to obtain wound control before proceeding with bone or soft-tissue reconstruction.
2. It is vital that attempts be made to keep things simple. Remember that the instrumentation available in the combat environment is necessarily limited. Kirschner wires are an excellent option for hand stabilization.
3. It is essential to obtain soft-tissue coverage at the time of reconstruction. The pedicle flap has been used successfully in combat support hospitals (CSHs) without requiring highly specialized instruments or a microscope necessary for free flap placement.

DAMAGE CONTROL

For patients evacuated to level V medical treatment facilities, initial debridement and irrigation—followed by wet-to-dry dressing changes—are adequate. Amputation of limbs with large wounds complicated by bone and soft-tissue loss may become a necessary consideration.

SUMMARY

This case is an example of using available resources to obtain an acceptable outcome. The surgeons were successful in an austere environment by using basic wound care management and relatively simple medical techniques.

SUGGESTED READING

Chapter 26: Injuries to the hand and feet. In: *Emergency War Surgery, Third United States Revision.* Washington, DC: Department of the Army, Office of The Surgeon General, Borden Institute; 2004.

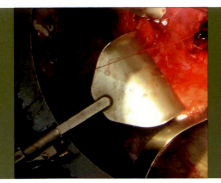

VII.5
Blast Injury of the Humerus

CASE PRESENTATION

This male patient sustained a blast injury from an improvised explosive device (IED), resulting in a large, lateral arm wound (Figs. 1 and 2) and an open humerus fracture. No loss of consciousness or other injuries were noted. Physical examination revealed a normal vascular examination of the upper extremity. Sensory and motor functions of the median and anterior interosseous nerves were preserved. The radial, posterior interosseous, and ulnar nerves were nonfunctional, with no evident light-touch sensation or motor function in their distribution. A large metallic fragment was palpable in the axilla. Plain radiographs revealed a severely comminuted humerus fracture (Fig. 3). In the operating room, the wound was irrigated and debrided. All necrotic tissue and loose bone were removed. The palpable fragment was excised through an incision in the axilla. Intraoperatively, the brachial plexus and brachial artery were palpable through the lateral arm wound. An external fixator was placed spanning the severely comminuted humerus fracture (Fig. 4). The wounds were packed with wet-to-dry dressings soaked with Dakin's solution. Intravenous antibiotics were administered. The patient was evacuated to a level IV medical treatment facility on postoperative day 1.

TEACHING POINTS

1. Fractures, nerve palsies, and vascular injuries often accompany seemingly minor soft-tissue injuries to the arm making a thorough evaluation critical. It is important to adequately assess the vascular status of the extremity after a humerus fracture with associated nerve palsies. The nerves of the brachial plexus lie immediately adjacent to the brachial artery at the medial side of the humerus. The artery can be injured by the same mechanism causing the fracture, or it can become injured during medical evacuation if initial splinting of the extremity was inadequate.

2. Nerve injuries require only documentation in theater. The extent of nerve injury can be evaluated and addressed more fully at a higher level treatment facility.

CLINICAL IMPLICATIONS

1. Initial neurovascular findings should be documented, and the examination should be frequently repeated, especially after any manipulation of the fractured extremity.

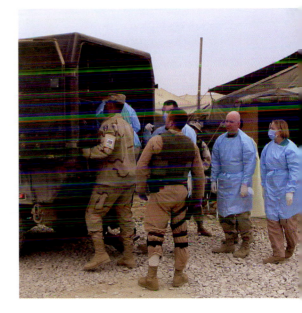

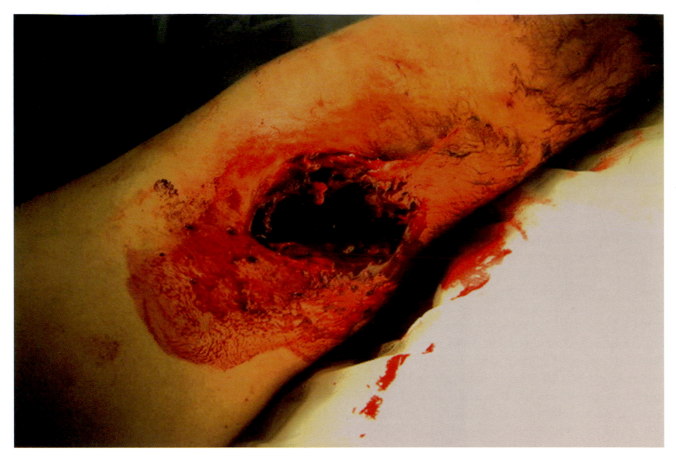

FIGURE 1. (Top)
*Large, lateral arm
wound on admission.*

FIGURE 2. (Bottom)
*Close-up of arm
wound in Fig. 1.*

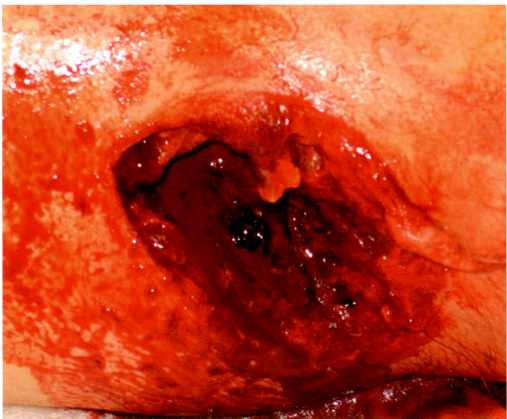

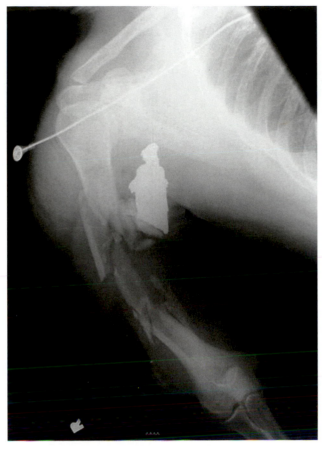

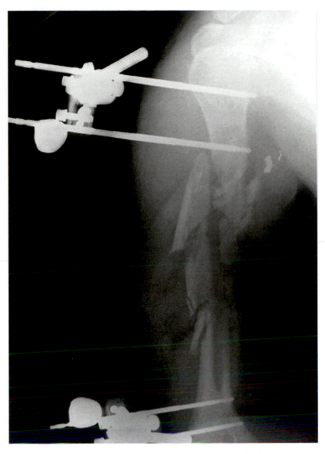

FIGURE 3. *Comminuted humeral fracture, large metal fragment, and limb shortening are evident.*

FIGURE 4. *Radiograph status post external fixation.*

2. Intravenous antibiotics should be started as soon as possible. Tetanus immunization should be considered based on the patient's immunization status and the nature of the wound.

3. If wound debridement is performed, bone fragments that are attached to viable soft tissue and large bone fragments should be retained.

DAMAGE CONTROL

Injuries to the upper extremity range from isolated bone, muscle, nerve, or vascular injuries to any combination of these. External fixation of the humerus poses a significant risk to vascular and neural structures. Transportation casts are an acceptable alternative to external fixation and are described in the *Emergency War Surgery* handbook. Complex vascular repairs are not appropriate in settings requiring damage control. An alternative (shunting, ligation) should be considered. Although the damage associated with the extremity alone (ie, any combination of vascular, nerve, bone, or muscle injuries) may necessi-

tate amputation, a lesser combination of these injuries in an otherwise severely wounded patient may warrant consideration of amputation as well.

SUMMARY

Open humerus fractures resulting from gunshot wounds or blast injuries are very common. It is highly likely that every orthopaedic surgeon deployed to a combat support hospital (CSH) will use an external fixator for this injury. It is also probable that every general surgeon deployed to a CSH will encounter a vascular injury to the brachial artery associated with a humerus fracture. A thorough understanding of these injuries and the range of options to treat them are important.

SUGGESTED READING

Chapter 23: Extremity fractures. In: *Emergency War Surgery, Third United States Revision*. Washington, DC: Department of the Army, Office of The Surgeon General, Borden Institute; 2004.

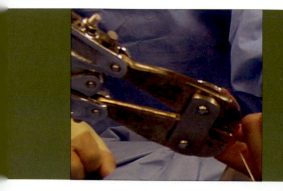

VII.6
Open Ulna Fracture

CASE PRESENTATION

This male patient, a host national, sustained multiple gunshot wounds to the chest, abdomen, right upper extremity, and left proximal forearm. He was admitted to the general surgery service of a combat support hospital (CSH) where he underwent laparotomy and multiple surgical procedures. A tube thoracostomy was inserted for management of hemopneumothorax. A right radial nerve palsy was noted. The orthopaedic surgery service was consulted intraoperatively for care of the soft-tissue wounds of his right arm and the open ulna fracture of his left arm (Fig. 1). Both were irrigated and debrided the day of injury. The ulna fracture was stabilized with an external fixator spanning the distal humerus to the ulna (Figs. 2 and 3). Treatment was prolonged and complicated. The arm wound and open ulna fracture were treated with wet-to-dry dressings soaked with Dakin's solution until the soft tissues were healed. Six weeks after injury, the patient returned to the operating room (OR) for definitive fracture care. Soft-tissue wounds were healed, the external fixator was removed, and an open reduction and internal fixation were performed. An iliac crest bone graft was harvested and placed at the fracture site (Fig. 4). The status of the patient's radial nerve palsy was followed on an outpatient basis. The patient performed range-of-motion exercises at home to keep his right elbow, wrist, and hand mobile. An orthoplast splint was fabricated to hold the wrist and fingers in extension. At last follow-up, the patient had a tingling sensation in the distribution of the superficial branch of the radial nerve.

TEACHING POINTS

1. This patient had multiple injuries requiring urgent surgery. Principles of Advanced Trauma Life Support (ATLS) were performed. He was then taken directly to the OR.
2. In this case of polytrauma, orthopaedic injuries are secondary. If the patient is considered stable enough to undergo further surgery, the orthopaedic surgeon is frequently called to address any orthopaedic injuries after the patient is already under anesthesia.
3. Wound control must be obtained before definitive fracture fixation is performed. The ability to cover orthopaedic implants is key to limiting wound contamination and infection of instrumentation.
4. The decision to operate on the extremity affected by radial nerve palsy injuries is difficult. There is no occupational therapy

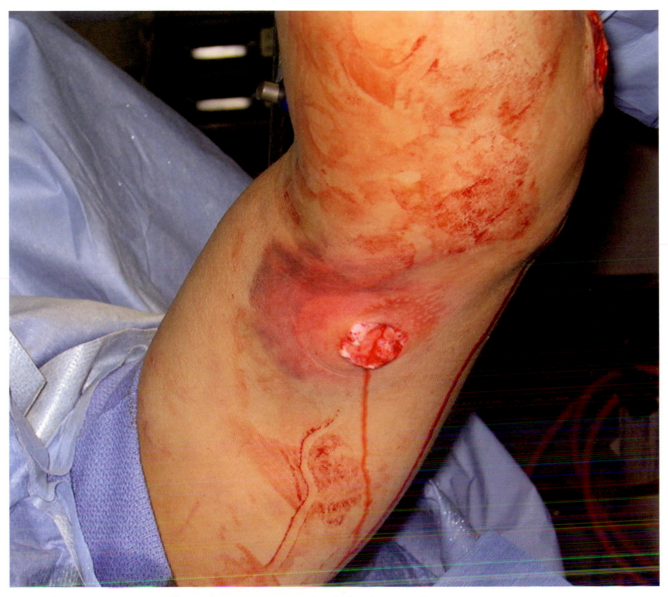

FIGURE 1. *Penetrating wounds are apparent proximal and distal to the elbow.*

provided by the host nation. Complex orthoses are not available. Considering these two factors, the decision to proceed with observation rather than perform an internal splinting procedure was made. The patient was informed that the nerve may recover, but it would take many months.

CLINICAL IMPLICATIONS

In the war zone, internal fixation of combat injuries is contraindicated. In this case, however, because the patient was a host national and was not evacuated, eventual definitive repair, which required internal fixation, became necessary. The following principles apply:

1. Wound control must be obtained before definitive fixation of fractures is performed.
2. The ability to cover the orthopaedic implants is key to limiting wound contamination and infection.

SUMMARY

This patient required prolonged inpatient and outpatient care. His treatment necessitated operative and postoperative management different from the typical patient treated at a CSH. Fractures that are the result of combat injuries are often complex and invariably open, making them difficult to treat in any circumstance. CSHs are not typically equipped

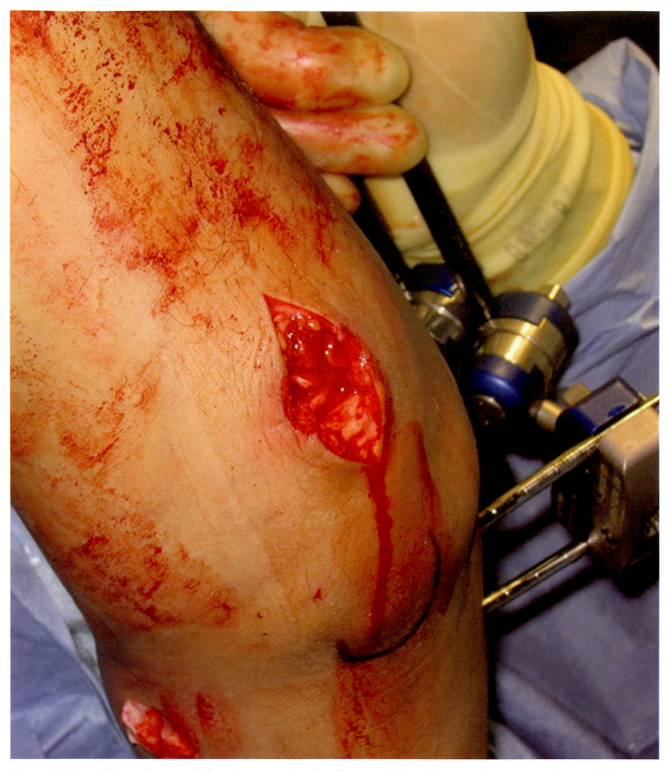

FIGURE 2. *Completion of external fixation spanning the elbow and joint. Entry and exit wounds are evident.*

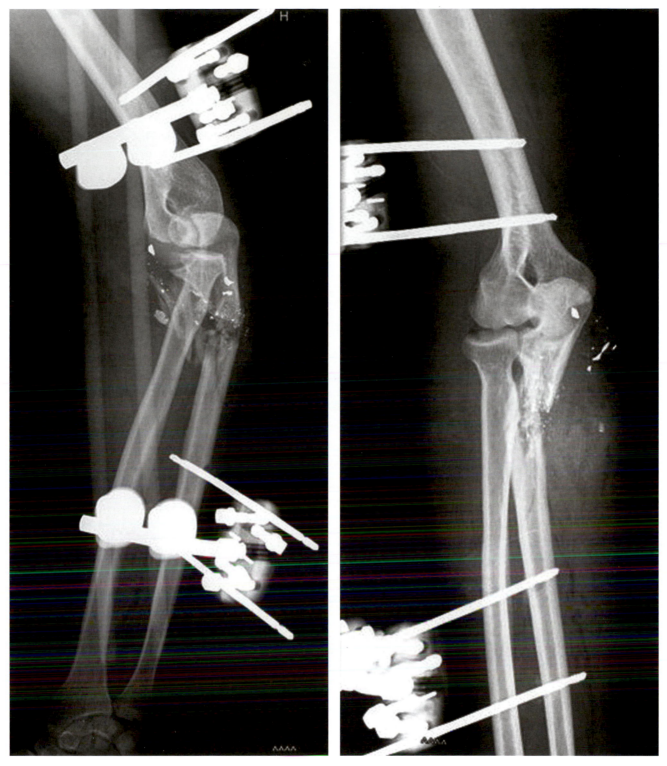

FIGURE 3. *Radiographs showing two views* (Left) *lateral;* (Right) *PA of distal humerus and forearm. Reduction accomplished by spanning the elbow with an external fixator.*

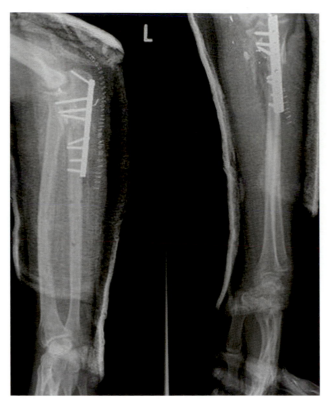

FIGURE 4. *Radiograph of fracture after internal fixation.*

with the resources, beds, and manpower necessary to render definitive repairs and comprehensive follow-up therapy. The surgeon must implement management in accordance with the given circumstances, with the understanding that his or her improvisation may differ considerably from stateside practice.

SUGGESTED READING

Chapter 23: Extremity fractures. In: *Emergency War Surgery, Third United States Revision.* Washington, DC: Department of the Army, Office of The Surgeon General, Borden Institute; 2004.

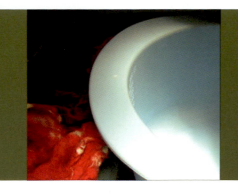

VII.7
Gunshot Wound of the Hand

CASE PRESENTATION

This male patient was cleaning a 9-mm handgun when the weapon discharged, resulting in a through-and-through injury to his left hand (Figs. 1 and 2). At the combat support hospital (CSH), the hand was neurologically intact, and no vascular injury was noted. There was an entrance wound in the palm and an exit wound on the dorsal side of the hand. Plain radiographs revealed a 2-cm bone loss of the fourth metacarpal (ring finger) (Fig. 3). The wound was irrigated and debrided. All loose bone fragments were removed. The ring finger metacarpal shaft was missing, as was the extensor mechanism. A Kirschner wire spacer was placed for stabilization (Fig. 4), and the wound was packed with wet-to-dry dressings soaked with Dakin's solution. A splint was applied, and intravenous antibiotics (cefazolin and gentamicin) were administered. On the hospital ward, the patient's hand was elevated in a stockinette. He was evacuated on postoperative day 1.

TEACHING POINTS

1. A hand wound must be thoroughly debrided and irrigated. All dead tissue and bone must be removed. Tissue, including skin, with marginal or questionable viability is left for subsequent evaluation to improve chances for an optimal outcome. A thorough physical examination is crucial to determine neurological and vascular status. At the time of surgery, it is important to document the damaged anatomical structures.

2. Bone defects in the hand are common injuries resulting from gunshot wounds or blast injuries. When attempting to stabilize fractures in the hand, a simple splint or Kirschner wire is usually sufficient. If multiple fingers are injured or if adjacent metacarpal bone defects are present, the fingers should be stabilized to help protect the soft tissue and vascular structures of the hand. If there is a substantial bone defect in the hand, the palm can fold over and compromise the blood supply to the fingers. This action could cause later injury, thereby limiting reconstructive options or necessitating amputation.

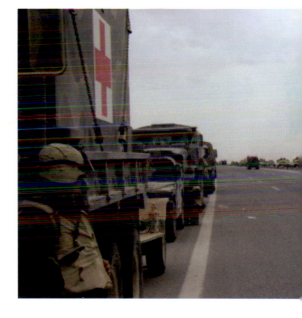

CLINICAL IMPLICATIONS

Even apparently minor wounds distal to the wrist crease may violate tendon sheaths and joints, resulting in serious deep space infection.

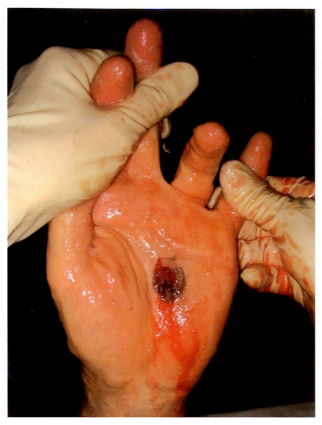

FIGURE 1. *Entrance wound on the palmar surface of the hand.*

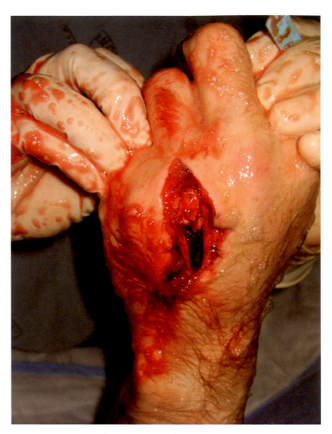

FIGURE 2. *Dorsal exit wound.*

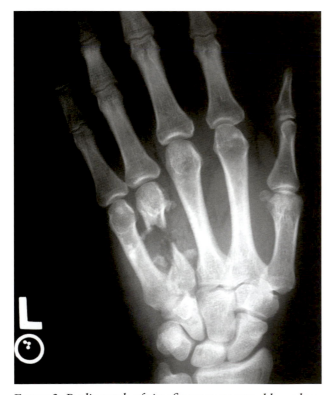

FIGURE 3. *Radiograph of ring finger metacarpal bone loss.*

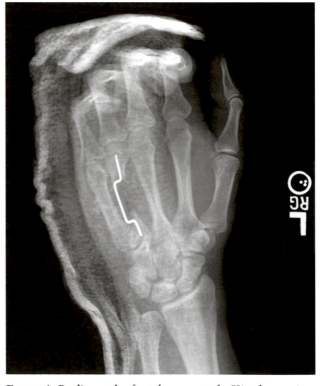

FIGURE 4. *Radiograph after placement of a Kirschner wire.*

IRRIGATION OF WAR WOUNDS

Irrigation of wounds is a common requirement of war surgery, and it prevents wound problems by removing debris, blood, and bacteria. Recent evidence challenges the current practice of routinely using high-pressure pulsatile lavage (HPPL) devices, and questions of fluids, additives, and volumes have been clarified.

Simple bulb irrigation or gravity irrigation is preferred. Although HPPL is fast, available, and easy to use in washing wounds, it also traumatizes tissue such that, at 2 days after HPPL, bacterial load rebounds more than gentler methods (eg, bulb syringe use). Gentler methods lead to the least rebound and are the least expensive and widely available. Large-bore, gravity-run tubing should be used, which is as gentle as bulb syringe, but is faster and accepts two bags at once. Traditional debridement should be performed in addition to irrigation. (See Chapter 22 of *Emergency War Surgery, Third United States Revision*.)

Research demonstrates that normal saline, sterile water, and potable tap water have similar usefulness and safety. The sterile isotonic solutions are readily available and remain the fluid of choice for irrigation. If unavailable, sterile water or potable tap water can be used.

No additive is recommended for routine irrigation of war wounds. Recommended, however, is warm saline in 3-L bags gravity-run as follows:
- 1 to 3 L for small-volume wounds,
- 4 to 8 L for moderate wounds, and
- 9 or more liters for large wounds with heavy contamination.

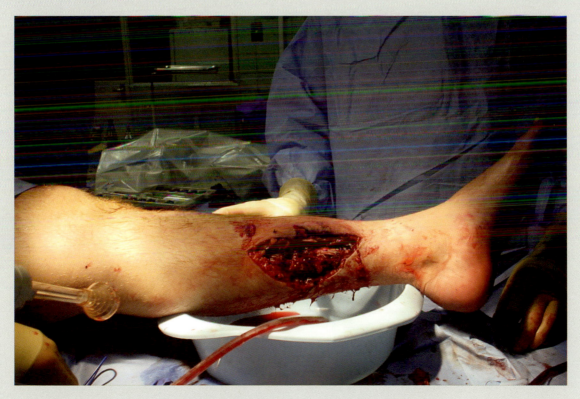

FIGURE 5. (Left)
*Compartments of
the hand.*

FIGURE 6. (Right)
*Hand fasciotomy
incisions.*

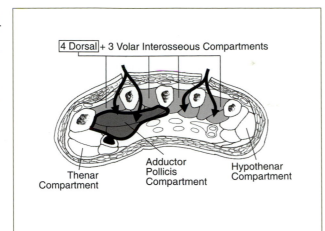

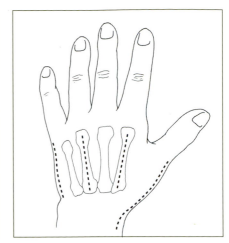

Infection involving the flexor synovial sheath of one finger can easily spread via the common synovial sheath to other fingers, the palm, and the thumb. The following principles are important in managing hand wounds:

1. Consider hand fasciotomies (Figs. 5 and 6) before evacuation.
2. Perform a thorough exploration of the area to define the extent of injury.
3. Preserve as much tissue as possible for future reconstruction.
4. Minimize debridement of tendons and preserve nerve tissue.
5. Do not amputate fingers, if possible.
6. Perform stabilization with Kirschner wires to preserve function, ensure patient comfort, and—if multiple fingers are involved—prevent injury during evacuation.
7. Cover exposed tendon, bone, and joints, if possible.

DAMAGE CONTROL

In patients who require urgent evacuation, careful splinting in a functional position is appropriate.

SUMMARY

Hand wounds are very common in the combat theater. Hands are unprotected by armor and are therefore exposed to wounding by gunshots, blasts, and thermal mechanisms. Early evaluation and appropriate treatment of these wounds can help preserve function and limit disability. Gloves can offer some protection against thermal injury.

SUGGESTED READING

Chapter 26: Injuries to the hands and feet. In: *Emergency War Surgery, Third United States Revision.* Washington, DC: Department of the Army, Office of The Surgeon General, Borden Institute; 2004.

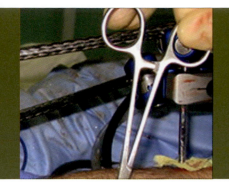

VII.8
Tibia Fracture With Compartment Syndrome

CASE PRESENTATION

This 20-year-old male sustained an open left tibia fracture as a result of a blast injury from a vehicle-borne, improvised explosive device (IED). He was taken to a combat support hospital (CSH), where a complete evaluation was performed. The only injuries identified were medial and lateral 3-cm wounds of the left leg (Figs. 1 and 2) with an underlying open tibia fracture (Fig. 3). No vascular or neurological injuries were noted on examination. The knee and ankle were nontender and without effusion. Leg compartments were soft, and there was no pain with passive range of motion of the toes. In the operating room, irrigation and debridement were performed using pulse lavage. Bone ends were curetted, and all loose bone was removed. An anteriorly positioned external fixator was placed using C-arm fluoroscopy guidance (Fig. 4). The leg compartments were tense. Subsequently, through two incisions, a four-compartment fasciotomy was performed. The medial and lateral incisions were connected to the traumatic wounds on both sides. Clinically, the diagnosis of compartment syndrome was confirmed, because the muscles bulged out when the compartments were released (Figs. 5 and 6). The wounds were dressed with wet-to-dry dressings soaked with Dakin's solution. Once on the hospital ward, the patient's leg was elevated. Intravenous antibiotics, including cefazolin and gentamicin, were administered. The operative dressing was not removed before the patient was evacuated on postoperative day 1. He underwent repeated irrigation and debridement at follow-on levels of care. Eventually, a wound infection was diagnosed at a stateside army medical center. Cultures were positive for *Acinetobacter baumannii* (most likely a battlefield contaminant obtained at the time of injury). This organism has been cultured repeatedly from wounds received in Iraq (see sidebar on page 284). Continued care was provided at the medical center.

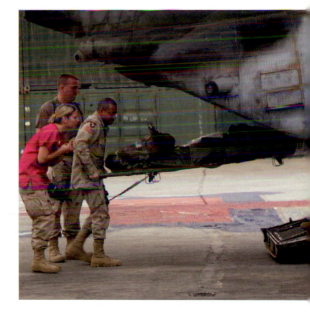

TEACHING POINTS

1. The injury this patient sustained is a very common one in the combat environment because the lower extremities are exposed and cannot be protected by body armor.
2. Compartment syndrome is a potentially catastrophic complication from a tibia fracture. If it is not diagnosed in a timely fashion, long-term disability will result. It is important to remember that physical examination of a trauma patient should be repeated frequently. The hallmarks of compartment syndrome are pain that is out of proportion

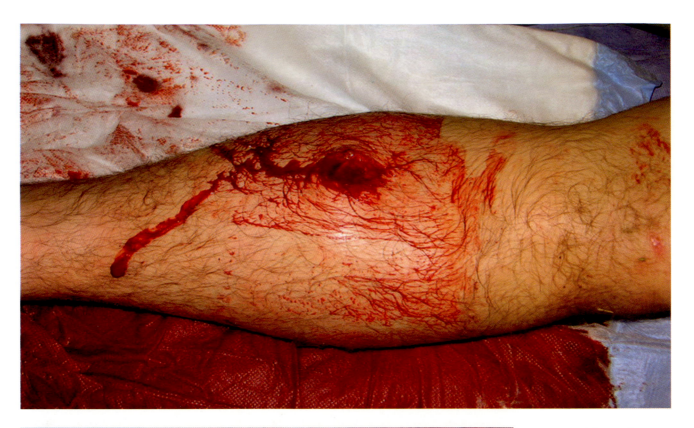

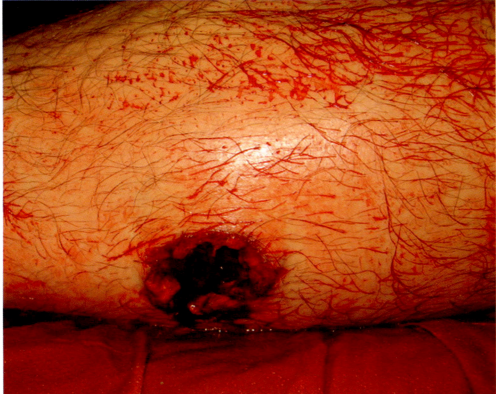

FIGURE 1. (Top Left)
Lower extremity wounds.

FIGURE 2. (Bottom Left)
Close-up of lower extremity wounds on admission.

FIGURE 3. (Top Right)
Radiographs of comminuted tibia fracture. Note soft-tissue free air.

FIGURE 4. (Bottom Right)
Radiographs of fracture reduced with external fixation.

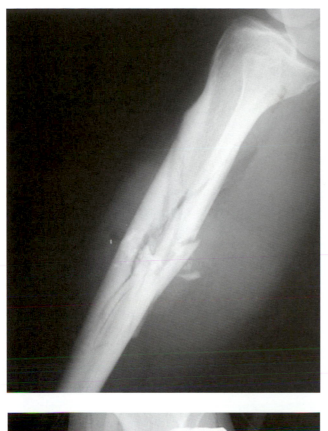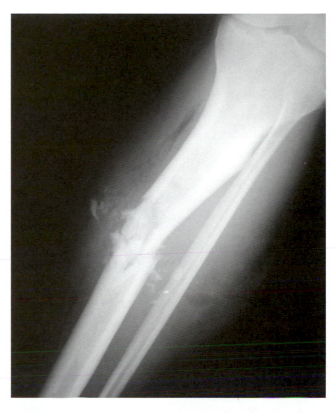

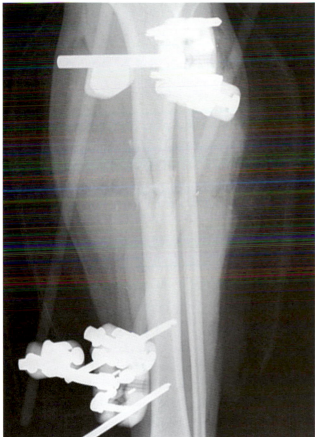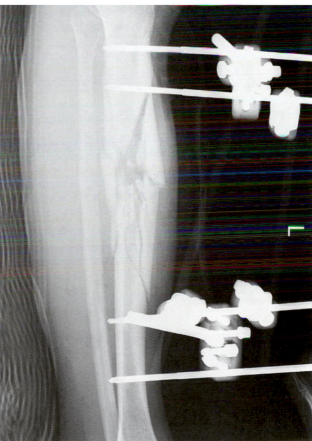

ACINETOBACTER AND WOUND INFECTIONS

Infection is a complication of battlefield injuries that can lead to significant morbidity and mortality. During the Vietnam War conflict, a 4% incidence of wound infection was reported despite 80% of wounds undergoing debridement/irrigation and 70% receiving antibiotics. Although the incidence of wound infection has not been determined for Operation Iraqi Freedom/Operation Enduring Freedom (OIF/OEF), it is unclear if it is higher than the 4% incidence noted during the Vietnam conflict.

First noted in April 2003, nosocomial, multidrug-resistant *Acinetobacter baumannii* infections have spread along the evacuation chain from medical facilities in Iraq, through hospitals in Europe, to the United States. After the onset of ground operations in Iraq, *A baumannii-calcoaceticus* complex (ABC) was recognized as an important bacterial pathogen infecting the wounds of casualties.

The initial report described 102 patients with ABC recovered from their blood cultures; 83% of these patients were from OIF/OEF. These numbers were in excess of historical norms.

Among patients admitted to Brooke Army Medical Center (San Antonio, Texas) from Iraq and Afghanistan, there were approximately 10 wound infections for every one patient with ABC bacteremia. Infections frequently involve burn casualties, as well as bone and soft-tissue infections. Although ABC is often considered a low virulent pathogen, its ability to develop broad-spectrum antimicrobial resistance to all modern antibiotics can lead to poor outcomes, especially in immunosuppressed patients. ABC is also of concern because it is often associated with nosocomial transmission of infection. Although the etiology of ABC has not been clearly elucidated, there is supporting evidence that nosocomial transmission was leading to the spread of the infection.

Although ABC's role as a pathogen was being determined among casualties of OIF/OEF, more virulent pathogens that had classically been associated with battlefield trauma—such as *Pseudomonas aeruginosa*, *Klebsiella pneumoniae*, and *Staphylococcus aureus*—were also being seen. These pathogens are notable for their more destructive properties and greater propensity to result in poor outcomes. Even more troubling, however, is the multidrug-resistant patterns of these pathogens, including methicillin-resistant *S aureus* (MRSA), extended-spectrum b-lactamase-producing *K pneumoniae*, and multidrug-resistant *P aeruginosa*.

—CLINTON K. MURRAY, MD, MAJ, MC, US Army

to the injury and pain with passive range of motion of the toes. In a combat environment, this is entirely a clinical diagnosis.

3. If at any time the examination results are consistent with compartment syndrome, an urgent fasciotomy must be performed. If all operating rooms are in use, this procedure can be done in the intensive care unit using local anesthesia and sedation. A person with impending compartment syndrome must never be moved via the medical evacuation system. If compartment syndrome is even a slight possibility, perform fasciotomies.

CLINICAL IMPLICATIONS

1. The possibility of compartment syndrome must be constantly reassessed at each stage of the evacuation process.
2. The need for repeated irrigation and debridement of wounds throughout the evacuation process is critical to keeping wounds clean.
3. Battlefield contaminants—such as *Acinetobacter*—may become apparent at any time and produce infection. These contaminants affect hospital treatment, timing of reconstructive procedures, and wound coverage.

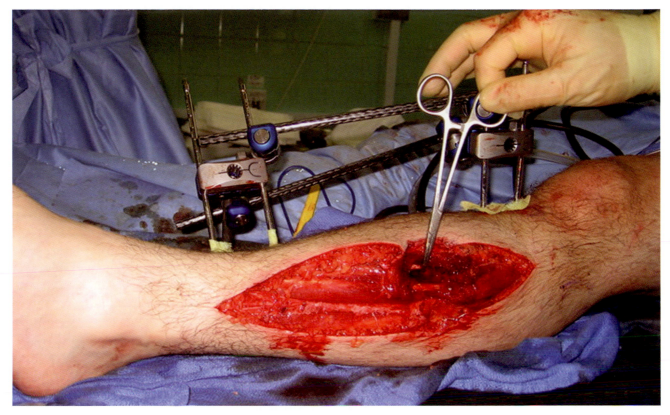

FIGURE 5. *Lateral view of extremity after a four-compartment fasciotomy.*

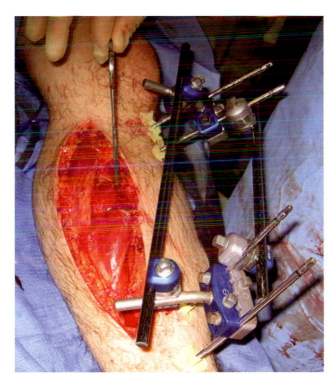

FIGURE 6. *Medial view of lower extremity after a four-compartment fasciotomy.*

DAMAGE CONTROL

Four-compartment fasciotomy is a primary damage control technique. All general and orthopaedic surgeons working at level II and level III medical treatment facilities should be able to perform this procedure.

SUMMARY

This case represents the standard approach to war wounds that results in an open tibia fracture, including irrigation and debridement, external fixation, and medial and lateral fasciotomies.

SUGGESTED READING

Chapter 22: Soft-tissue injuries. In: *Emergency War Surgery, Third United States Revision*. Washington, DC: Department of the Army, Office of The Surgeon General, Borden Institute; 2004: 22.12–22.13.

Chapter 23: Extreme fractures. In: *Emergency War Surgery, Third United States Revision*. Washington, DC: Department of the Army, Office of The Surgeon General, Borden Institute; 2004.

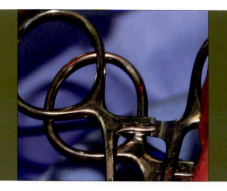

VII.9
Traumatic Below-Knee Amputation

CASE PRESENTATION

This 28-year-old male sustained an injury to his right leg from a high-energy blast. A field tourniquet (Combat Application Tourniquet System [CATS]; see sidebar on page 288) was placed above the injury. His clothing was saturated with blood. Removal of his combat boots revealed a significant, grossly contaminated, soft-tissue injury and a poorly perfused foot. Physical examination revealed a cool, paralyzed, insensate foot with no palpable or Doppler pulses (Figs. 1 and 2). An initial survey revealed no other injuries. Plain radiographs revealed fractures of the tibia and fibula, with extensive comminution and bone loss. The patient underwent surgery 1 hour and 40 minutes after the tourniquet had been placed. A pneumatic thigh tourniquet was then applied, and the field tourniquet was removed. Further exploration revealed that all major nerves and vessels supplying the foot had been severed. The decision was then made to proceed with a formal, below-knee amputation (Fig. 3). An open, length-preserving amputation was performed at the most distal level of viable soft tissue. After appropriate muscle debulking and hemostasis, skin traction was achieved by using three loosely applied 0-Prolene trauma sutures (Fig. 4). The limb was then covered with a soft dressing, and the knee was held in full extension with a long leg splint that supported the distal end and secured the knee anteriorly and posteriorly. The patient was evacuated to a level IV medical treatment facility within 12 hours of initial presentation.

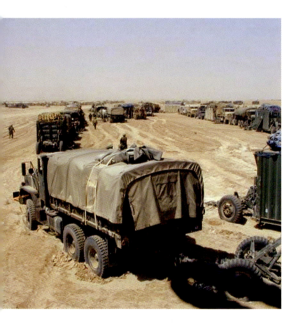

TEACHING POINTS

1. High-energy blast and gunshot wounds commonly result in severe soft-tissue loss. These wounds are often dramatic, so much so as to distract medical personnel from other life-threatening wounds. Adequate patient exposure and careful attention are necessary to determine the full extent of all injuries.

2. In this case, an exploration that reveals transection of major arteries and nerves is an absolute indication for amputation. Often, surgeons will undertake heroic measures to salvage a limb that will ultimately cause the patient more severe problems or result in death. Vascular grafts should not be performed on a paralyzed, insensate extremity with extensive soft-tissue loss.

3. Amputation is a common battlefield operation. All general and orthopaedic surgeons should be familiar with upper and lower extremity anatomy and amputation techniques.

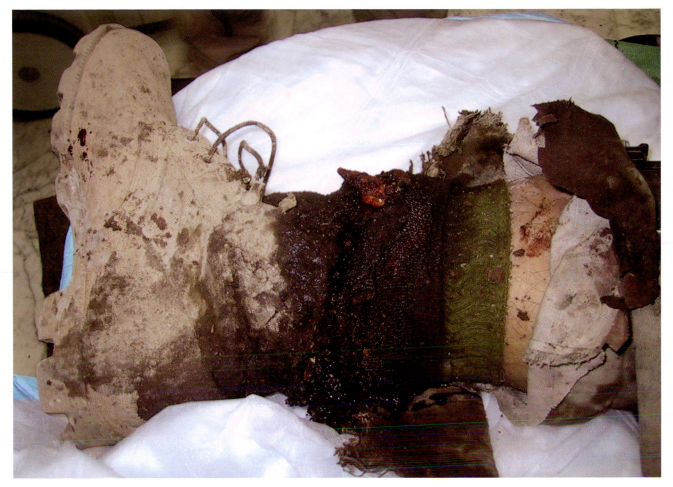

FIGURE 1. *Presentation of a seriously injured extremity.*

CLINICAL IMPLICATIONS

Surgeons in combat operations will see high-energy blast injuries that result in traumatic amputation. In treating these kinds of injuries, combat surgeons should be cognizant of the following principles:

1. High-energy blast or gunshot wounds commonly result in severe, soft-tissue loss.
2. Adequate patient exposure is necessary to determine the full extent of injury.
3. Field tourniquets applied correctly can save a patient's life.
4. Noting the timing when applying a field tourniquet is an important consideration in patient management, because it can have an effect on limb salvage.
5. An examination that shows irreparable transection of major arteries is an indication for amputation.
6. Severe soft-tissue and bony injuries to the extremity precluding functional recovery are indications for amputation.
7. All dead or necrotic tissue must be removed.
8. Hemostasis is achieved by double-tying the major vessels.
9. Some form of skin traction should be used to preserve skin length.
10. The knee should be immobilized in extension.
11. Debridement should be performed at the lowest viable level of soft tissue, leaving determination of the definitive or revised level of amputation to staff at a higher level facility.

DAMAGE CONTROL

In these types of cases, appropriately applied field tourniquets are lifesaving (see sidebar on page 288).

SUMMARY

Unfortunately, traumatic amputations are common and are the most severe limb injuries seen. This case illustrates the basic techniques of caring for a patient with a traumatic below-knee amputation.

COMBAT APPLICATION TOURNIQUET SYSTEM (CATS)

CATS is a one-handed tourniquet that completely occludes arterial and venous blood flow of an extremity in the event of a traumatic wound with significant hemorrhage. The CATS uses a windlass system with a free-moving internal band to provide circumferential pressure to the extremity. Once tightened and bleeding has stopped, the windlass is locked in place. A Velcro strap is then applied to secure the windlass during casualty evacuation. The combat application tourniquet (CAT)—also known as the one-hand tourniquet— differs from traditional tourniquets because it can be put on by the soldier with one hand and does not require the use of sticks for tightening.

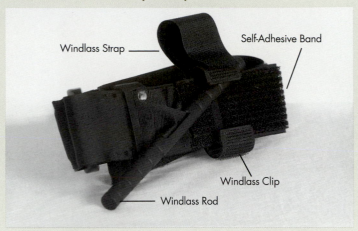

Courtesy of Phil Durango, LLC (Golden, Colorado).

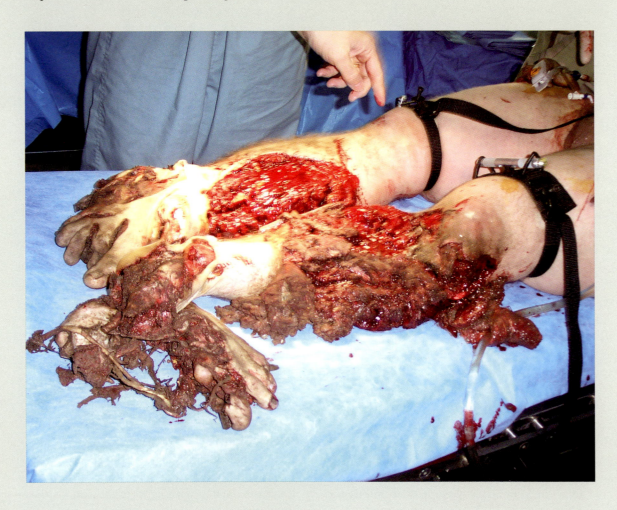

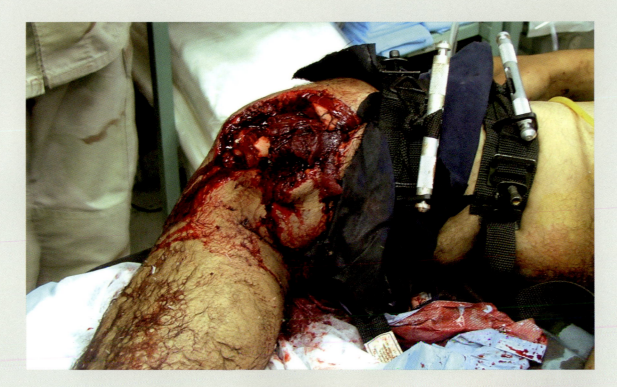

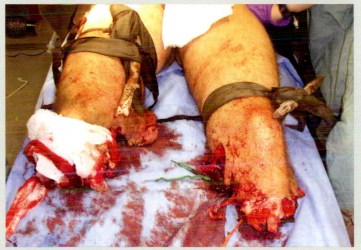

This patient survived.

Tourniquet use in Operation Iraqi Freedom has been lifesaving for combat casualties. The CAT has been the most effective field tourniquet, both in laboratory testing and clinical experience. Improvised tourniquets are less effective and are only recommended when no scientifically designed tourniquets are available, as evidenced in the casualty data. Prehospital tourniquet use has improved survival 23%, relative to emergency department use, and use before shock onset has improved survival 90% relative to use after shock onset. The rates of complications (eg, compartment syndrome) have been low. Despite the policy of encouragement of tourniquet use for limb bleeding, in 1 year 10 patients arrived dead at a Baghdad combat support hospital (CSH) with isolated limb exsanguinations. Use before extrication and transportation is recommended. For limbs of greater girth and tourniquets of lesser width, side-by-side use of additional tourniquets improved effectiveness if one tourniquet was not effective. Historically, there was only one first-aid device, the Thomas splint, that improved survival for limb-injured patients. Now there are data from Operation Iraqi Freedom that show that tourniquets also save lives.

—JOHN F. KRAGH, MD, COL, MC, US Army

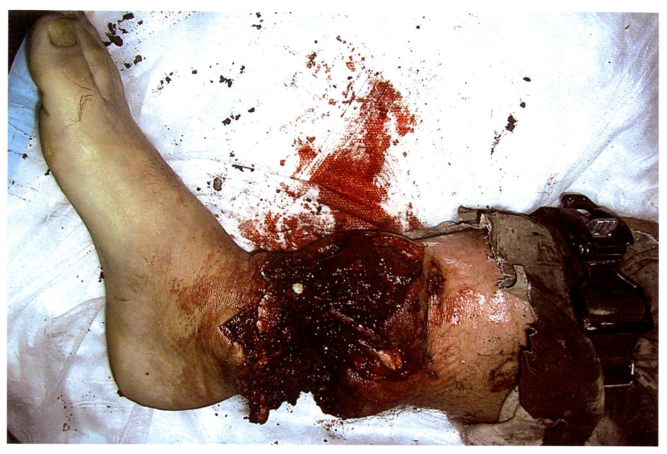

FIGURE 2. *Tissue damage is apparent. Note that the tourniquet is still in place before surgery.*

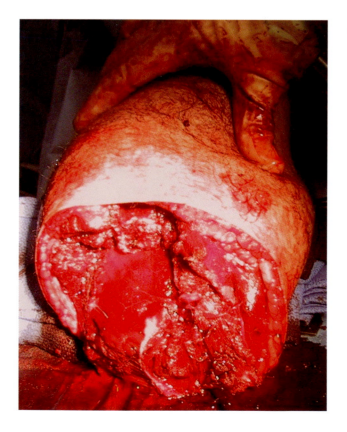

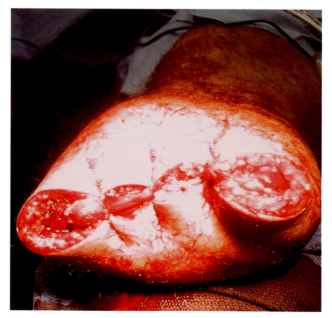

FIGURE 3. (Left) *End-on view of leg at the lowest level of viable soft tissue.*

FIGURE 4. (Right) *Skin traction obtained by using three interrupted sutures.*

SUGGESTED READING

Bosse MJ, MacKenzie E, et al. A prospective evaluation of the clinical utility of the lower-extremity injury-severity scores. *J Bone Joint Surg Am*. 2001;83-A:3–14.

Beekley AC, Sebesta JA, et al. Prehospital tourniquet use in Operation Iraqi Freedon: Effect on hemorrhage control and outcomes. *J Trauma*. 2008;64:S28–S37.

Chapter 22: Soft-tissue injuries. In: *Emergency War Surgery, Third United States Revision*. Washington, DC: Department of the Army, Office of The Surgeon General, Borden Institute; 2004.

Chapter 25: Amputations. In: *Emergency War Surgery, Third United States Revision*. Washington, DC: Department of the Army, Office of The Surgeon General, Borden Institute; 2004.

Dougherty PJ. Wartime amputee care. In: Smith DG, Michael JW, Bowker JH, eds. *Atlas of Amputations and Limb Deficiencies*. Rosemont, IL: American Academy of Orthopaedic Surgeons; 2004: 77–97.

Heppenstall RB, Scott R, et al. A comparative study of the tolerance of skeletal muscle to ischemia. Tourniquet application compared with acute compartment syndrome. *J Bone Joint Surg Am*. 1986;68:820–828.

Kragh JF, Walters TJ, et al. Practical use of emergency tourniquets to stop bleeding in major limb trauma. *J Trauma*. 2008;64:S38–S50.

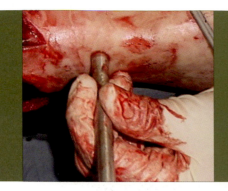

VII.10
Umbrella Effect of a Landmine Blast

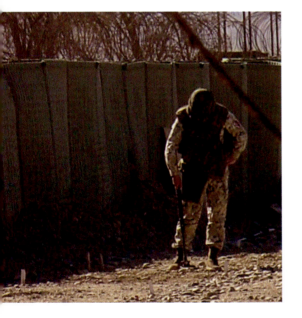

CASE PRESENTATION

A 23-year-old male arrived at the Forward Surgical Team (FST) facility after a landmine blast to his right upper extremity. Exact details surrounding this blast were unknown, but the injury was most likely caused by manipulation of the device. On initial evaluation, the patient's airway was patent, and breath sounds were equal bilaterally. His pulse was 118 beats per minute, and his blood pressure was 110/98 mm Hg. With the exception of the right upper extremity, he was fully intact neurologically. Complete exposure revealed a mangled right upper extremity with profuse arterial and venous bleeding (Figs. 1 and 2). Direct pressure failed to control the bleeding, and a brachial artery pressure point was applied. Following this action, a standard blood pressure cuff was placed on the upper arm and inflated to 150 mm Hg. With bleeding temporarily controlled, attention was focused on the secondary examination, which revealed no other injuries. While the patient was being resuscitated with isotonic crystalloid, the arm was examined carefully. Given that this was a high-velocity injury—with significant involvement of soft tissue (skin and muscle), bone, nerves, and blood vessels—the surgeon proceeded with primary amputation, using an approach that preserved as much soft tissue as possible. This procedure was followed with daily operative debridements for 4 days. Once the wound had fully demarcated and was completely clean, the amputation was closed just proximal to the elbow joint.

TEACHING POINTS

1. Typically, landmines are associated with an umbrella effect, in which the blast tears the muscle and soft tissue off the bone. This results in the injury extending more proximally than clinically apparent. This is illustrated in Fig. 3 with a lower extremity injury.
2. Decreased pulse pressure indicated the presence of class II hemorrhagic shock. A common mistake is to consider only the systolic blood pressure, which does not typically decrease until class III or class IV shock (see Table 1). Early initiation of aggressive resuscitation prevented the development of a more complex state of shock and is associated with a less intense systemic inflammatory response and improved outcome.
3. Historically, direct pressure over a wound is the first step in obtaining control of hemorrhage in all types of extremity trauma. The

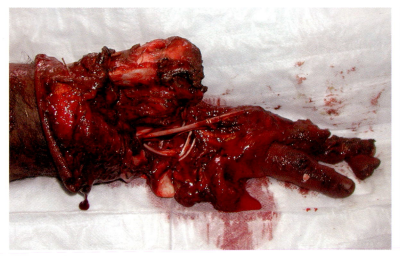

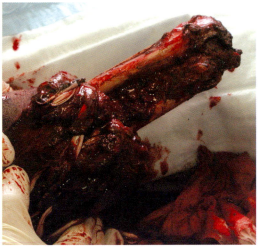

FIGURE 1. *Condition of right forearm on admission.*

FIGURE 2. *Severely mangled forearm with profuse arterial and venous bleeding.*

umbrella effect from a landmine blast frequently renders this action ineffective. The use of a blood pressure cuff proximal to the injury inflated to a pressure above the patient's systolic pressure is an effective means of control. In the forward setting, a simple tourniquet is also effective.

4. Although every reasonable attempt should be made to salvage an arm and hand, a primary amputation should be considered, when there is extensive involvement of three of the following components:

   a. Skin and soft tissue.
   b. Bone.
   c. Nerve.
   d. Blood vessel.

The presence of significant shock and the inability to provide complex rehabilitative care should also be considered.

5. Because the injury is typically more proximal, a radiograph should be obtained early in order to ensure that the level of amputation does not leave a proximal bony injury.

CLINICAL IMPLICATIONS

1. Historically, these types of injuries have been treated with guillotine amputation in a circular fashion, leaving a flat-ended stump that can be revised at a later date by using standard amputation closure techniques. In the setting of blast injuries, this technique results in a significantly shorter residual limb and more limited function. The current technique of amputation is the open-length preserving amputation, in which all viable soft tissue is preserved. To save length, any shape or form of a viable muscle or skin flap should be preserved. Therefore, the surgeon should save all potentially viable tissue. Further debridement can be performed during subsequent operations. Once the wound is clean, the amputation is closed using an approach that makes use of all residual tissue.

2. A common mistake is premature closure of the amputation site. The wound should never be closed during the first operation. Frequently, it requires serial operative debridements over a period of several days to a week.

DAMAGE CONTROL

In the unstable patient, immediate primary amputation may be lifesaving. If it appears that the extremity can be salvaged, blood supply to the extremity can be reestablished rapidly using a vascular shunt. This technique allows time for harvest of a vein graft and bony fixation without incurring a greater ischemic insult.

SUMMARY

A landmine blast leads to an umbrella effect in which the soft tissues, vessels, and nerves are stripped from the bone. This shredding results in a more proximal injury than may be clinically apparent and requires a reasoned approach to amputation.

HETEROTOPIC OSSIFICATION IN COMBAT-RELATED AMPUTATIONS

Heterotopic ossification (HO) refers to the formation of mature, lamellar bone in nonosseous tissue. It has proven to be a common specter in combat-injured soldiers from Operation Enduring Freedom (Afghanistan) and Operation Iraqi Freedom. Although occasionally noted following open fractures and complex soft-tissue injuries, HO most frequently occurs and becomes clinically problematic in traumatic and combat-related amputations because of the often compromised soft-tissue envelope and the forces transmitted to affected regions of the residual limb (Fig. 1). Previous mentions of HO in combat-related amputations are limited to anecdotal reports from historical conflicts, and it appears to have been conspicuously absent in American casualties of the Vietnam War.

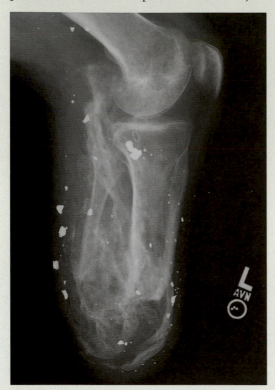

FIGURE 1. *Lateral radiograph of a traumatic transtibial amputation secondary to an improvised explosive device (IED) demonstrating severe HO throughout the residual limb.*

More than one-half of all combat-related amputees from the current conflicts in Southwest Asia have developed HO in their terminal residual limbs. The prevalence of HO is 63% in amputations with adequate radiographic follow-up.[1] The critical risk factors for HO formation in this population are a blast mechanism of injury and a final amputation level within the initial zone of injury. Amputation level within the zone of injury is also predictive of HO magnitude and severity (Fig. 2). However, frequent concomitant injury proximal to amputations, coupled with a desire to maintain functional residual limb length and joint levels, make proximal revision above the zone of injury impractical. For these reasons, we do not advocate it as a routine practice. Prolonged exposure to subatmospheric pressure dressings (wound VACs), serial pulsatile lavage, occult traumatic brain injury, and gross bacterial contamination of wounds have all been theorized as potential inciting factors to HO formation in amputees.

Given this high prevalence of HO, utilization of both clinically proven modalities (eg, nonsteroidal antiinflammatory drugs [NSAIDs] and radiotherapy) and theoretical prophylactic modalities (eg, etidronate, vitamin K antagonists, and corticosteroids) is appealing in the treatment of combat-related amputees. However, at present, medical contraindications (eg, concomitant multisystem trauma or long bone fractures, bleeding risks, and compromised immune system) and logistical barriers preclude their routine utilization early in the postinjury process of care when they would be most efficacious.

Once HO is present in a residual limb, no treatment is required for asymptomatic lesions. When present, symptoms usually consist of focal residual limb pain with activity, with or without associated skin breakdown. Symptomatic HO is virtually always palpable within the residual limb. Nonoperative management of symptomatic ectopic bone consists of medication adjustments, activity modification, and serial liner and socket modifications in an effort to off-load affected regions. Lesions remain asymptomatic, and conservative measures are successful in approximately 85% of amputees with HO.

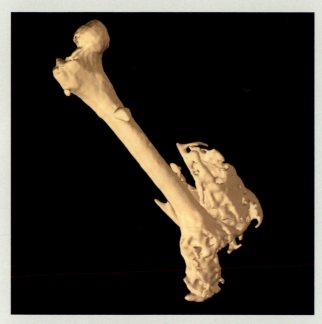

When nonoperative management fails, surgical candidates should be counseled on the frequent need for myodesis takedown and formal amputation revision in conjunction with surgical excision of lesions, as well as an approximately 25% incidence of postoperative wound complications. Nonetheless, relatively early (median: 6 months) operative excision of symptomatic lesions has been successful, with good clinical results and no symptomatic recurrences to date in more than 40 excisions. Although our low overall recurrence rate precludes a statistical demonstration of efficacy, we advocate perioperative recurrence prophylaxis with NSAIDs and/or external beam radiation. Ongoing and future research may further elucidate causative factors, the specific cells and chemokine signals responsible, and a practicable primary prophylactic regimen for the prevention of HO in amputations.

—MAJ BENJAMIN KYLE POTTER, MD

FIGURE 2. *Three-dimensional CT reconstruction of a transfemoral amputation, within the zone of injury, secondary to blunt trauma. Severe HO is present in the terminal residual limb.*

1. Potter BK, Burns TC, et al. Heterotopic ossification following traumatic and combat-related amputations. Prevalence, risk factors, and preliminary results of excision. *J Bone Joint Surg Am.* 2007;89:476–486.

TABLE 1. *Classes of Shock*

CLINICAL SIGNS	CLASS I	CLASS II	CLASS III	CLASS IV
Heart rate	< 100	> 100	> 120	> 140
Systolic blood pressure	Normal	Normal	Decreased	Decreased
Pulse pressure	Normal/increased	Decreased	Decreased	Decreased
Respiratory rate	14–20	20–30	30–40	> 35
Urine output (mL/hr)	> 30	20–30	5–15	Negligible
Mental status	Slightly anxious	Mildly anxious	Anxious, confused	Confused lethargic
% Blood volume loss	Up to 15%	15%–30%	30%–40%	> 40%
Blood loss (mL, 70-kg adult)	Up to 750 mL	750–1,000 mL	1,500–2,000 mL	> 2,000 mL

Adapted with permission from the American College of Surgeons, Committee on Trauma. Advanced Trauma Life Support for Doctors—Student Course Manual. 6th ed. Chicago, Ill: ACS; 1997: 98.

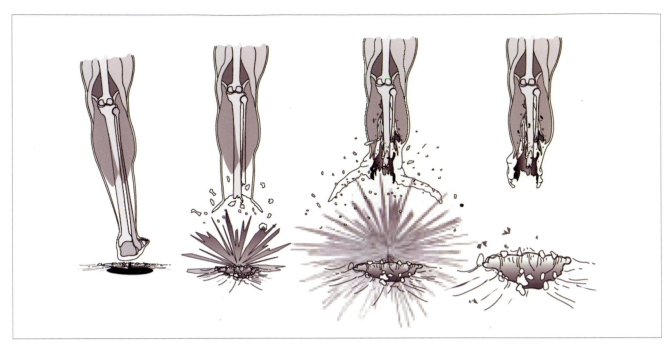

FIGURE 3. *"Umbrella" mechanisms of injuries caused by antipersonnel landmines.*

SUGGESTED READING

Chapter 1: Weapons effects and parachute injuries. In: *Emergency War Surgery, Third United States Revision.* Washington, DC: Department of the Army, Office of The Surgeon General, Borden Institute; 2004.

Chapter 6: Hemorrhage control. In: *Emergency War Surgery, Third United States Revision.* Washington, DC: Department of the Army, Office of The Surgeon General, Borden Institute; 2004.

Chapter 25: Amputations. In: *Emergency War Surgery, Third United States Revision.* Washington, DC: Depart-ment of the Army, Office of The Surgeon General, Borden Institute; 2004.

Gray R. *War Wounds: Basic Surgical Management—The Principles and Practice of the Surgical Management of Wounds Produced by Missiles or Explosions.* Geneva, Switzerland: International Committee of the Red Cross; 1994.

Johansen K, Daines M, et al. Objective criteria accurately predict amputation following lower extremity trauma. *J Trauma.* 1990;30:568.

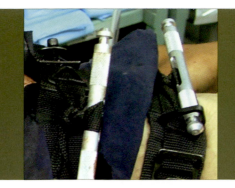

VII.11
Penetrating Injury of the Left Foot

CASE PRESENTATION

An 11-year-old host nation male presented 36 hours after sustaining a blast injury to his left foot during combat operations in a remote area of the country. On evaluation, there was significant gross contamination and soft-tissue damage with a medial longitudinal laceration deep to the first metatarsal. There was also a plantar soft-tissue avulsion through the plantar fascia and a lateral transverse laceration deep to the base of the fifth metatarsal (Figs. 1 and 2). Vascular and neurological integrity were demonstrated on physical examination with the assistance of a translator. Radiographs revealed no bony injury. The patient was taken to the operating room where he underwent meticulous debridement and irrigation, as well as undermining of soft tissues to adequately cover bony and fascial structures. Initially, a wound VAC device was placed medially. He was given intravenous antibiotics with broad-spectrum aerobic and anaerobe coverage for 72 hours. After 3 days, more debridement and irrigation were performed, and wet-to-dry dressing changes were initiated. The patient was then placed on oral antibiotics for 14 days. At 3 months, the foot showed excellent healing, was sensate, and was well perfused (Figs. 3 and 4).

TEACHING POINTS

1. Soft-tissue injuries are very common either as the result of blast injuries or gunshot wounds. All contaminating debris and devascularized tissue must be removed and the wound irrigated liberally. Exposed fibrous and collagenous tissues must be covered ultimately to prevent chronic infection. Wound VACs are excellent devices to promote healing and granulation tissue. However, in the case of small irregular wounds, wound VACs may cause maceration if improperly placed. Wet-to-dry dressings can promote excellent healing. Epithelialization will ultimately result in minimal scarring.

2. In this patient, the initial concern was the prolonged exposure to gross contamination, the extent of soft-tissue injury, and the exposed structures. Strict adherence to accepted principles produced excellent clinical results.

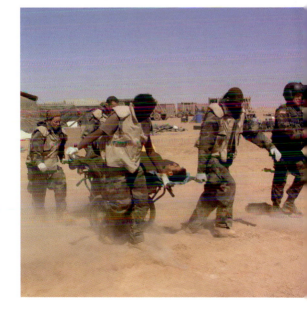

CLINICAL IMPLICATIONS

1. Combat surgeons frequently see soft-tissue injuries with varying degrees of contamination, sometimes many days following the acute injury.

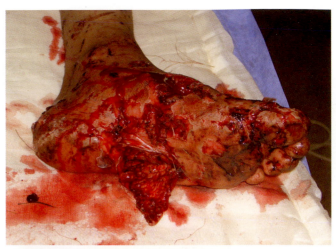

FIGURE 1. (Top)
The foot on presentation had significant soft-tissue injury.

FIGURE 2. (Middle)
Another view of the foot on presentation.

FIGURE 3. (Bottom)
Foot is healing.

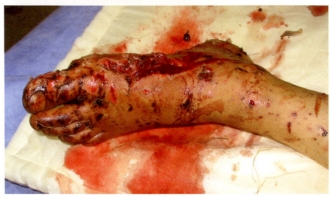

2. Generally, host nation patients require definitive treatment. Therefore, soft-tissue stabilization and healing are entirely managed at a level III medical treatment facility.

3. Surgeons need to perform meticulous debridement of the wounds, as well as manage the healing processes.

DAMAGE CONTROL

Often patients with life-threatening injuries concurrently present with these types of soft-tissue injuries. Washout with debridement and wet-to-dry dressing changes remains a safe, effective treatment for these injuries.

SUMMARY

This case demonstrates the effectiveness of secondary intention healing in soft-tissue injuries. In this case, a patient with a serious foot injury made a good, functional recovery with adequate washout, debridement, and dressing changes.

SUGGESTED READING

Chapter 22: Soft-tissue injuries. In: *Emergency War Surgery, Third United States Revision*. Washington, DC: Department of the Army, Office of The Surgeon General, Borden Institute; 2004.

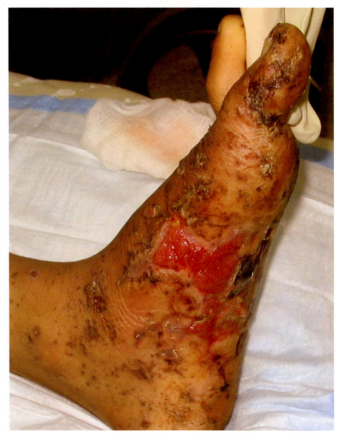

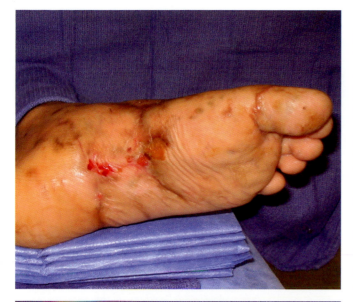

WET-TO-DRY DRESSINGS AND WOUND HEALING

Wet-to-dry dressings are used if the wound is infected or if it is not stitched closed. Wet dressings (gauze that is usually saline soaked) are put inside the wound, and dry dressings are put on top of the wound to prevent drying and contamination. When the wet dressing dries, it sticks to the debris in the wound. When the dressing is pulled off, it cleans out the wound. In this way, wet-to-dry dressings can be used to help promote wound healing because they:

- support autolytic debridement (the body's own capacity to lyse and dissolve necrotic tissue),
- absorb exudate, and
- trap bacteria in the gauze.

Moist environments have been proven to aid in:

- reepithelialization,
- wound healing, and
- shortened healing time.

Wet-to-dry dressings:

- require more intense wound care,
- can adhere to healthy granulation tissue if dries,
- can injure healthy epithelial cells and slow down the healing process, and
- may leave lint or fiber residue in the wound.

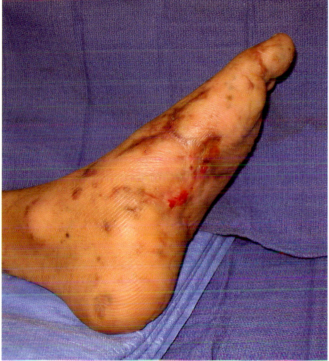

FIGURE 4. (Top and Bottom) *Later stages of healing.*

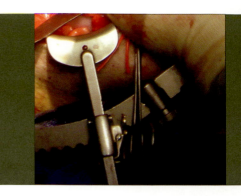

VII.12
High-Energy Gunshot Wound to the Forearm

CASE PRESENTATION

An Iraqi Army male sustained a high-velocity (see sidebar on page 23) gunshot wound to the right forearm. On presentation, he reported pain in the right forearm and denied any numbness or paresthesias. Examination revealed an 8 x 6 cm oval wound on the dorsoradial right forearm, with a thin skin bridge in the middle (Fig. 1), as well as a subcentimeter wound over the proximal-ulnar border of the forearm. There were numerous bone fragments visible in the wound, and he was unable to radially deviate his wrist. The radial, ulnar, median, and anterior interosseous nerves had intact motor function. Sensation was grossly intact, except for a small area on the dorsoradial aspect of the hand. There was a 2+ radial pulse, and the hand was well perfused. Radiographs of the right forearm showed a severely comminuted mid-to-distal one third radial shaft fracture with approximately 8 to 10 cm of segmental bone loss. In addition, there was an oblique midshaft ulna fracture with some shortening and displacement (Fig. 2). In the emergency department, the patient was given intravenous antibiotics and tetanus. He was taken to the operating room where he underwent debridement and irrigation of the open fractures. The small skin bridge was excised, and the wound was extended to enhance exposure in the zone of injury. Numerous bone fragments were removed from the wound bed because they were not attached to any soft tissue. The extensor carpi radialis longus and brevis tendons were transected and primarily repaired. The radial artery was patent, and the dorsal sensory branch of the radial nerve was also intact. A wrist spanning external fixator was placed with two pins in the index finger metacarpal and two pins in the radial shaft (Fig. 3). The surgically created wound was loosely closed over a drain, and the remaining soft tissue defect was covered with a soft dressing. Postoperative radiographs showed that the radius had a 10-cm segmental defect. The patient returned to the operating room on hospital day 3 for definitive treatment of the forearm fractures. The ulna fracture was approached along the subcutaneous border of the ulna, and open reduction internal fixation was performed with a nine-hole Synthes, 3.5-mm locking limited contact dynamic compression plate. Following stable osteosynthesis of the ulna fracture, a volar Henry approach was performed to address the distal radius fracture. The distal radius was examined, and there was intraarticular extension of the fracture into the scaphoid fossa. A single 3.5-mm cortical screw

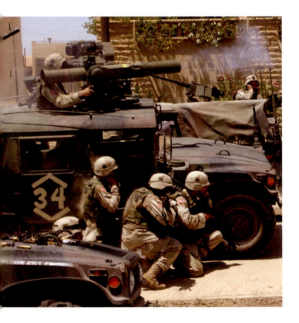

was placed in lag fashion to stabilize the radial styloid fragment prior to additional internal fixation. The distal portion of the ulna was exposed, and a distal ulna osteotomy was performed proximal to the distal radioulnar joint. The osteotomized portion of the distal ulna was tapered to enhance fixation of the ulna to the radius. The forearm was placed in neutral position, and bony continuity, radial height, and volar tilt were reestablished. A seven-hole Synthes, low-profile distal radius locking plate was used to secure the residual distal radius to the ulnar shaft, thereby creating a one-bone forearm (Figs. 4 and 5). The external fixator was removed, and the dorsal soft-tissue wound was closed with interrupted sutures. The remaining volar soft-tissue defect was covered with a split-thickness skin graft (STSG) taken from the ipsilateral thigh. A wound VAC was placed over the STSG and was set to 75 mm Hg in continuous mode. Dressings were removed 5 days after surgery, and there was 100% take of the STSG. The patient was discharged from the hospital, and he elected to follow-up with a physician in the Iraqi healthcare system.

TEACHING POINTS

1. A thorough physical examination must include detailed evaluation of wrist and hand function. In addition, a complete neurovascular examination must be performed to evaluate for any potential deficits, because they can potentially alter treatment decisions.
2. Radiographs of the injured extremity should be obtained in orthogonal planes, and the proximal and distal joints should be completely visualized.
3. Complex reconstruction of segmental bone defects in the forearm is challenging in the best conditions, let alone in an austere environment. Use of vascularized free bone transfers is technically demanding and prolonged operative times and extensive exposures increase the risk of complications, as well as donor site morbidity. Vascularized transfer is indicated in segmental bone defects larger than 6 to 8 cm.
4. Although bone stabilization with rigid internal fixation is relatively easy to obtain, the decision to proceed with a vascularized fibula graft or one-bone forearm should be made with great caution. It is important to talk with the patient about the risks and benefits of both treatment options. Furthermore, the surgeon must understand his/her own capabilities, as well as the resources available at his/her disposal.

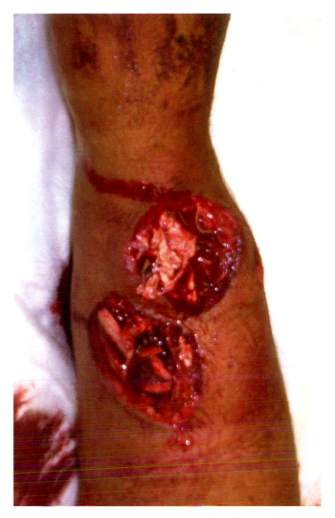

FIGURE 1. *Gunshot wound to the distal right forearm. Bone fragments are visible in the wound.*

CLINICAL IMPLICATIONS

High-energy open fractures of the forearm should be treated with staged procedures to facilitate management of bone and soft-tissue defects. The following treatment principles should be applied:

1. Administration of intravenous antibiotics and tetanus in the emergency department.
2. Emergent debridement and irrigation in the operating room, with removal of any loose bone fragments or devitalized soft tissue.
3. Extension of the wound proximally and distally to completely expose and evaluate the zone of injury.
4. Placement of a wrist spanning external fixator for bone defects involving the distal one third of the forearm.
5. Primary repair of transected tendons or nerves, if possible.

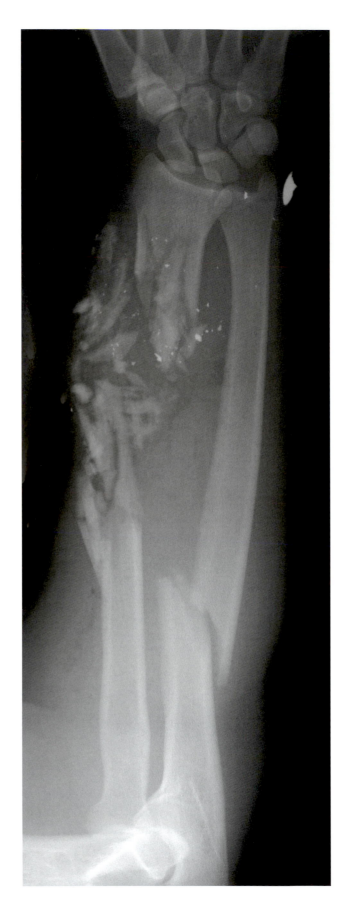
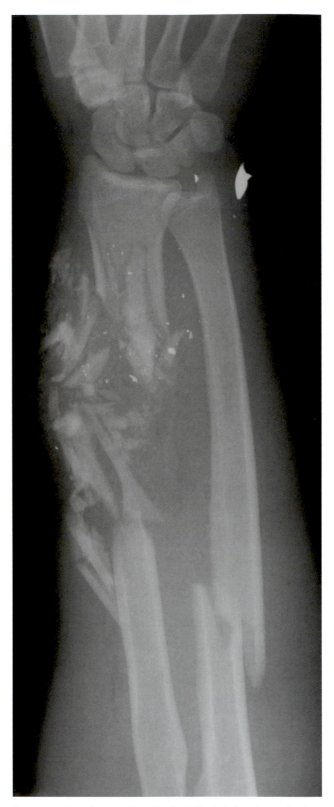

FIGURE 2. *Radiographs:* (Left) *PA;* (Right) *lateral of right forearm. Comminuted fracture of the distal third of the radius and displaced fracture of the ulna are evident.*

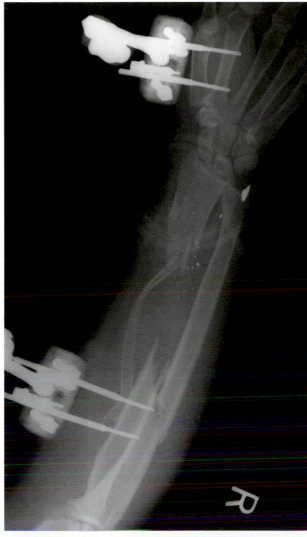

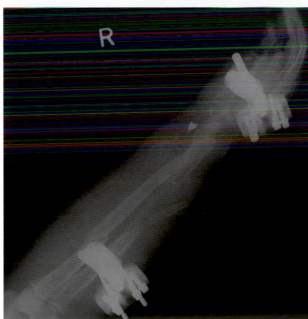

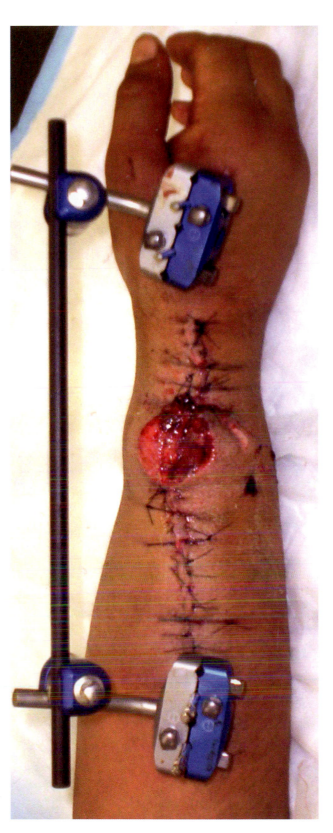

FIGURE 3. *Radiographs:* (Top Left) *PA;* (Bottom Left) *lateral of right forearm. An external fixator, spanning the wrist, is in place* (Right).

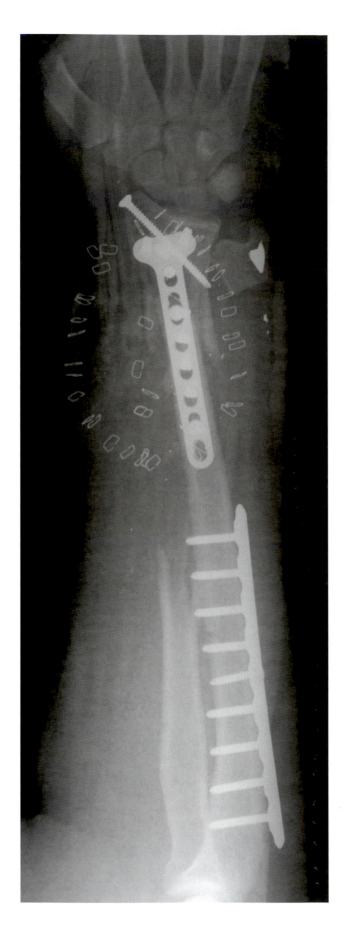

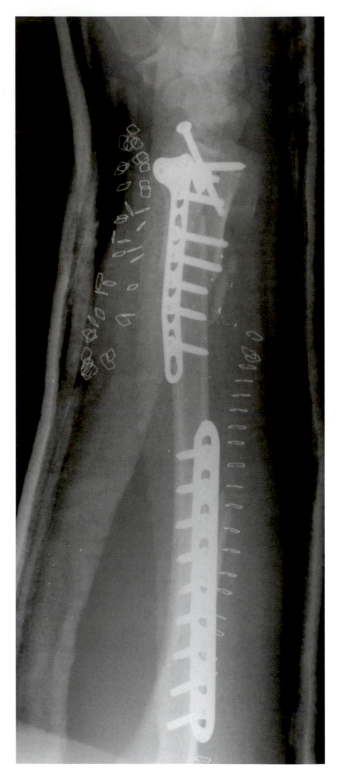

FIGURE 4. (Left) *Radiograph* (lateral view), *hospital day 3, s/p open reduction and internal fixation. See text for more details.*

FIGURE 5. (Right) *Radiograph* (AP view) *of one-bone forearm.*

6. The use of an ulna-to-radius osteotomy to bridge bone defects greater than 6 to 8 cm.

7. Definitive osteosynthesis with rigid internal fixation.

8. Soft-tissue coverage within 3 to 7 days to minimize infection and provide a stable envelope for bone healing.

DAMAGE CONTROL

Open forearm fractures with extensive segmental bone loss can be temporarily managed with intravenous antibiotics, tetanus toxin, and a well-padded sugar-tong splint (so named because it resembles the sugar tong used for handling cubes of sugar). Rapid transport to a facility with an orthopaedic surgeon and the appropriate equipment should be arranged.

SUMMARY

This case demonstrates that open forearm fractures with extensive segmental bone and soft-tissue loss are challenging clinical problems. It is important to obtain initial skeletal stabilization with an external fixator to restore the anatomy and prevent further damage to the soft-tissue envelope. In addition, placement of an external fixator facilitates staging the procedures and allows for further evaluation of the evolving injury. Definitive fixation of forearm fractures with segmental bone loss should take into account the patient's desires, technical skill of the surgeon, environmental factors, and facility resources.

SUGGESTED READING

Chapter 23: Extremity fractures. In: *Emergency War Surgery, Third United States Revision*. Washington, DC: Department of the Army, Office of The Surgeon General, Borden Institute; 2004.

Green DP, Hotchkiss RN, et al, eds. *Green's Operative Hand Surgery*. 5th ed. Philadelphia, Pa: Elsevier; 2005.

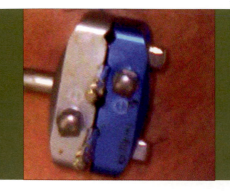

VII.13
High-Energy Orthopaedic Polytrauma

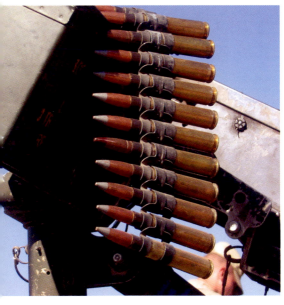

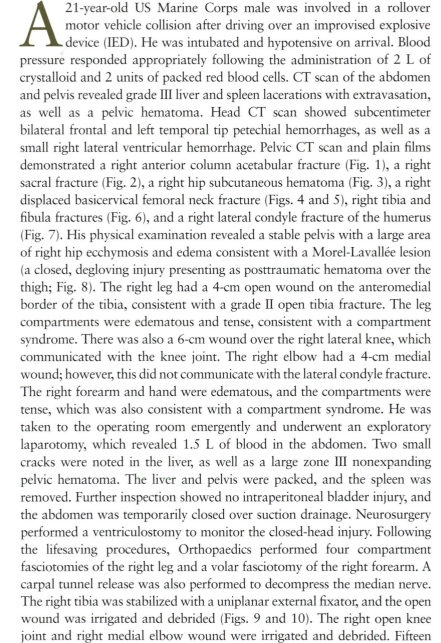

CASE PRESENTATION

A 21-year-old US Marine Corps male was involved in a rollover motor vehicle collision after driving over an improvised explosive device (IED). He was intubated and hypotensive on arrival. Blood pressure responded appropriately following the administration of 2 L of crystalloid and 2 units of packed red blood cells. CT scan of the abdomen and pelvis revealed grade III liver and spleen lacerations with extravasation, as well as a pelvic hematoma. Head CT scan showed subcentimeter bilateral frontal and left temporal tip petechial hemorrhages, as well as a small right lateral ventricular hemorrhage. Pelvic CT scan and plain films demonstrated a right anterior column acetabular fracture (Fig. 1), a right sacral fracture (Fig. 2), a right hip subcutaneous hematoma (Fig. 3), a right displaced basicervical femoral neck fracture (Figs. 4 and 5), right tibia and fibula fractures (Fig. 6), and a right lateral condyle fracture of the humerus (Fig. 7). His physical examination revealed a stable pelvis with a large area of right hip ecchymosis and edema consistent with a Morel-Lavallée lesion (a closed, degloving injury presenting as posttraumatic hematoma over the thigh; Fig. 8). The right leg had a 4-cm open wound on the anteromedial border of the tibia, consistent with a grade II open tibia fracture. The leg compartments were edematous and tense, consistent with a compartment syndrome. There was also a 6-cm wound over the right lateral knee, which communicated with the knee joint. The right elbow had a 4-cm medial wound; however, this did not communicate with the lateral condyle fracture. The right forearm and hand were edematous, and the compartments were tense, which was also consistent with a compartment syndrome. He was taken to the operating room emergently and underwent an exploratory laparotomy, which revealed 1.5 L of blood in the abdomen. Two small cracks were noted in the liver, as well as a large zone III nonexpanding pelvic hematoma. The liver and pelvis were packed, and the spleen was removed. Further inspection showed no intraperitoneal bladder injury, and the abdomen was temporarily closed over suction drainage. Neurosurgery performed a ventriculostomy to monitor the closed-head injury. Following the lifesaving procedures, Orthopaedics performed four compartment fasciotomies of the right leg and a volar fasciotomy of the right forearm. A carpal tunnel release was also performed to decompress the median nerve. The right tibia was stabilized with a uniplanar external fixator, and the open wound was irrigated and debrided (Figs. 9 and 10). The right open knee joint and right medial elbow wound were irrigated and debrided. Fifteen

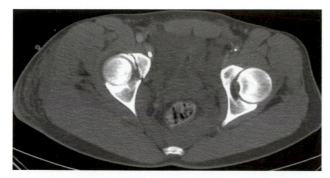

FIGURE 1. *Pelvis CT. Note right acetabular fracture.*

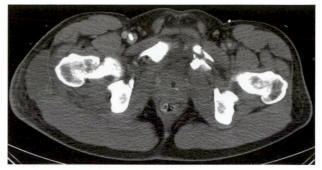

FIGURE 3. *Pelvis CT. There is marked edema and hematoma adjacent to the right hip. Note fracture of left pelvic ramus.*

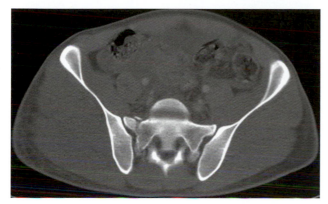

FIGURE 2. *Pelvis CT. There is a displaced fracture of the right sacrum.*

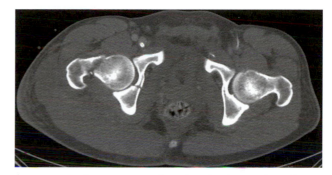

FIGURE 4. *Pelvis CT. Displaced right femoral neck fracture and acetabular fracture are evident.*

pounds of traction were applied to the external fixator frame, and the right basicervical femoral neck fracture was treated with a closed reduction and percutaneous screw fixation using three 7.0 mm cannulated screws (Fig. 11). All of the patient's wounds were placed in soft dressings, and the right upper extremity was placed into a posterior splint. He was taken to the intensive care unit for further monitoring and then transferred to a higher echelon of care the following day.

TEACHING POINTS

1. A complete examination of the spine, chest, pelvis, and extremities is an essential part of the secondary survey in patients sustaining blunt trauma. All body surfaces should be exposed and thoroughly palpated. In addition, all major joints should be put through a full range of motion and assessed for potential ligamentous injury.

2. Radiographs should be obtained of any painful extremity or if there is any deformity, ecchymosis, or crepitus. It is important to make sure that good quality radiographs are obtained in two orthogonal planes and that the entire bone, to include the proximal and distal joints, is visualized.

3. Compartment syndrome is a clinical diagnosis and usually manifests with pain out of proportion on physical examination and pain that is not controlled with pain medication. In addition, patients can note paresthesias and will have pain on passive stretch of the affected extremity.

4. In patients without a reliable clinical examination (eg, an intubated or head injured patient), compartment pressure measurements can be obtained. Diagnosis of a compartment syndrome is made when either the absolute pressure is greater than 30 mm Hg or the pressure is within 30 mm Hg of the diastolic blood pressure (delta P < 30 mm Hg). Once the diagnosis is made, emergent fasciotomy is indicated.

5. In cases in which the diagnosis of an open joint is not clinically obvious, a saline load test can be performed. Following sterile preparation of the skin, a large bolus of normal saline (ie, 60 cc for the knee and 30 cc for the elbow/ankle) can be injected into the joint. If fluid leaks from the open wound, then

the joint has been violated, and surgery is indicated. To further enhance visualization, methylene blue can be added to normal saline.

CLINICAL IMPLICATIONS

In patients with multiple extremity injuries (orthopaedic polytrauma), it is important to prioritize which injuries should be treated first. This patient has multiple orthopaedic emergencies to include upper and lower extremity compartment syndromes, open tibia fracture, open knee joint, and femoral neck fracture. The following treatment principles should be applied:

1. Administration of intravenous antibiotics and tetanus in the emergency department.
2. **Compartment syndromes should be released first** to minimize ischemia and preserve muscle and nerve function. Large incisions should be used to completely visualize and release the muscular fascia. In the leg, the anterior and lateral compartments are released through a lateral incision, and the superficial and deep posterior compartments are released through a medial incision. The volar forearm compartment can be released through a number of different incisions, and a carpal tunnel release can also be performed by extending the incision across the wrist flexion crease at an oblique angle. If necessary, the mobile wad can be released through the volar forearm incision, and the dorsal forearm compartment can be released through a separate dorsal incision.

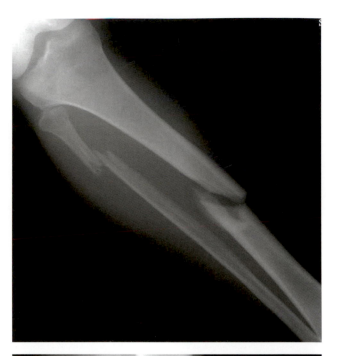

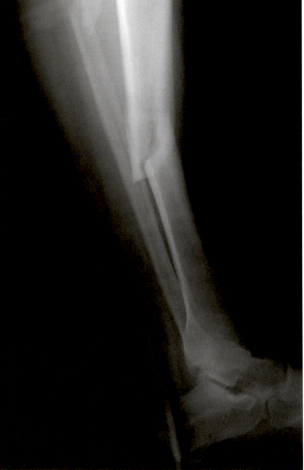

FIGURE 6. *Radiographs of right tibia and fibula fractures.*

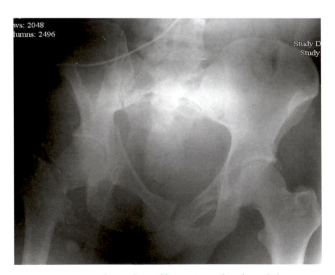

FIGURE 5. *AP pelvis plain film. Note displaced fracture of the right femoral neck and right acetabulum fracture and right sacrum.*

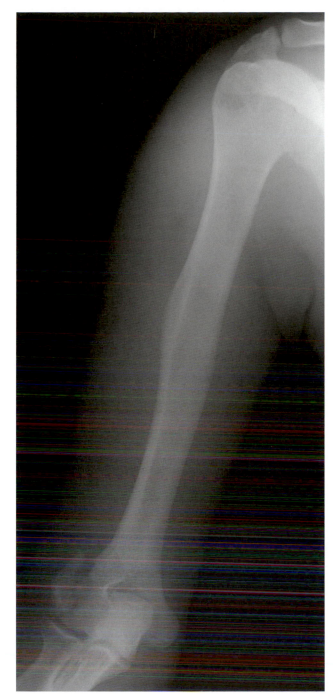

FIGURE 7. *Radiograph of right humerus. Note fracture of lateral epicondyle.*

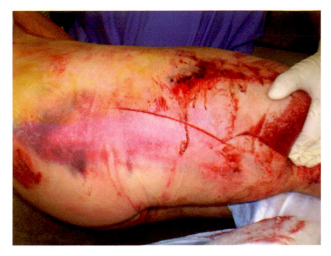

FIGURE 8. *Note edema and ecchymosis of right hip.*

3. Open fractures should be addressed next, and traumatic wounds should be extended proximally and distally to expose the fracture and zone of injury. All devitalized soft tissue and loose bone fragments should be removed first, and this is followed by copious irrigation using pulse lavage (typically 9 L of normal saline for high-energy fractures).

4. Long bone fractures should be initially stabilized with external fixators. The fracture should be reduced and the external fixator frame tightened. Intraoperative fluoroscopy is a useful adjunct to ensure proper pin placement and to confirm fracture reduction. In addition to stabilizing fractures, external fixators help decrease pain, prevent further soft-tissue damage, and allow for access to complex soft-tissue wounds. Definitive management of fractures with internal fixation devices is carried out after soldiers return to higher echelon facilities in the continental United States.

5. An open joint is also a surgical emergency and requires prompt treatment with debridement and copious irrigation. Once the joint has been adequately lavaged, the arthrotomy should be closed to prevent further contamination of the joint space.

6. Displaced femoral neck fractures in young adults are surgical emergencies because of the potential for blood flow compromise to the femoral head and the development of osteonecrosis. Prompt anatomical reduction and internal fixation with three large cannulated screws were performed on this patient and is the preferred method of treatment.

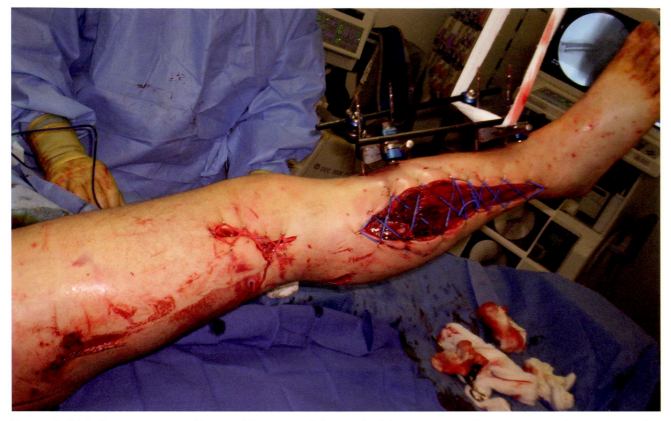

FIGURE 9. *Right lower extremity. External fixators stabilize a tibial fracture. Lateral compartment fasciotomy and lateral knee wound are evident.*

7. Many upper extremity fractures are amenable to stabilization with well-padded splints. In this instance, the lateral condyle fracture of the distal humerus was treated in a posterior splint, rather than subjecting the patient to the additional surgical time and morbidity of an external fixator.

8. Treatment of Morel-Lavallée lesions is controversial and consists of either observation or percutaneous drainage. The main concern with these injuries is an increased risk for infection related to surgical approaches through the zone of injury. This patient was treated by leaving the skin envelope intact, except for the small incision that was made to fix the femoral neck fracture.

DAMAGE CONTROL

If an orthopaedic surgeon is not available when a patient presents with complex extremity injuries, a general surgeon can perform limb-saving fasciotomies. Orthopaedic damage control involves early intravenous antibiotics, irrigation of open fractures at the bedside, and placement of well-padded splints for transport to a facility with the necessary personnel and equipment. General surgeons deploying to a combat theater should familiarize themselves with the use and application of external fixators.

SUMMARY

This case demonstrates the severity of musculoskeletal injuries from high-energy blunt trauma (see *Emergency War Surgery, Third United States Revision*, Fig. 1-9, page 1.12). In this instance, priority was given to his potentially life-threatening intraabdominal injuries, followed by attention to multiple complex extremity injuries. A systematic treatment plan was used to address, respectively, the compartment syndromes, open fracture, open knee joint, displaced femoral neck fracture, and lateral condyle fracture of the distal humerus. All of the patient's injuries were promptly treated, and he was stabilized for transport to a higher echelon of care.

SUGGESTED READING

Browner BD, Jupiter JB, et al. *Skeletal Trauma*. 3rd ed. Philadelphia, Pa: Saunders; 2003.

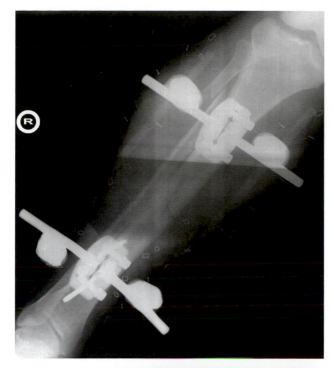

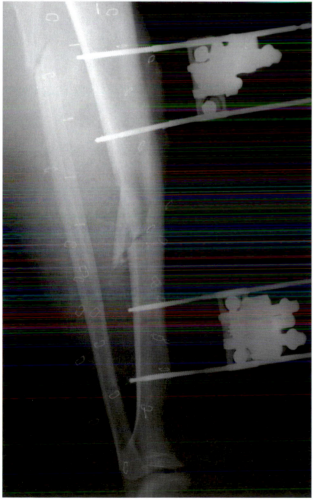

FIGURE 10. *AP* (Top Left) *and lateral* (Bottom Left) *radiographs of right leg with external fixator in place.*

FIGURE 11. (Right) *Radiograph of right hip. Three cannulated screws are in place to reduce femoral neck fracture.*

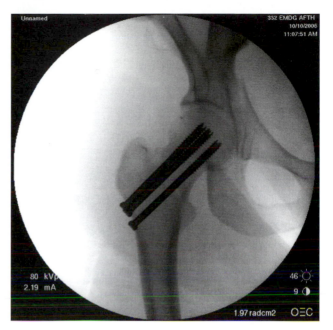

Bucholz RW, Heckman JD, eds. *Rockwood & Green's Fractures in Adults.* 5th ed. Philadelphia, Pa: Lippincott Williams & Wilkins; 2002.

Canale ST. Campbell's *Operative Orthopaedics.* 10th ed. St. Louis, Mo: Mosby; 2003.

Chapter 13: Face and neck injuries. In: *Emergency War Surgery, Third United States Revision.* Washington, DC: Department of the Army, Office of The Surgeon General, Borden Institute; 2004.

Chapter 22: Soft-tissue injuries. In: *Emergency War Surgery, Third United States Revision.* Washington, DC: Department of the Army, Office of The Surgeon General, Borden Institute; 2004.

Chapter 23: Extremity fractures. In: *Emergency War Surgery, Third United States Revision.* Washington, DC: Department of the Army, Office of The Surgeon General, Borden Institute; 2004.

Orthopaedic Trauma

by COL James Ficke, MD

Since September 11, 2001, US and coalition troops have been actively engaged in the largest conflict since Vietnam. As of January 2008, more than 4,300 US soldiers have died in this conflict, and more than 30,000 have been injured.[1] Of these casualties, approximately 54% sustained open wounds to the extremities and 26% sustained fractures. Of even greater impact, 82% of all of these fractures were open[2] and required urgent, in-theater debridement, often necessitating stabilization. The cases presented in this chapter encompass a thorough survey of typical injuries currently seen in contemporary combat. Leading civilian and military orthopaedic surgeons have collaborated on two annual Extremity War Injury Symposia[3] to identify management principles and challenges faced by surgeons who treat combat injuries. These principles include:

- improvement of prehospital care for extremity injuries,
- initial debridement and stabilization,
- management of massive bone and soft-tissue defects,
- treatment and prevention of wound infections, and
- prevention of heterotopic ossification.[3]

The following additional comments are warranted.

CIVILIAN (HOST NATIONAL) CARE

Often, the only potential for definitive reconstruction rests on the capabilities of the CSH. Definitive care for a host national patient can be accomplished safely without sophisticated techniques. With minimal additional technology, successful wound management and staged reconstruction may be possible. Early fixation and bone grafting in this situation may be deleterious, however, in the face of inadequate soft-tissue coverage. Although microvascular free tissue transfer is not commonly practiced in theater, alternatives such as pedicle flaps and negative pressure wound therapy (wound VAC) can significantly reduce in-hospital stay, while still permitting appropriate definitive fixation.

EXTERNAL FIXATION AND TRANSPORT

The field external fixator has largely replaced a transportation cast. The disadvantage of casting is primarily related to wound access, weight, and time to apply. In nearly all lower extremity injuries, an external fixator can be safely applied, allowing wound access, comfort, and minimal additional soft-tissue trauma. When periarticular fractures are stabilized with joint-spanning external fixators, these should be placed anteriorly whenever possible in order to facilitate transport.

EXTREMITY COMPARTMENT SYNDROME

Tibia fractures as a result of blast injury are fairly common, and this chapter demonstrates essential principles in their management. Open tibia fractures lack the abundant soft-tissue envelope of the femur, and complications (eg, infection or compartment syndrome) tend to occur with higher frequency. This necessitates serial examinations and low threshold for performing four-compartment fasciotomy through two incisions. Recent evidence for incomplete release demonstrates the imperative for long incisions, release from 5 cm below the knee joint distally to the musculotendinous junction, and assurance of release of all four compartments. This is best accomplished for the deep posterior compartment by the ability to directly touch the posteromedial fibula from the medial incision, and performing an "H" between the separate longitudinal releases of the anterior and lateral compartments directly visualizing the intermuscular septum with the horizontal incision. Some surgeons would disagree that simple bulging of muscle confirms the diagnosis of compartment syndrome. More importantly,

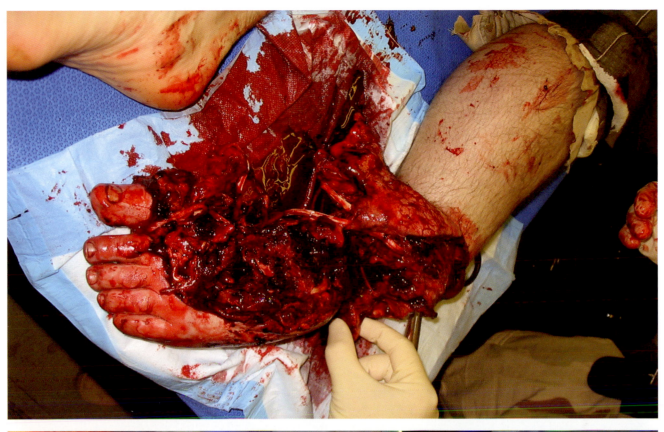

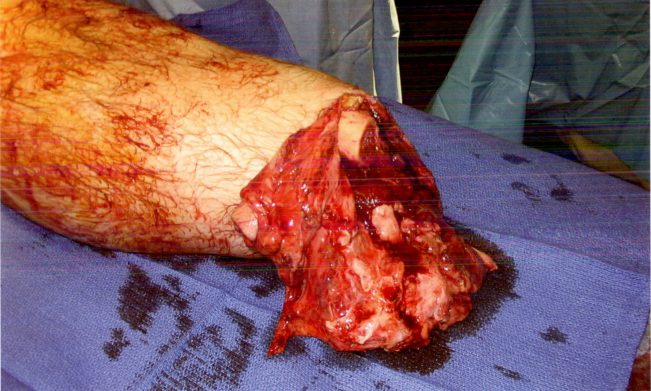

FIGURE 1. (Top) *Distal leg wound at presentation.* (Bottom) *Postoperative view of wound. The irregular soft-tissue margins are intentional.*

DEPARTMENT OF THE ARMY

CONSENSUS STATEMENT ON LENGTH PRESERVING AMPUTATIONS

Goal: Provide standardization of care for the performance of life saving amputations which provide maximum limb length preservation for optimal rehabilitative function.

Background: The notion of the "zone of injury" is dependent upon the mechanism of injury, i.e. blast, gunshot, and crush injuries, as well as comorbidities such as severe blood loss with massive resuscitation, burns, compartment syndrome, and tourniquet use which may extend the amount of tissue damage. The wounds will evolve over time and merit frequent wound inspection and evaluation. Indications for amputation include traumatic amputations, vascular injury not amenable to repair, and limb infection with uncontrolled sepsis. Current consensus on battle injured nonsalvageable limbs is to preserve limb length, and conserve viable tissue for reconstruction in a definitive level V facility. The former open circular technique eliminates many potential options and should be avoided when possible.

Initial Surgical Management: Thorough inspection of the wounds with liberal use of surgical wound extension to inspect all levels of tissue including examination of fascial planes.

A meticulous debridement of all nonviable tissue including skin, fat, fascia, muscle, and bone should be performed. All gross contamination must be debrided.

The amputation level should be performed at the most distal level which provides viable bone and soft tissues for later closure. If an amputation is completed, but a fracture exists proximally, stabilize this segment with pins or external fixation, and preserve length.

Vascular structures should be ligated proximal to the bone resection and separated from nerves.

Be prepared to accept atypical skin and tissue flaps so long as the tissue is viable.

If the limb distal to the wound is viable, but there is a fracture, this should be preserved and the bone stabilized. This is most often accomplished with an external fixator. Amputation can and should be made at the definite treatment facility.

Avoid open circular, or guillotine amputations if possible. If needed then perform the amputation at the most distal level. All wounds must be left open.

Post Operative Management: Soft dry dressing should be applied. Circumferential wraps with gauze rolls and ace wraps must be applied in a figure of 8 fashion without excessive compression.

The limb may be placed in a splint or bivalved cast to prevent joint contractures and provide soft tissue support. There should be simple access for wound inspection.

In the event of the short skin flaps, be prepared to place the limb with skin traction to prevent soft tissue retraction. Alternatively, consider negative pressure dressing when conditions permit.

Avoid placement of pillows under the knee to prevent contractures in the below knee level to prevent hip contractures in the above knee level. Plan on repeat debridement generally within 48-72 hours; however these wounds must be watched closely.

Coordinate dressing changes/repeat debridement with evacuation schedule to avoid extended periods without wound care or inspection. *Closure is not recommended until arrival at the definitive care facility*, and then myodesis should be accomplished whenever possible.

muscle viability and contractility must be assessed, and complete release ensured. Additionally, a fasciotomy with normal muscle should not be criticized; rather, the dire consequences of missed compartment syndrome far outweigh an occasional fasciotomy without compartment syndrome. In the face of evolving compartment status, ongoing resuscitation, or significant coagulopathy, delaying evacuation to ensure limb viability is justified and preferable to delaying fasciotomy.

AMPUTATION

The overall amputation rate in the present conflicts in Southwest Asia appears to remain fairly constant and is more related to immediate nonreconstructible trauma than to any other cause. The principles of open-length preserving amputation include removing clearly devitalized tissue (skin, fat, muscle, and bone) and leaving the wound open (Fig. 1; also see Consensus Statement on facing page). Wound debridement is more important than formal flaps. The ideal incision follows the lines of injury, thus providing greater latitude in the definitive care decision process. Loose approximation to prevent skin retraction may have the same effect without increasing the infection rates. At present, formal skin traction is rarely used. An open circular amputation does not preserve length, and leads to unnecessary challenges in healing and rehabilitation of the residual limb. For these reasons, open circular amputation is no longer recommended.

PELVIC STABILIZATION

Pelvic ring injuries need to be assessed early for stability, and stabilized as part of the damage control and resuscitation process. This is one of the critical roles an orthopaedic surgeon plays in lifesaving hemostasis. A contained retroperitoneal hematoma can be controlled with external fixation. Use of a pelvic binder, although often effective in short term, is not advisable for prolonged transport. Packing can result in hemodynamic stability (as in the case presented). Early or prophylactic fasciotomies should be considered in the face of massive resuscitation and unclear clinical picture. Recent evidence suggests that delayed fasciotomy is associated with increased mortality and amputation rates.[4] However, more rigid

analysis of clinical outcomes data is required. Present practice of lower extremity, four-compartment fasciotomy through two separate wide incisions (including release of the entire extent of the muscle) appears to be most preventive of additional muscular injury. It should be emphasized that the vast majority of fractures should not be definitively internally fixed in theater. Femoral neck fractures, however, are one of the very few strong indications for definitive internal fixation in the combat zone. The risk of osteonecrosis of the femoral head outweighs the infection risk in this injury, and pinning with reduction can be safely performed if fluoroscopy is available. Intraarticular foreign bodies constitute a contaminated joint and mandate open debridement.

These 13 cases catalog a wide diversity of extremity trauma, as well as their spectrum of severity. Principles of surgery are learned with practice and study; and a comprehensive review is not in the scope of this book. However, wound debridement, soft-tissue coverage, and consideration of the necessary differences between care of host national patients who often require prolonged and definitive management versus damage control stabilization and transport of US patients are well described. A deployed surgeon of any discipline must know the technique for fasciotomy and the indications for the procedure, as well as be able to anticipate and prevent the drastic consequences of compartment syndrome.

REFERENCES

1. DefenseLINK Casualty Report. Available at: http://www.defenselink.mil/news/casualty.pdf. Accessed May 25, 2006.
2. Owens BD, Kragh JF, et al. Characterization of extremity wounds in Operation Iraqi Freedom and Operation Enduring Freedom. *J Orthop Trauma.* 2007;21:254–257.
3. Pollak AN, Calhoun J. Extremity war injuries: State of the art and future directions. Prioritized future research objectives. *J Am Acad Orthop Surg.* 2006;14:S212–S214.
4. ALARACT-106/2007. *Management of OIF/OEF Casualties Requiring Extremity Fasciotomy.* Washington, DC: Department of the Army Military Operations/Department of the Army Surgeon General; 2007.

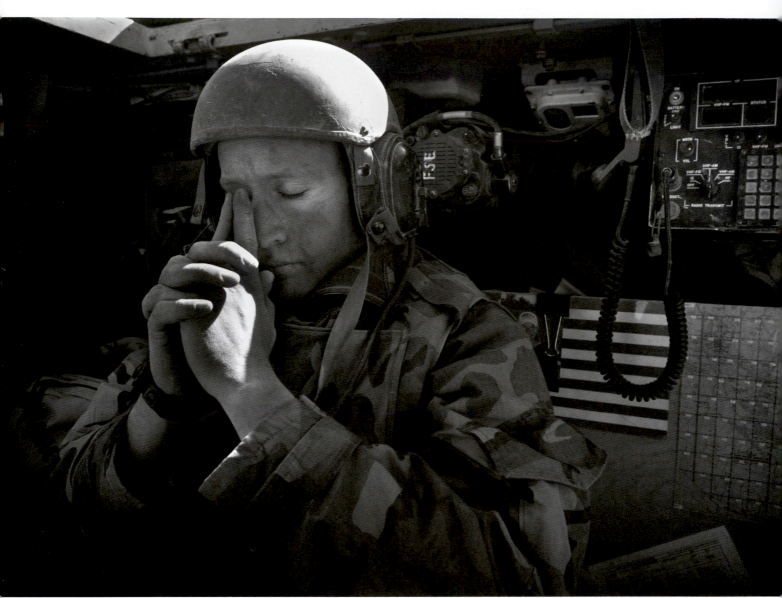

Courtesy David Leeson, *The Dallas Morning News*

Chapter VIII
VASCULAR TRAUMA

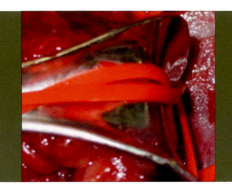

VIII.1
Innominate Vein Injury

CASE PRESENTATION

This 20-year-old male soldier was injured in the right neck when his 40-mm grenade launcher misfired and exploded as he attempted to clear it. The patient presented completely alert with normal vital signs. He did complain of mild hoarseness. Examination revealed that a fragment entered through the right neck in zone II. There were no overt signs of vascular injury. On chest X-ray (CXR), the fragment appeared to be lodged behind the sternoclavicular joint (Fig. 1). During neck exploration, profuse bleeding was encountered. Resection of the medial left clavicle failed to allow access to the area of bleeding where a large fragment was palpable, prompting median sternotomy. This maneuver adequately exposed the fragment embedded in the innominate vein. The fragment was removed (Fig. 2) and the injury controlled with digital pressure. It was repaired using a running 5-0 Prolene suture (Figs. 3 and 4). No other vascular injuries were noted. After washout of a concurrent hand injury and a period of observation, the patient was evacuated from the combat support hospital (CSH) without difficulty to a level IV medical treatment center.

TEACHING POINTS

1. This is an example of a symptomatic (hoarseness), but stable, patient with a possible zone I and/or zone II neck injury. The size of the fragment and the mechanism of injury increased the concern of serious injury, but all zone II neck injuries with penetration of the platysma should be explored in the combat environment. Symptomatic zone I and III injuries should be explored if an arteriogram is not available (Fig. 5).

2. Zone II injuries are relatively easy to expose by a standard approach anterior to the sternocleidomastoid muscle. Occasionally, local wound exploration will identify the wound tract and fragment. In this case, exploration was limited. Frequently, a fragment cannot be identified, and the surgeon must specifically rule out injury to the carotid artery, internal jugular vein, trachea, or esophagus. In this case, zone II exploration was negative. Resection of the medial portion of the left clavicle revealed the fragment was in the innominate vein. However, this approach inadequately exposed the fragment and vessel necessitating median sternotomy (Fig. 6). Once the specific injury was identified and properly exposed, it was relatively easily repaired.

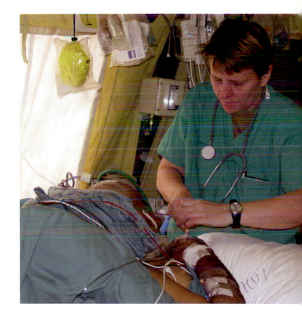

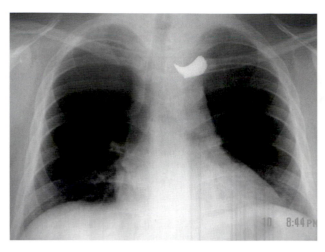

FIGURE 1. *This CXR was obtained preoperatively and demonstrates a large fragment from a 40-mm grenade overlying the left sternoclavicular joint on single frontal view.*

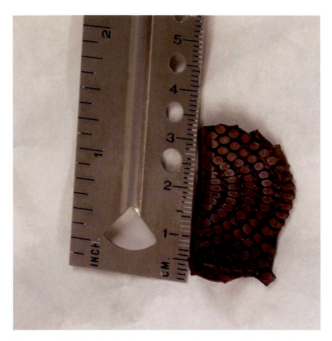

FIGURE 2. *This is the fragment that was lying in the innominate vein.*

3. This case emphasizes the importance of ruling out vascular injury in all neck injuries prior to evacuation. It is not possible to intervene surgically if this type of patient becomes unstable in flight.
4. This type of case is technically more difficult to perform at the Forward Surgical Team (FST) facility and emphasizes the importance of bringing stable patients from the point of injury directly to level III whenever possible.
5. Distal injury of the subclavian arteries is more difficult to address and may require a supraclavicular approach or resection of the proximal clavicle to allow adequate exposure (Fig. 7). The combination of a median sternotomy with an anterior thoracotomy and supraclavicular incision (trapdoor) can also be used.

CLINICAL IMPLICATIONS

Twenty percent of penetrating neck injuries result in vascular injury. Mortality may occur from exsanguination or less commonly from esophageal injury that progresses to mediastinitis. Tracheal injuries must be excluded. The presence of any of the following symptoms mandates exploration:

1. Obvious bleeding.
2. Expanding hematoma.
3. Bruit or thrill in the neck.
4. Hypotension.
5. Dyspnea, hoarseness, or stridor.
6. Absent or decreased pulses in the neck or arm.
7. Focal neurological deficit or mental status changes.
8. CXR with hemothorax or widened mediastinum.

Signs of esophageal or tracheal injury include the following:

1. Crepitus or subcutaneous emphysema.
2. Dyspnea or stridor.
3. Air bubbles in wound.
4. Tenderness or pain over trachea.
5. Odynophagia (pain on swallowing).
6. Hoarseness.
7. Hematemesis or hemoptysis.

DAMAGE CONTROL

Hypotensive patients with suspected zone I injury of the common carotid artery or subclavian artery and vein can be approached through a median sternotomy or an extended left anterior thoracotomy (clamshell incision). Generally, the median sternotomy is an optimal approach for the aorta, innominate, and proximal

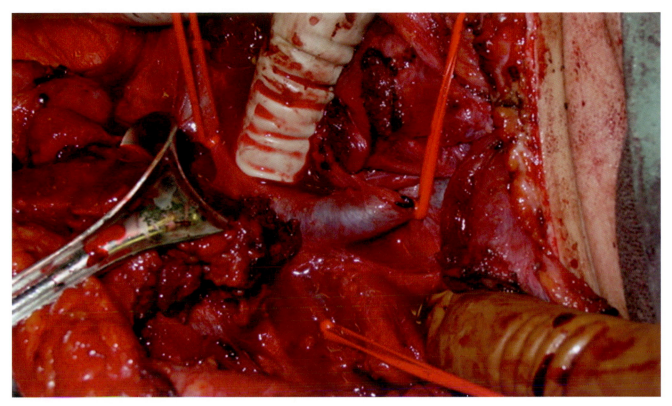

FIGURE 3. *The gloved finger at the top is occluding the hole in the innominate vein.*

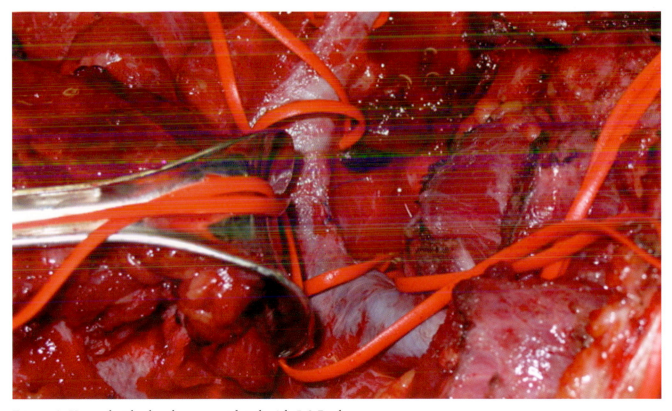

FIGURE 4. *Venorrhaphy has been completed with 5-0 Prolene.*

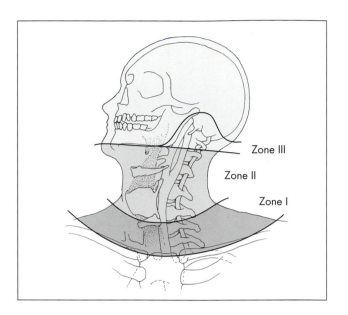

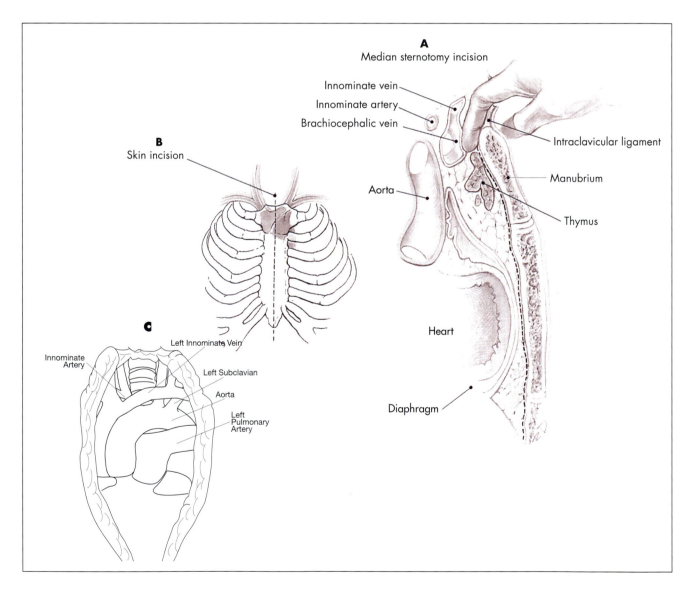

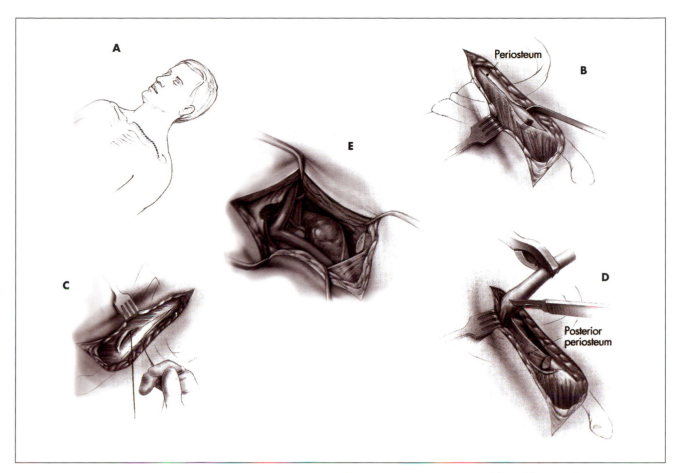

FIGURE 7. (A) *Supraclavicular incision.* (B) *Exposing the clavicle.* (C) *Dividing clavicle with a Gigli saw.* (D) *Dividing posterior periosteum.* (E) *Exposed left subclavian and common carotid arteries.* Reprinted with permission from Thal ER, Weigelt JA, Carrico J. *Operative Trauma Management: An Atlas.* 2nd ed. New York, NY: McGraw-Hill Professional; 2002. Copyright © 2002 The McGraw-Hill Companies, Inc.

PENETRATING NECK TRAUMA

Introduction
- Vascular injuries occur in 20% and aerodigestive tract in 10% of cases.
- Mortality is primarily due to exsanguinating hemorrhage.
- Esophageal injury, which results in mediastinitis and intractable sepsis, may also be fatal.

Anatomy
The neck is divided into three zones to aid in decision-making for diagnostic tests and surgical strategy. In each zone, the primary structures at risk of injury are different (see Fig. 5).
- ZONE I (clavicle to cricoid membrane): The structures of concern include large vessels of the thoracic outlet (subclavian artery and vein, common carotid artery), the lung, and the brachial plexus.
- ZONE II (cricoid membrane to angle of mandible): Structures of concern include the common carotid artery, internal jugular vein, esophagus, and trachea.
- ZONE III (angle of mandible to base of skull): The structure of concern is primarily the internal carotid artery.

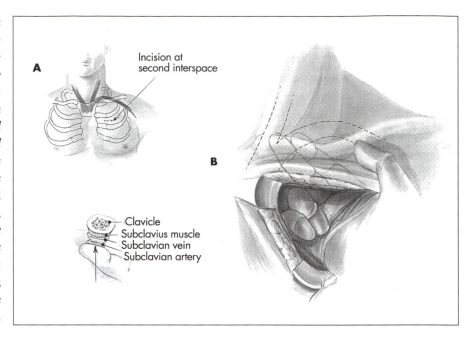

FIGURE 8. *Temporary occlusion of a subclavian injury through a limited left thoracotomy. This is a temporary control measure to allow greater exposure. (A) Temporary control of subclavian artery injury may be obtained through a second intercostal incision. (B) Digital pressure is applied to the subclavian artery and vein.* Reprinted with permission from Thal ER, Weigelt JA, Carrico J. *Operative Trauma Management: An Atlas.* 2nd ed. New York, NY: McGraw-Hill Professional; 2002. Copyright © 2002 The McGraw-Hill Companies, Inc.

subclavian arteries. An anterior thoracotomy through the second intercostal space may allow digital pressure to be applied upward and medially (compressing the subclavian artery and vein against the clavicle) as a temporary measure to control bleeding (Fig. 8).

SUMMARY

This is a case in which suspected zone I and zone II neck injuries (see Fig. 5) required the combination of right neck exploration and ultimately median sternotomy to identify and repair the vascular injury suggested by the patient's hoarseness, mechanism of injury, entrance wound, and CXR.

Note: See discussion of this case on page 359.

SUGGESTED READING

Chapter 27: Vascular injuries. In: *Emergency War Surgery, Third United States Revision.* Washington, DC: Department of the Army, Office of The Surgeon General, Borden Institute; 2004.

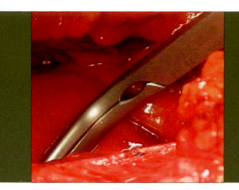

VIII.2
External Iliac Vein Injury, Exposure and Control

CASE PRESENTATION

This 23-year-old male soldier presented after an insurgent attack. He was traveling inside an armored vehicle when he was injured by a shoulder-fired, rocket-propelled–shaped charge missile that penetrated the vehicle but ultimately failed to explode. He arrived at the combat support hospital (CSH) hypotensive and actively bleeding from a large, left groin wound with an obvious femur fracture. Upon arrival in the emergency medical treatment area, direct pressure was applied to the wound, and pressure was applied to the left femoral pressure point. This decreased the bleeding and allowed visualization of the severed end of the superficial femoral artery (SFA) and the profunda femoris artery (PFA), which was clamped (Fig. 1). These maneuvers initially decreased the bleeding. Further resuscitation increased the blood pressure, resulting in diffuse bleeding from multiple locations. The patient was transported to the operating room and prepped from neck to feet of both extremities. No attempt at limb salvage was contemplated for this unstable patient with ongoing hemorrhage because of massive injury to the femoral artery, vein, and nerve associated with a large soft-tissue wound and femur fracture—an injury that essentially constituted a traumatic, near-complete amputation (Fig. 2). A high above-the-knee amputation was quickly performed. Ligation of the PFA was performed distal to its first branch in the hopes of preserving enough blood supply to avoid an eventual hip disarticulation. The superficial femoral vein (SFV) and branches were ligated as distal as possible to allow drainage (Fig. 3). With the amputation complete, bleeding from the ilioinguinal ligament region was noted. Despite retraction, the source of bleeding could not be identified. However, direct pressure over the ligament controlled visible bleeding, which was dark and consistent with a venous origin. It was determined that exposure of the external iliac vessels was necessary. Options for exposure included division of the inguinal ligament, laparotomy, or an iliac fossa (kidney transplant) incision. Division of the inguinal ligament was ruled out because pressure over the ligament was temporarily controlling the bleeding and exposure may have been inadequate. Similarly, it was felt that laparotomy may not allow adequate exposure of the distal external iliac artery and vein. Therefore, the transplant incision was used in this case because it provided the best exposure to the distal iliac vessels and would allow proximal control of the distal aorta, if necessary. This approach allowed proximal control of the iliac vein at the bifurcation and that stopped the bleeding. A 2-cm posterior laceration of the external iliac vein was identified and lateral

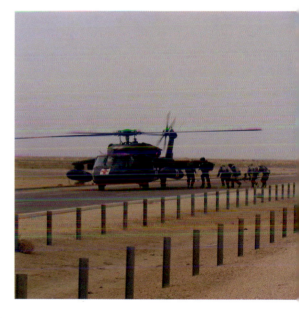

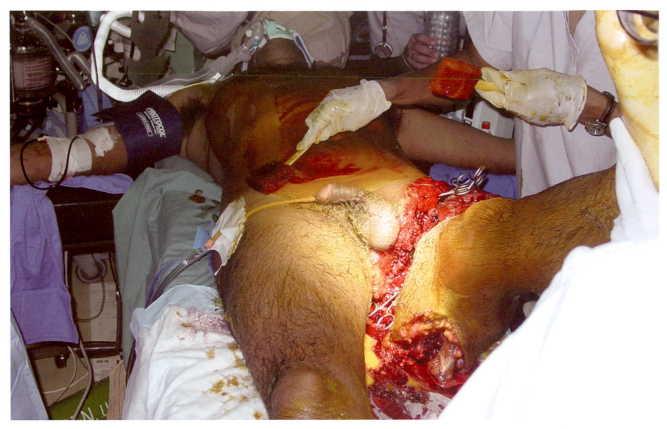

FIGURE 1. *Large proximal left lower extremity injury. Vascular clamps are in place.*

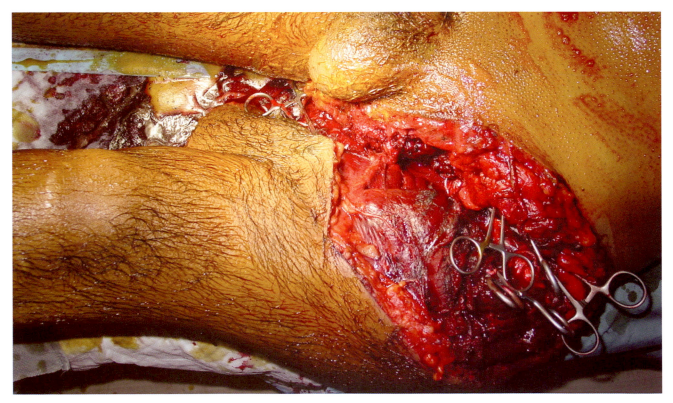

FIGURE 2. *Extensive tissue injury.*

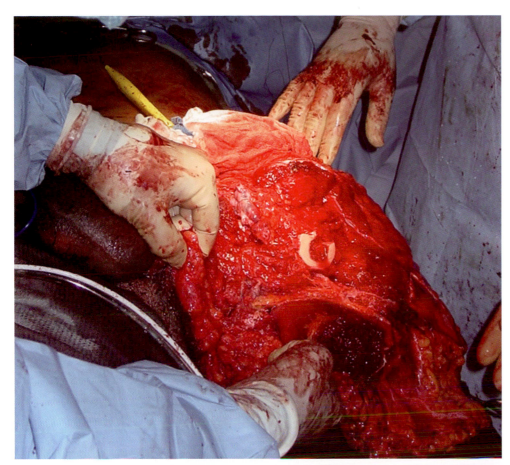

FIGURE 3. (Top)
*Initial amputation
has been performed.*

FIGURE 4. (Bottom)
*The external iliac
vein is dissected,
and an injury is
repaired.*

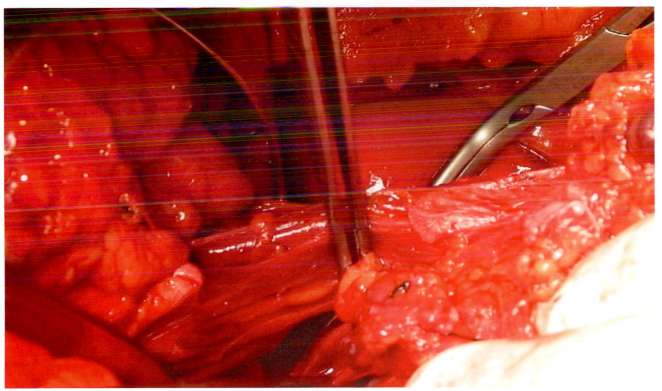

venorraphy performed (Fig. 4). With hemorrhage finally controlled, the wound was debrided with preservation of as much tissue as possible. The patient was evacuated to a level IV medical treatment facility. There, he underwent proctoscopy and an exploratory laparotomy for a rectal contusion and underwent diversion colostomy. The patient ultimately required a hip disarticulation. He progressed well with aggressive physical therapy and was able to ambulate with assistance upon discharge from Walter Reed Army Medical Center.

TEACHING POINTS

1. Nothing stops bleeding like direct pressure. In this case, direct pressure allowed enough control of the bleeding that direct clamping of the visualized vessels could be performed. The dictum not to use blind clamping is correct. However, if a vessel can be visualized, a clamp can provide excellent hemostasis.

2. Proctoscopy is warranted for injuries in this location due to the proximity of the wound to the rectum. Because of the urgency of bleeding, this step was correctly omitted at the patient's initial evaluation to address the life-threatening injury at hand. Once life-threatening injuries have been stabilized, it is important that the patient be completely reevaluated for other injuries that may have been initially missed or ignored and that may result in subsequent deterioration. Similarly, it is important that, at each level along the evacuation chain, the patient is completely reevaluated.

3. Use of the transplant incision (Fig. 5) gives excellent exposure of the iliac and hypogastric vessels and aorta. In this case, the transplant incision allowed for isolation and repair of this injury and examination of the proximal vessels to rule out injury.

CLINICAL IMPLICATIONS

1. Early control of external bleeding is critical. A patient with compressible hemorrhage can be temporized with direct pressure until surgical control of hemorrhage is possible.

2. The surgeon must balance the realistic likelihood of ultimate functional reconstruction against the risk of death associated with attempts to preserve a limb.

DAMAGE CONTROL

It is critical to recognize the need to institute damage control techniques at initial presentation. This case demonstrates the immediate recognition of the need for amputation as opposed to prolonged attempts at limb

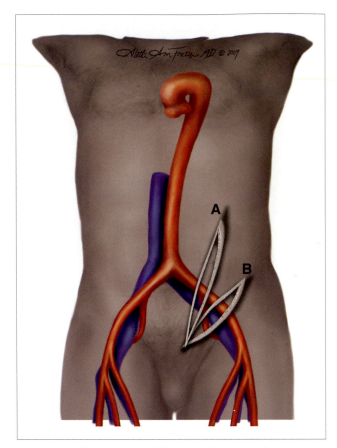

FIGURE 5. *Illustration of iliac vessel (transplant) incisions.*

salvage. It is likely that this soldier survives today because of this initial decision.

SUMMARY

This is a case in which traumatic near amputation is completed operatively. Persistent hemorrhage was identified from above the inguinal ligament and required exposure of the external iliac vessels. The transplant incision was used with good results.

Note: See discussion of this case on page 359.

SUGGESTED READING

Chapter 25: Amputations. In: *Emergency War Surgery, Third United States Revision.* Washington, DC: Department of the Army, Office of The Surgeon General, Borden Institute; 2004.

Chapter 27: Vascular injuries. In: *Emergency War Surgery, Third United States Revision.* Washington, DC: Department of the Army, Office of The Surgeon General, Borden Institute; 2004.

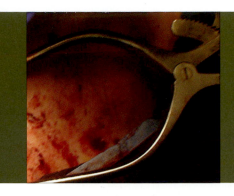

VIII.3
Penetrating Subclavian Artery Injury

CASE PRESENTATION

While on guard duty, this male patient was injured by a blast from a vehicle-borne, improvised explosive device (IED). On hospital admission, he was neurologically and hemodynamically uncompromised. His wounds were multiple, superficial fragment injuries. One such injury was in the right supraclavicular fossa. The wound was approximately 3 mm in length, but no evidence of distal neurovascular compromise was evident. A plain chest X-ray revealed a widened mediastinum, and a fragment could be seen superior to the right clavicle. CT scan revealed a hematoma around the subclavian vessels. The fragment was located along the posterior-superior margin of the subclavian artery. Consideration was given to evacuating the patient to a vascular surgeon at a level IV medical treatment facility. However, the risk of rebleeding during the 6-hour evacuation process was deemed to be significant. In the operating room, he was placed in the supine position. His chest was prepared and draped. Both lower extremities were prepped to provide an autologous vein, if needed. An incision was made superior and parallel to the clavicle. Proximal and distal control of the subclavian artery was obtained. The injury was in the most superior aspect of the subclavian artery. Proximal control was obtained distal to the origin of the vertebral artery. Distal control was obtained after transecting the anterior scalene muscle. The fragment had produced a tangential injury along the superior-posterior aspect of the artery. The vessel injury was only about 2 mm in length. The fragment destroyed only a very small portion of the vessel wall. The 3-mm fragment was removed from the surgical field, and primary repair was performed using polytetrafluoroethylene (PTFE) pledgets as bolsters for the fine Prolene suture. Hemostatic closure of the injury was achieved, and excellent distal pulses were present to palpation after repair. The Doppler signal of the radial artery was normal. The wound was closed after a small drain was placed in the area of dissection.

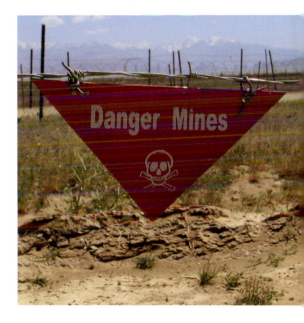

TEACHING POINTS

1. Subclavian artery injuries are treacherous because vascular control can be difficult to obtain. Injuries to the origin of the right subclavian artery require a median sternotomy to obtain proximal vascular control. A median sternotomy, with a trapdoor along the fourth left intercostal space, might be necessary to access the proximal left subclavian artery.

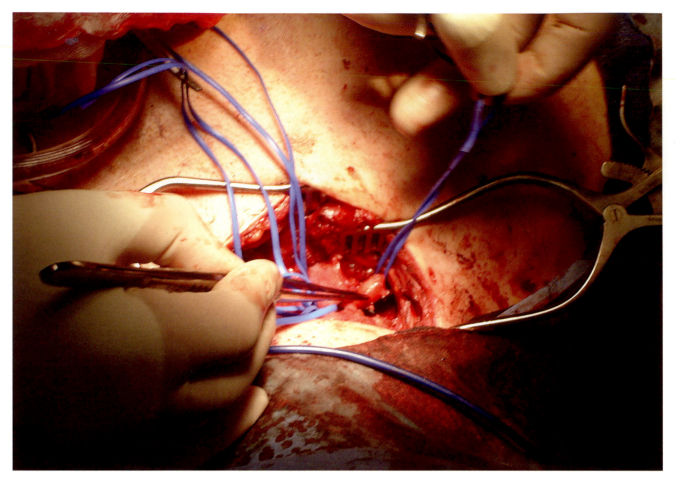

FIGURE 1. *The surgeon is grasping the right subclavian artery just proximal to the site of injury. Injury is not visible because it is on the dorsal aspect of the artery.*

2. In this case, the injury was near the middle of the right subclavian artery. Proximal and distal control were readily obtained using the supraclavicular approach. The chest had been prepared. A sternotomy set was available if more proximal control had been required.

3. A good working knowledge of the thoracic inlet is necessary to make sound decisions for the optimal surgical approach. The hemodynamically compromised patient, with injury to the thoracic inlet, requires immediate vascular control. A median sternotomy would be the most expeditious route to control hemorrhage.

4. The only evidence of significant hemorrhage on presentation may be radiographic findings that include extrapleural densities, pleural effusion, or mediastinal widening.

5. Autologous vein grafts are preferred for traumatic vascular repairs. In cases where an autologous vein is either inadequate or not available, prosthetic graft should be used for an expeditious repair or if a significant size discrepancy exists. In this case, PTFE was not used as an interposition graft, but as a pledget. Minimizing foreign material is an objective in combat wounds. However, in this patient, the injury was from a 3-mm fragment that was removed from the surgical site. Also, adjacent tissue destruction was minimal. Because the subclavian artery has a fragile texture, a buttressed repair was required.

CLINICAL IMPLICATIONS

Surgeons must be prepared to provide vascular exposure in areas not frequently approached. Under certain circumstances, prosthetic material is acceptable in vascular repairs. Basic vascular principles always apply and include the following:

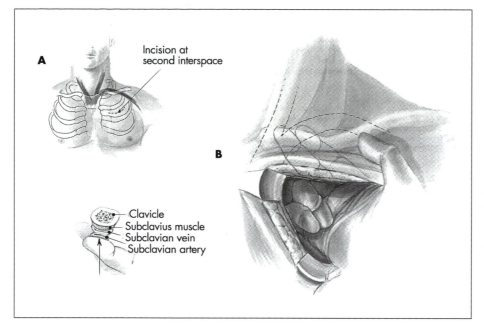

FIGURE 2. (A) *Temporary control of subclavian artery injury may be obtained through a second intercostal space incision.* (B) *Digital pressure is applied to the subclavian artery and vein.* Reprinted with permission from Thal ER, Weigelt JA, Carrico J. *Operative Trauma Management: An Atlas.* 2nd ed. New York, NY: McGraw-Hill Professional; 2002. Copyright © 2002 The McGraw-Hill Companies, Inc.

1. Hard signs of vascular injury may not be present (as in this case), but surgeons should remain alert to subtle injury changes. A missed subclavian artery injury has a high mortality rate.

2. Soft signs of arterial injury that require additional diagnostic evaluation—eg, proximity of wounds to major vessels, shock, diminished pulse, or nerve injury—should prompt further evaluation or exploration.

DAMAGE CONTROL

The key to controlling hemorrhage from a subclavian artery injury is adequate exposure. This may require a median sternotomy, a supraclavicular approach, or an infraclavicular approach to the vessel. The proximal clavicle can be resected if needed. A trapdoor incision can be used, if necessary. Once exposure is obtained, placement of a shunt is appropriate until definitive repair can be achieved.

SUMMARY

This is a case in which clinical vigilance led to the diagnosis and repair of a subclavian artery injury. This case demonstrates the importance of maintaining appropriate clinical concern and identifying subtle vascular injuries. Evacuation of this patient from theater without identifying his particular injury could have easily resulted in loss of an extremity or a fatal outcome.

Note: See discussion of this case on page 359.

SUGGESTED READING

Chapter 27: Vascular injuries. In: *Emergency War Surgery, Third United States Revision.* Washington, DC: Department of the Army, Office of The Surgeon General, Borden Institute; 2004.

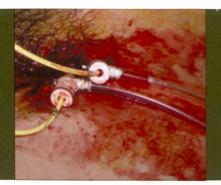

VIII.4
Shunts in Vascular Injuries

CASE PRESENTATION

This 16-year-old female presented to a Forward Surgical Team (FST) after a gunshot wound to the right groin. The groin area was examined. Several centimeters of the common femoral artery were destroyed. A no. 10 French Argyle shunt was placed in the proximal and distal lumens of the injured artery and secured in position with 0 silk ties. The wound was approximated in a single layer, and the dressing was clearly marked to indicate the shunt. The patient was then intubated, sedated, and transferred (via helicopter) to the combat support hospital (CSH; Fig. 1). Distal pulses were intact. Resuscitation was continued, and the patient was taken to the operating room for reexploration (Fig. 2). The shunt was patent. The contralateral greater saphenous vein was harvested, and an interposition graft was performed (Figs. 3 and 4). The patient was not anticoagulated because of her ongoing coagulopathy from relative hypothermia and blood loss. She was admitted postoperatively to the intensive care unit, where the graft remained patent. Her recovery was prolonged, but she was eventually returned home.

TEACHING POINTS

1. Well-positioned arterial shunts can be lifesaving and limbsaving. A functional shunt allows perfusion, while resuscitation is ongoing. The patient can then be evacuated to a higher echelon of care without compromising the extremity.
2. Dressings should be marked clearly to indicate a shunt is in place.
3. Systemic anticoagulation is not recommended for cases of arterial trauma unless the injury is isolated, there is no ongoing hemorrhage, and the patient does not have a coagulopathy.

CLINICAL IMPLICATIONS

1. Arterial injuries are common on the battlefield.
2. Usually, patients have suffered significant hemorrhage before arriving at the first echelon of care.
3. Shunt placement allows perfusion of the injured extremity while the patient is being resuscitated or transferred. The Argyle shunt, Javid shunt, and Sundt shunt are all acceptable. The proximal end of the shunt is placed first, then the distal end. The shunt is secured in position with 0 silk ties. Once flow has been confirmed by the

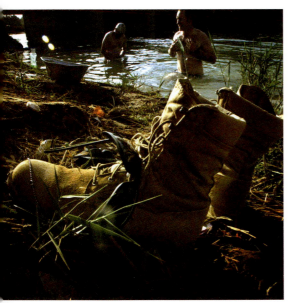

Courtesy David Leeson, *The Dallas Morning News*

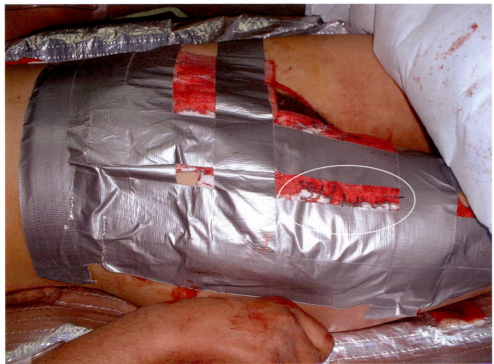

FIGURE 1. (Top) *Transfer of patients between military treatment facilities can result in confusion because of the lack of communication. In this case, the dressing has been marked (as "shunt" [white circle]) so the receiving team knows that further surgery is required.*

FIGURE 2. (Bottom) *Shunt bridging the arterial injury.*

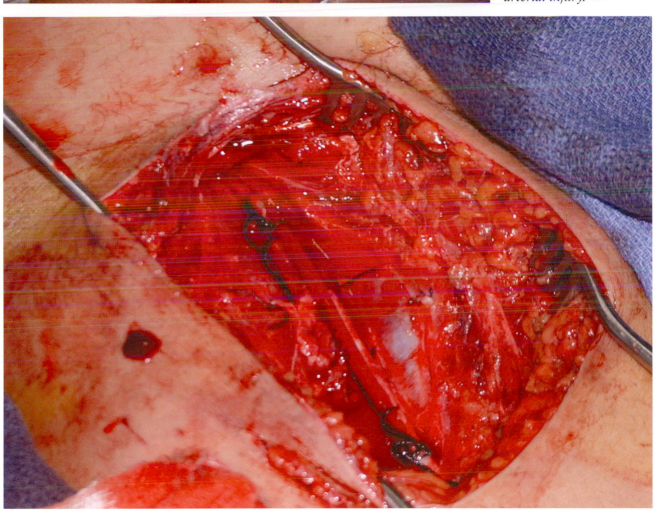

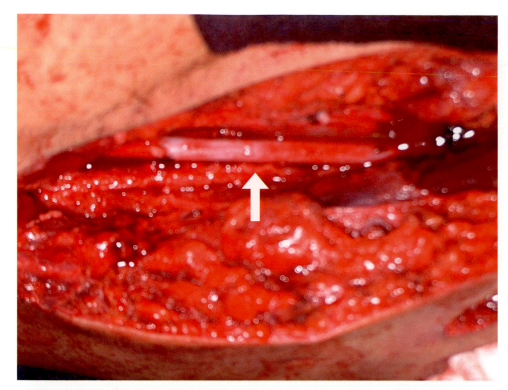

FIGURE 3. (Top Left) *Saphenous interposition graft in place.*

FIGURE 4. *Vascular shunt in another patient.* (Bottom Left) *Patient presenting to CSH with shunt in left brachial artery.* (Top Right) *Shunt in place.* (Bottom Right) *Saphenous interposition graft in place.*

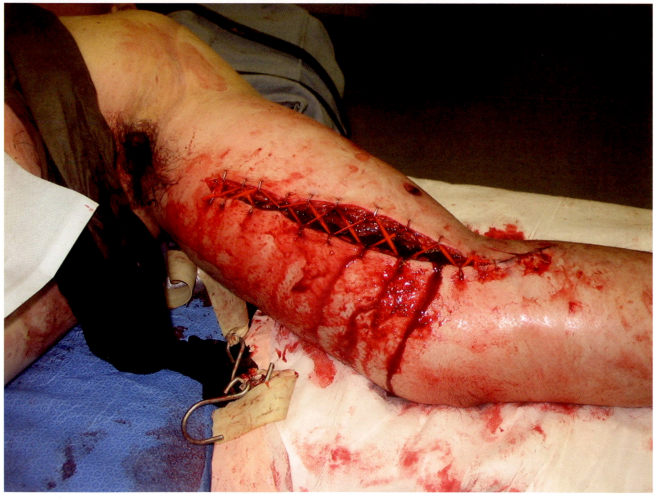

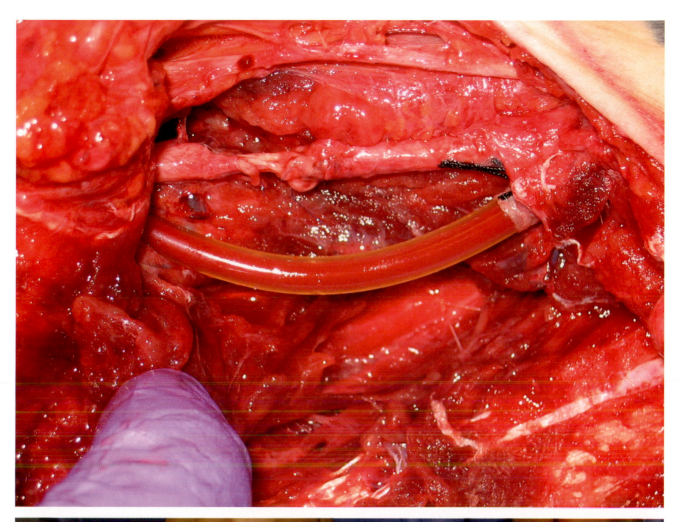

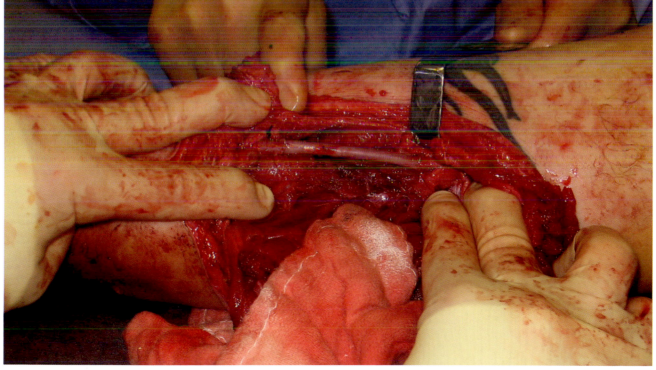

SHUNTS

A shunt diverts or permits flow of a body fluid from one pathway or region to another by surgical means. There are various types of shunts, but they usually have two similar elements: a catheter (the tubing) and the shunt (which regulates pressure/flow). Usually for the shunt being used, the surgeon selects a range of pressure and bases that decision on the patient's needs. Note: Interestingly, the various parts of the shunt system are named according to where they are placed in the body. In addition, these parts are normally made from materials that are well-tolerated by the human body.

Javid Shunt

A Javid or Argyle shunt is frequently used for shunting cerebral blood flow.
Javid shunts:
— are soft, kink-resistant, and tapered
— have extra length that allows looping
— have smooth, polished tips for easy insertion

Sundt Shunt

This shunt is also known as the Sundt carotid endarterectomy shunt. During carotid endarterectomy procedures, the shunt provides temporary carotid bypass for cerebral circulation. Dr Thoralf M. Sundt (1930–1992) developed the Sundt shunt for carotid surgery.

presence of distal pulses or Doppler signal, the shunt is covered with viable tissue, dressed, and marked.

DAMAGE CONTROL

Placement of an arterial shunt is a damage control technique. The use of prosthetic grafts can hasten the completion of a procedure in unstable patients where expeditious surgery is required. Prosthetics can also be used in areas of extensive soft-tissue debridement as a "prolonged shunt," where planned revision days to weeks later, out of theater, will be undertaken.

SUMMARY

This case is a common scenario in which a patient with an arterial injury is first seen at an FST facility that has minimal capability to provide massive resuscitation and definitive repair. The shunt allowed the patient to be evacuated safely to a higher level of care without compromise of the extremity.

Note: See discussion of this case on pages 359–360.

SUGGESTED READING

Chapter 6: Hemorrhage control. In: *Emergency War Surgery, Third United States Revision*. Washington, DC: Department of the Army, Office of The Surgeon General, Borden Institute; 2004.

Chapter 7: Shock and resuscitation. In: *Emergency War Surgery, Third United States Revision*. Washington, DC: Department of the Army, Office of The Surgeon General, Borden Institute; 2004.

Chapter 27: Vascular injuries. In: *Emergency War Surgery, Third United States Revision*. Washington, DC: Department of the Army, Office of The Surgeon General, Borden Institute; 2004.

Moore WS. *Vascular Surgery: A Comprehensive Review*. 6th ed. Philadelphia: WB Saunders Company; 2002.

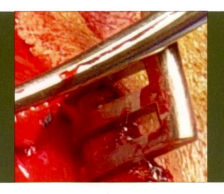

VIII.5
Arteriovenous Fistula, Delayed Effect of Blast

CASE PRESENTATION

This 26-year-old male presented with complaints of swelling in the right temple, buzzing in his right ear, and a feeling of fullness on his face. Two months previously, he sustained minor injuries to his right side, the result of a blast from an improvised explosive device (IED). On physical examination, he had a 6 x 4 cm soft mass anterior to his right ear, with engorgement of the superficial veins (Fig. 1). There was a bruit over the mass. Plain radiographs showed multiple, small radiopaque foreign bodies in the soft tissues on the right side of the head and neck. An ultrasound scan confirmed an arteriovenous fistula between the superficial temporal artery and an overlying vein (Fig. 2). In the operating room, the fistula was exposed, and the vein branches were ligated (Fig. 3). Once the superficial artery was exposed, the arteriotomy was closed with a single 6-0 Prolene suture. The patient made a full recovery.

TEACHING POINTS

1. Arteriovenous fistulae and pseudoaneurysms are the result of arterial injury that can manifest in a delayed manner days, months, or even years after injury.

2. An arteriovenous fistula develops when an artery and vein in close proximity are both injured. The higher pressure in the artery keeps the connection between the two vessels open.

3. Many smaller arteriovenous fistulae are asymptomatic, but tend to enlarge over time, thus increasing flow through the fistula. Larger fistulae can cause symptomatic venous insufficiency or congestive heart failure. As the fistula enlarges, the artery becomes tortuous and is at risk for thrombosis.

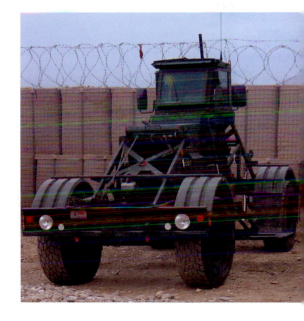

CLINICAL IMPLICATIONS

1. Consequences of arterial injury may present long after other wounds have healed and can be the result of a seemingly innocuous injury.

2. Arterial injuries should be repaired when diagnosed to prevent complications of arteriovenous fistulae.

SUMMARY

Arteriovenous fistulae and pseudoaneurysms most often present in a delayed manner, well after the initial injury. Generally, these conditions

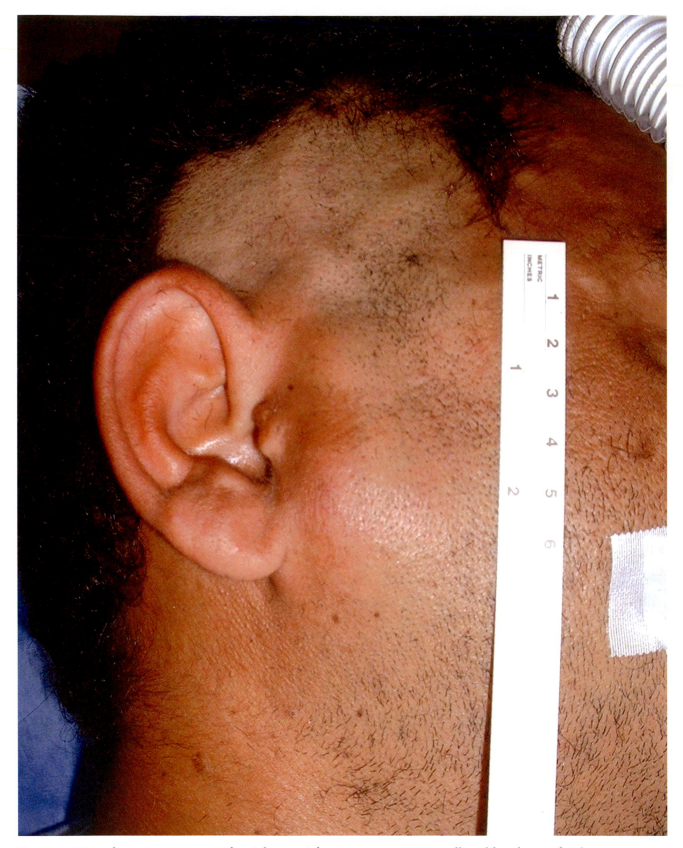

FIGURE 1. *Note the mass anterior to the right ear. A bruit was present, as well as dilated superficial veins.*

FIGURE 2. (Right) *Exposure of the arteriovenous fistula.*

FIGURE 3. (Left) *Fistula treated with vein ligation and closure of the arterial injury.*

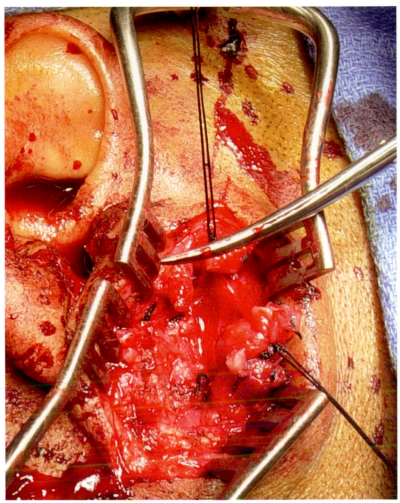

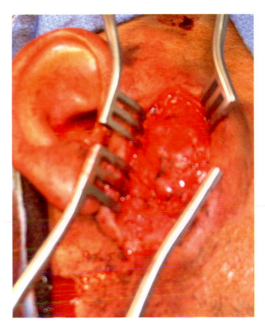

become apparent after the patient has been evacuated home. In this case, the arteriovenous fistula was repaired to alleviate the patient's symptoms and to prevent further complications.

Note: See discussion of this case on page 360.

SUGGESTED READING

Chapter 13: Face and neck injuries. In: *Emergency War Surgery, Third United States Revision.* Washington, DC: Department of the Army, Office of The Surgeon General, Borden Institute; 2004.

Chapter 15: Head injuries. In: *Emergency War Surgery, Third United States Revision.* Washington, DC: Department of the Army, Office of The Surgeon General, Borden Institute; 2004.

Chapter 27: Vascular injuries. In: *Emergency War Surgery, Third United States Revision.* Washington, DC: Department of the Army, Office of The Surgeon General, Borden Institute; 2004.

Moore WS. *Vascular Surgery: A Comprehensive Review.* 6th ed. Philadelphia: WB Saunders Company; 2002.

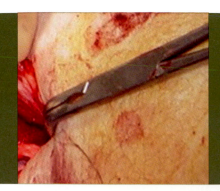

VIII.6
Brachial Artery Injury, Transection

CASE PRESENTATION

This 24-year-old male was injured by a blast from an improvised explosive device (IED). On presentation, he had a compressive dressing around his right arm and had no pulses in the extremity. The dressing was removed in the operating room and the wound explored. The brachial artery, basilic vein, and portions of the brachial plexus were transected (Fig. 1). Control of the proximal and distal ends of the brachial artery was obtained with vascular clamps. The patient was given 5,000 units of heparin, and the basilic vein was ligated. The right groin and thigh were prepped, and the greater saphenous vein harvested and inserted as a reversed interposition graft. Once flow was restored, the brachial plexus was explored, and the transected ends were tagged with Prolene suture. Viable muscle tissue was closed over the brachial artery repair and the wound dressed open. Within 48 hours, the patient was evacuated with pulses intact.

TEACHING POINTS

1. Even in the event of major nerve injury, upper extremity arterial injuries should be repaired. Tagging the injured nerves if primary repair is not possible allows easier identification for future repair or grafting. Systemic anticoagulation should only be given if there is an isolated injury.

2. In any battlefield vascular injury, autologous vein is the conduit of choice. The incidence of infected grafts following use of synthetic material mandates replacement of these type grafts at the earliest possible time.

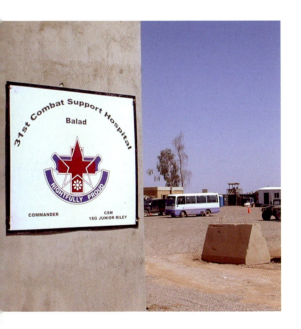

CLINICAL IMPLICATIONS

1. Typically, surgical training in vascular procedures is based on the treatment of atherosclerotic disease. As such, the upper extremity is poorly represented during a surgeon's residency and in garrison practice. On the battlefield, the upper extremity is often wounded, and the surgeon needs to know how to care for such injuries. When proximal control is not easily obtained through the wound, the axillary artery should be exposed and clamped through an infraclavicular incision.

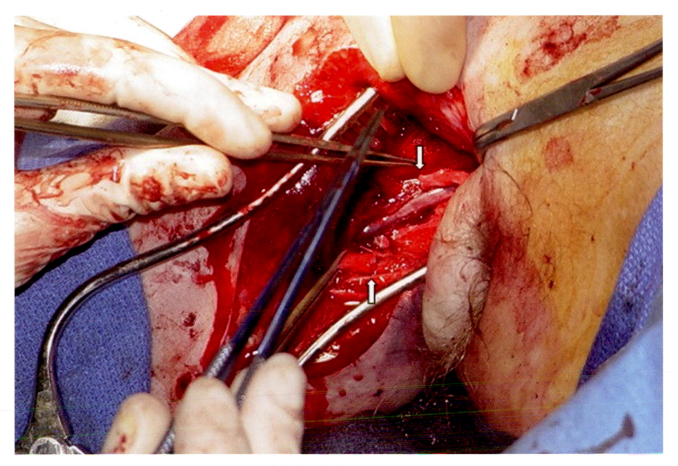

FIGURE 1. *Arrows indicate transected ends of the brachial artery.*

2. Proximal and distal control of extremity injuries can be obtained through the primary wound or an extension of that wound. When that is not possible, it may be necessary to obtain proximal control through a separate incision.

3. Exposed vein grafts will dessicate, leading to graft blowout and potential exsanguination. They must be covered by soft tissue or muscle. Superficial muscles, such as the sartorious or gracilis in the thigh, may be mobilized to cover a graft.

DAMAGE CONTROL

If a definitive repair cannot be performed, a shunt may be placed in the brachial artery to perfuse the limb during evacuation, resuscitation, or for conversion of an emergent case to a less urgent one while other cases are being attended. If the brachial artery is injured distal to the profunda brachii, the artery can be ligated, and perfusion to the hand can be maintained.

SUMMARY

This case presents a typical battlefield wound. The patient had injuries to his brachial artery, basilic vein, and brachial plexus. Using basic vascular techniques, the brachial artery was repaired with a saphenous vein interposition graft.

Note: See discussion of this case on page 360.

SUGGESTED READING

Chapter 8: Vascular access. In: *Emergency War Surgery, Third United States Revision*. Washington, DC: Department of the Army, Office of The Surgeon General, Borden Institute; 2004.

Chapter 27: Vascular injuries. In: *Emergency War Surgery, Third United States Revision*. Washington, DC: Department of the Army, Office of The Surgeon General, Borden Institute; 2004.

Moore WS. *Vascular Surgery: A Comprehensive Review*. 6th ed. Philadelphia: WB Saunders Company; 2002.

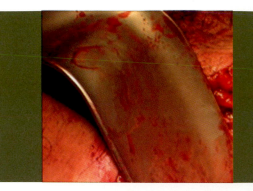

VIII.7
Femoral Vein Injury

CASE PRESENTATION

A 27-year-old male sustained a gunshot wound to the right buttock that exited the right groin just below the inguinal ligament. He presented with severe hemorrhaging from the exit wound. His initial blood pressure was 65/42 mm Hg, and his heart rate was 88 beats per minute. The patient's Glasgow Coma Scale score was 15, but the patient was somnolent. Significantly, his pH was 7.11, and his base deficit was 14. Resuscitation was started in the trauma bay, and the patient was taken immediately to the operating room. After the patient was prepped—from the nipples to the ankles circumferentially—a lower abdominal incision was made, and control of the right external iliac artery and vein was obtained with vessel loops. Vascular control of the femoral artery and vein distal to the injury was obtained (Fig. 1). Constant pressure had been maintained on the wound during this time. Despite this maneuver, some bleeding continued, but decreased when the patient was given recombinant factor VII. With bleeding controlled, a large medial wound to the femoral vein without complete transection was identified. Significant back bleeding through the venous tributaries continued, and this bleeding was controlled with ligation. Vascular clamps were then placed proximal and distal to the wound, and arterial flow was reestablished. Lateral venorrhaphy was then performed. Back bleeding was excellent, with no clotting noted. All clamps were removed, with good flow noted in the vein. Exploration of the abdomen revealed no further injuries, and all surgical wounds were closed. Throughout treatment, the patient received 7,500 mL of crystalloid fluid, 11 units of packed red blood cells, 2 units of fresh frozen plasma, and 100 mL of albumin. During the operation, the patient's pH improved to 7.29, and his base deficit decreased to 6. Postoperatively, the patient's foot remained well perfused, with no evidence of neurological injury. He was evacuated awake and alert to a level III medical treatment facility.

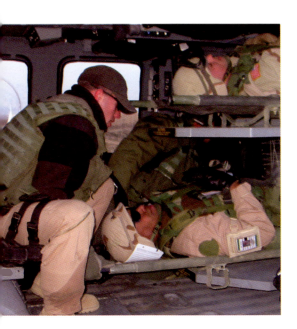

TEACHING POINTS

1. Vascular control of proximal lower extremity injuries can be extremely difficult to obtain, especially when associated with large wounds. In this case, proximal control was obtained first in the abdomen, and distal control was obtained below the wound.

2. Patients in combat environments frequently present acidotic and coagulopathic. They require a multidisciplined approach that ad-

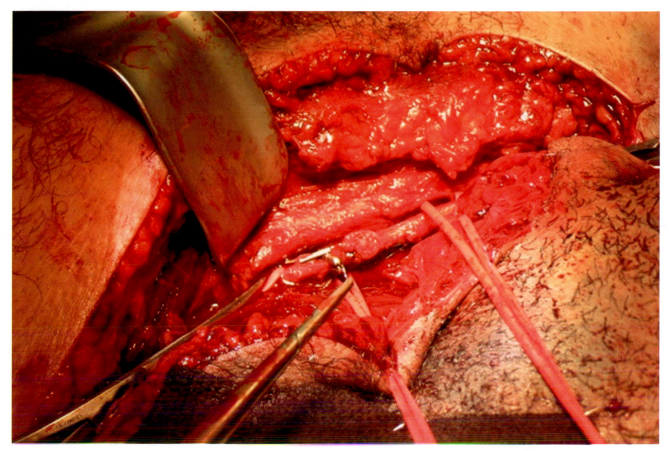

FIGURE 1. *Common femoral vein injury after control has been obtained.*

dresses control of hemorrhage and resuscitation simultaneously. Also, patients must be kept warm during the evacuation and resuscitation processes.

3. Patients can exsanguinate from isolated, major venous injury, especially proximal extremity injuries. It is difficult to place tourniquets on these wounds. Usually, the bleeding can be initially controlled with direct pressure (Fig. 2).

4. Forward Surgical Teams (FSTs) must be able to expertly administer packed red blood cells, whole blood, recombinant factor VII, and fresh frozen plasma.

CLINICAL IMPLICATIONS

Patients with vascular injuries present in a variety of ways. Once the diagnosis of vascular injury is made or suspected, some basic tenets apply:

1. Control external bleeding by direct pressure, if possible. Avoid blind clamping with vascular clamps. If possible, applying a temporary tourniquet proximal to the wound is often helpful.

2. Administer intravenous antibiotics, tetanus toxoid, and analgesia.

3. Note that reduction of long bone fractures may reestablish blood flow.

4. Prepare and drape both the injured and contralateral extremities in case vein grafting is required.

5. Debride the injured vessel (once control is obtained) to normal-appearing tissue, pass balloon catheters proximally and distally to remove thrombus, and flush with heparinized saline.

6. Repair the artery first to decrease ischemia time, if both artery and vein are injured, and no shunt is used.

7. Note that major veins should be repaired in stable patients, but may be ligated in life-threatening situations. Limb arteries can also be ligated in life-threatening situations, but limb loss will be likely.

8. Consider fasciotomy after all vascular repairs.

9. Document a neurological examination before and after surgery.

10. Monitor distal pulses hourly.

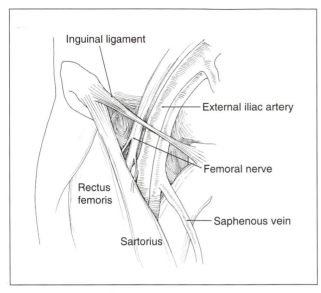

FIGURE 2. *Inguinal anatomy.*

DAMAGE CONTROL

Major veins should be repaired in stable patients, but may be ligated in life-threatening situations. Consider shunting injured vessels, especially if both artery and vein are injured, extensive debridement is required, there is concurrent long bone fracture, or the patient is not stable and requires ongoing resuscitation. Vascular shunts can be placed in unstable patients for up to 72 hours. Shunts should be secured firmly with silk sutures. Heparin is not required. Make sure that the receiving facility knows that the shunts are in place, if the patient is evacuated for definitive repair.

SUMMARY

This patient presented with a major venous injury that required large-volume resuscitation. Initial control was obtained using direct pressure. Surgical control was also obtained. With the patient stabilized, lateral venorrhaphy was performed with good results.

Note: See discussion of this case on page 360.

SUGGESTED READING

Biss TT, Hanley JP. Recombinant activated factor VII (rFVIIa/NovoSeven) in intractable haemorrhage: Use of a clinical scoring system to predict outcome. *Vox Sang.* 2006;90(1):45–52.

Boffard KD, Riou B, et al. Recombinant factor VIIa as adjunctive therapy for bleeding control in severely injured trauma patients: Two parallel randomized, placebo-controlled, double-blind clinical trials. *J Trauma.* 2005;59(1):8–15; discussion 15–18.

Chapter 7: Shock and resuscitation. In: *Emergency War Surgery, Third United States Revision.* Washington, DC: Department of the Army, Office of The Surgeon General, Borden Institute; 2004.

Chapter 23: Extremity fractures. In: *Emergency War Surgery, Third United States Revision.* Washington, DC: Department of the Army, Office of The Surgeon General, Borden Institute; 2004.

Chapter 27: Vascular injuries: In: *Emergency War Surgery, Third United States Revision.* Washington, DC: Department of the Army, Office of The Surgeon General, Borden Institute; 2004.

Clark AD, Gordon WC, et al. "Last-ditch" use of recombinant factor VIIa in patients with massive haemorrhage is ineffective. *Vox Sang.* 2004;86:120–124.

Kenet G, Walden R, et al. Treatment of traumatic bleeding with recombinant factor VIIa. *Lancet.* 1999;354:1879.

Levy JH, Fingerhut A, et al. Recombinant factor VIIa in patients with coagulopathy secondary to anticoagulant therapy, cirrhosis, or severe traumatic injury: Review of safety profile. *Transfusion.* 2006;46:919–933.

Meng Z, Wolberg A, et al. The effect of temperature and pH on the activity of factor VIIa: Implications for the efficacy of high-dose factor VIIa in hypothermic and acidotic patients. *J Trauma.* 2003;55:886–891.

Perkins JG, Schreiber MA, et al. Early versus late recombinant factor VIIa in combat trauma patients requiring massive transfusion. *J Trauma.* 2007;62:1095–1099; discussion 1099–1101.

Spinella PC, et al. The effect of recombinant activated Factor VIIa on mortality in combat-related casualties with severe trauma and massive transfusion. Forthcoming.

Stein DM, Dutton RP, et al. Determinants of futility of administration of recombinant factor VIIa in trauma. *J Trauma.* 2005;59(3):609–615.

RECOMBINANT FACTOR VIIa

Recombinant factor VIIa (rFVIIa) is currently only FDA approved for the prevention of bleeding during surgery or episodes of severe hemorrhage in patients with congenital FVIIa deficiency and hemophilia A or B with inhibitors. Since its FDA approval, rFVIIa has been proposed as a potential intervention to limit bleeding in surgery and trauma. The first case report of rFVIIa use in trauma was in 1999 and was soon followed by a series of controlled experimental animal studies published using swine models of liver trauma, many of which showed decreased blood loss. These initial studies coincided with a number of subsequent case reports and case series of rFVIIa in trauma and uncontrolled hemorrhage. The majority of publications suggested decreased blood loss and/or decreased transfusion requirements for patients, although some offered cautionary notes and limitations of rFVIIa—especially in acidosis and refractory coagulopathy. The only randomized controlled trial (RCT) to date on the use of rFVIIa in the setting of trauma was published in 2005. This study randomized patients suffering both blunt and penetrating injuries with rFVIIa administered after the 8th unit of blood. This trial showed no survival benefit, although it did show a reduction of 2.6 red blood cell (RBC) transfusions for the blunt trauma subgroup, and a similar—though nonsignificant—trend in the penetrating injury subgroup.

Thromboembolic complications associated with rFVIIa have been a serious concern given the valid biological plausibility for such events. A metaanalysis of RCTs published in 2006, however, suggested that there is no overall increase in adverse events. Retrospective military studies have shown that early administration of rFVIIa reduced transfusion requirements when compared with late administration. Severely injured patients requiring massive transfusion who received rFVIIa had a lower mortality at 12 and 24 hours and at 30 days without a significant increase in adverse events, including deep venous thrombosis. Ongoing clinical trials of the use of rFVIIa in trauma will help to clarify risk:benefit ratios.

In a recent prospective, randomized human trauma study, rFVIIa was shown to be effective in decreasing transfusion requirements, to include those patients requiring massive transfusion (RBCs $\geq$ 10 units/24 hours), in humans with life-threatening hemorrhage, including patients with hypothermia (30°–33°C; pH > 7.1). However, rFVIIa is 90% inactivated in patients with profound acidosis (pH < 7.1), based on in vitro data.

A retrospective review of combat casualty patients with severe trauma (ISS > 15) and massive transfusion (RBCs $\geq$ 10 units/24 hours) admitted to one Combat Support Hospital in Baghdad, Iraq, was conducted. Admission vital signs and laboratory data, blood products, ISS, 24-hour and 30-day mortality, and severe thrombotic events were compared between patients who received rFVIIa and those who did not receive rFVIIa. Of 124 patients who received massive transfusion, 49 patients received rFVIIa and 75 patients did not. ISS scores and vital signs did not differ between the two groups. A statistically significant decrease in mortality was demonstrated in the group who received rFVIIa at 12 hours, 24 hours, and 30 days. When rFVIIa was given at a median of 2 hours from admission, an association with decreased mortality was seen. There was no statistical difference in the incidence of severe thrombotic events (DVT, PE, stroke) between the study groups. There is currently an ongoing Phase III trauma trial of rFVIIa that addresses the question of whether earlier administration of rFVIIa improves the outcome of severely injured patients.

Guidelines for administration in the deployed surgical setting: rFVIIa should be considered for administration to trauma patients or patients in shock who have the following signs associated with hemorrhage:

a. Hypotensive from blood loss.
b. Base deficit > 6.
c. Difficult to control bleeding associated with hypothermia (T < 96°F).
d. Coagulopathic bleeding (clinically or an INR > 1.5).
e. Require damage control maneuvers.
f. Require fresh whole blood.
g. Anticipated or actual transfusion of > 4 units of PRBCs.
h. Anticipated significant operative hemorrhage.

Adapted, in part, from JTTS, CPG for Recombinant Factor VIIa, October 2007. See CPG for references and dosing.

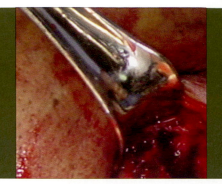

VIII.8
Brachial Artery Injury, Blunt Trauma

CASE PRESENTATION

This 30-year-old male patient was involved in a motor vehicle accident (Fig. 1). The vehicle he was traveling in was struck by a dump truck, and he was the only person in the vehicle to survive the accident. He presented with a fractured scapula, a proximal humerus fracture (Fig. 2), and a left pneumothorax. Tube thoracostomy was performed, and the patient was taken to the operating room. Exploration revealed the bicep and triceps muscles were avulsed from the bone, resulting in an internal amputation. The patient's distal upper extremity pulses were absent. Arteriogram using a C-arm showed cutoff of arterial flow near the humerus fracture. Exploration of the artery showed clear cutoff at the injury (Fig. 3). The artery containing the intimal flap was resected, and a shunt was placed (Fig. 4). Internal fixation was then performed by the orthopaedic surgeons. A successful end-to-end anastomosis was performed to repair the artery (Fig. 5).

TEACHING POINTS

1. Although penetrating injury is a more common mechanism of arterial injury in combat zones, blunt arterial injury does occur. Blunt arterial injury parallels civilian trauma experiences and is usually associated with concurrent long bone fracture, as in this case.
2. Diagnosis can be difficult, and arteriography may not be available. However, it is reasonable to assume that the arterial injury will be near the fracture. In this case, the injury was apparent. Penetrating injuries to arteries do not usually represent a diagnostic challenge.
3. A common approach in concurrent arterial and long bone fracture is to reestablish perfusion by placing a shunt and completing the repair after fixation of the fracture, as in this case.

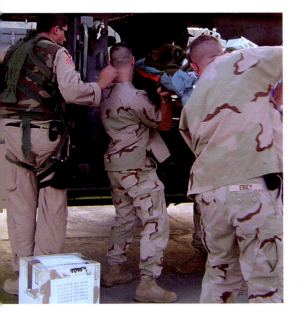

CLINICAL IMPLICATIONS

Hard signs of vascular injury that suggest the need for immediate exploration include the following:

1. Pulsatile external bleeding.
2. Enlarging hematoma.
3. Absent distal pulses.
4. Thrill or bruit.
5. Ischemia.

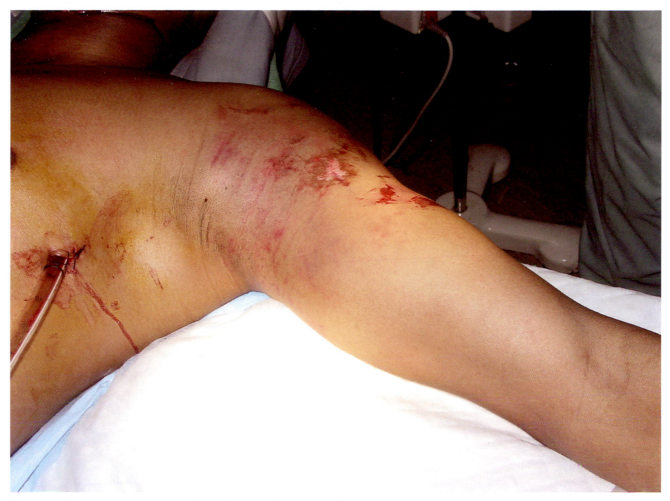

FIGURE 1. *Patient as he appeared at the time of presentation.*

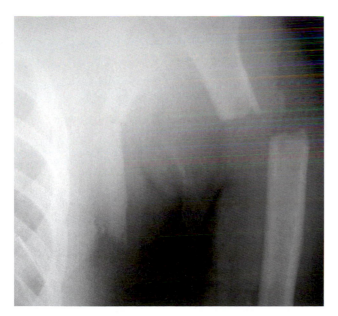

FIGURE 2. *Humerus fracture and scapula fracture are seen in this radiograph.*

Signs of ischemia include the following:

1. Pain.
2. Pallor.
3. Pulselessness.
4. Poikilothermia.
5. Paresthesia.
6. Paralysis.

DAMAGE CONTROL

Vascular shunts can be placed in unstable patients for up to 72 hours. Shunts should be secured firmly with silk sutures. Heparin is not required. Distal pulses should be monitored hourly. If the patient is evacuated for definitive repair, the receiving facility should know that the shunt is in place.

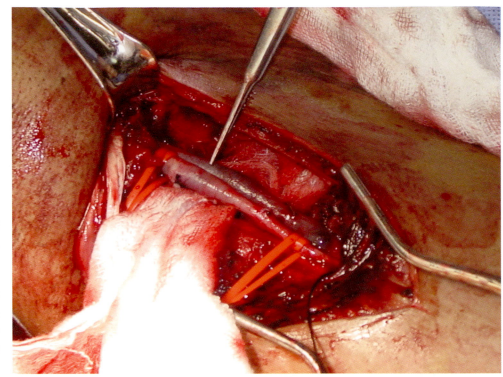

FIGURE 3. (Top) *Area of arterial injury.*

FIGURE 4. (Bottom) *A shunt has been placed to reestablish flow while the humerus is stabilized.*

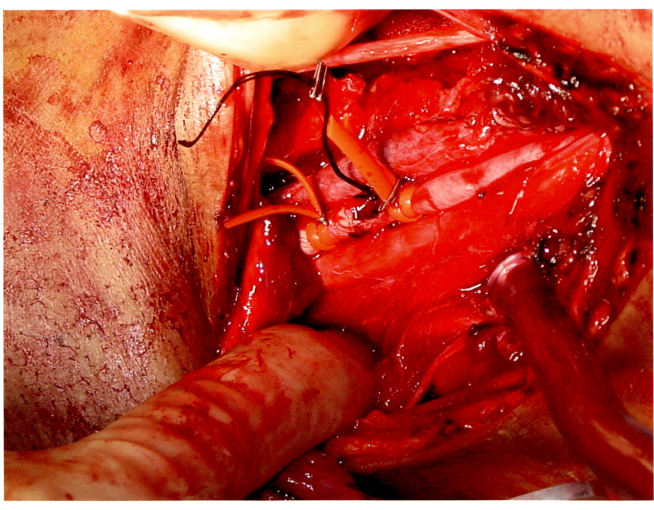

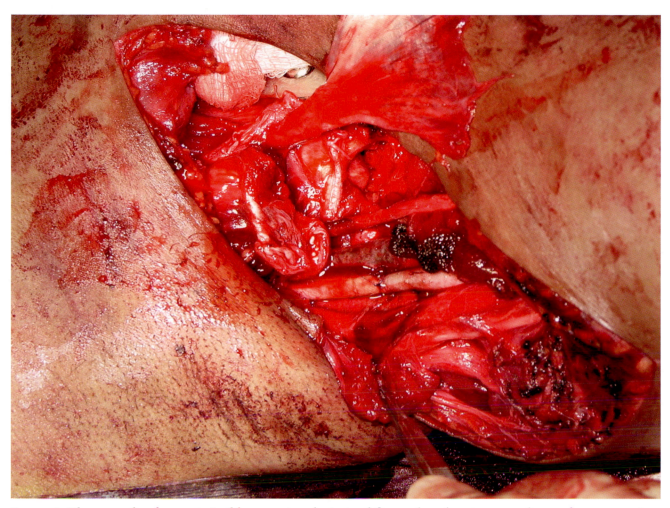

Figure 5. *The artery has been repaired by resecting the intimal flap and performing an end-to-end anastomosis.*

SUMMARY

This patient presented with a pulseless upper extremity after blunt trauma resulted in a proximal humerus fracture. Initial placement of a shunt allowed reperfusion of the extremity while the fracture was fixated. Vascular repair was completed with good result.

Note: See discussion of this case on page 360.

SUGGESTED READING

Chapter 23: Extremity fractures. In: *Emergency War Surgery, Third United States Revision*. Washington, DC: Department of the Army, Office of The Surgeon General, Borden Institute; 2004.

Chapter 27: Vascular injuries. In: *Emergency War Surgery, Third United States Revision*. Washington, DC: Department of the Army, Office of The Surgeon General, Borden Institute; 2004.

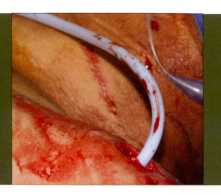

VIII.9
Left Subclavian Artery Gunshot Wound

CASE PRESENTATION

This 23-year-old host nation male presented to the combat support hospital (CSH) after sustaining a single gunshot wound to the upper anterior chest, medial to the left shoulder. On arrival, the patient was in extremis with minimal bleeding from the wound. He was intubated immediately without difficulty, and a left-sided chest tube was placed with drainage of approximately 600 mL of blood. After intravenous access was gained via a right subclavian vein central line and a fluid bolus was started, new profuse bleeding from the left chest wound was noted. Attempts at direct pressure on the wound were unsuccessful. To obtain control of this bleeding, a large urinary catheter was placed in the wound, and the balloon was inflated with water (Fig. 1). The proximal end of the urinary catheter was also clamped to prevent bleeding from the lumen of the catheter. With bleeding controlled and the patient responding to fluid infusion, the remainder of the primary and secondary surveys was completed. No other injuries were identified. The patient was then transported directly to the operating room, where the chest and left groin were prepped and draped. A left anterolateral thoracotomy was performed. This classic incision was also extended fairly far posteriorly. Bleeding from the subclavian artery was first controlled by compression with a sponge stick. Next, proximal and distal control were obtained using vascular clamps. Injury to the subclavian artery involved approximately 50% to 75% of the vessel circumference. The vessel was mobilized, and the area of injury was resected to include the surrounding blast-affected areas. The subclavian artery was repaired primarily using end-to-end anastomosis. Following this repair, there was excellent capillary refill of the fingers and strong radial and ulnar pulses. The thorax was irrigated to remove any retained clots, a new chest tube was placed, and the incision was closed. The edges of the gunshot wound were debrided, and the entrance wound was left open and closed by secondary intension. This postoperative course was uneventful, and the patient was transferred to a host nation facility after removal of the chest tube.

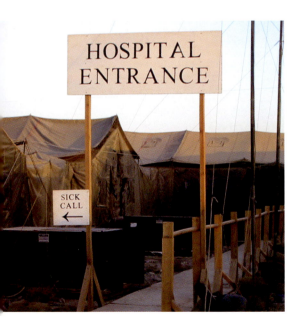

TEACHING POINTS

1. Direct pressure should be the first method used to control hemorrhage. Unfortunately, there are regions of the body where this approach will not be successful (eg, subclavian and groin

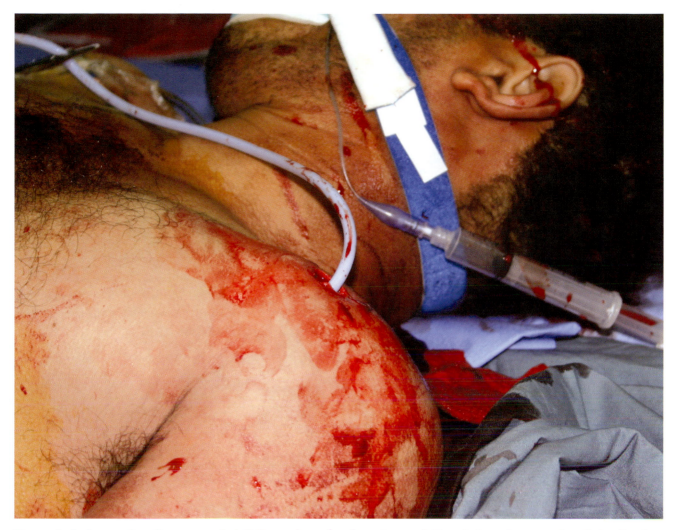

FIGURE 1. *Left superior chest wound. A Foley catheter has been inserted directly into the wound and the distal balloon inflated with water to staunch uncontrolled hemorrhage.*

injuries). In these circumstances, insertion of a urinary catheter and inflation of the balloon with water will frequently tamponade bleeding under bony or ligamentous structures. It is important to clamp the proximal end of the catheter to prevent bleeding from the lumen.

2. Use of a urinary catheter with a 30-mL balloon works best. If that is not immediately available, then several smaller urinary catheters may also be effective.

3. This technique is also useful in controlling hepatic bleeding, when there is bleeding from the tunnel created by a bullet.

4. The choice of operative incision for penetrating thoracic trauma may be difficult because the side of injury dictates the type of incision used. The surgeon should be prepared to make a second or even third incision in 25% to 30% of cases.

5. In this case (left-sided injury), an anterolateral thoracotomy incision with a posterior extension provided both proximal and distal control. Use of a median sternotomy would have been inappropriate because the left subclavian vessels are posterior and cannot be reached from this incision. In addition, a clavicular incision is ill-advised because it is frequently difficult to gain proximal control. Another approach combines all three of these incisions into a trapdoor incision, also known as a "book" thoracotomy. However, this incision is frequently associated with causalgia in the postoperative period.

6. When exposing a right-sided subclavian injury, a median sternotomy with cervical extension should be the incision of choice.

7. Great care must be taken to avoid injury to the brachial plexus during this operation.
8. Concurrent or isolated injury to the subclavian vein may be treated with either lateral venorrhaphy or ligation.

CLINICAL IMPLICATIONS

Unlike this case, most missile injuries of the subclavian artery will require interposition graft (vein or prosthetic) and will not be amenable to primary repair.

DAMAGE CONTROL

Insertion of a urinary catheter to staunch noncompressible subclavian vessel hemorrhage is an acute temporizing measure only. This may be used for intratheater transport prior to definitive repair. It is not recommended for prolonged treatment.

SUMMARY

Obtaining initial control of bleeding from a vessel under a bony or ligamentous structure can be difficult. Use of a urinary catheter is an effective method (as in this case). Incision choice after a subclavian wound may also be difficult, because the approach to a right-sided injury is different from a left-sided injury. Once the incision has been made, the surgeon needs to be prepared to extend the incision or make another incision, if required.

Note: See discussion of this case on pages 360–361.

SUGGESTED READING

Chapter 16: Thoracic injuries. In: *Emergency War Surgery, Third United States Revision.* Washington, DC: Department of the Army, Office of The Surgeon General, Borden Institute; 2004.

Chapter 27: Vascular injuries. In: *Emergency War Surgery, Third United States Revision.* Washington, DC: Department of the Army, Office of The Surgeon General, Borden Institute; 2004.

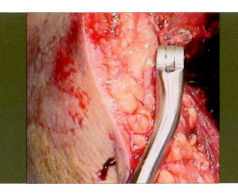

VIII.10
Gluteal Compartment Syndrome

CASE PRESENTATION

A 19-year-old US Marine Corps male vehicle driver was involved in a blast injury after driving over an improvised explosive device (IED). He presented with a Glasgow Coma Scale score of 15, but was hypotensive with a systolic blood pressure in the 80s and a pulse in the 120s. He reported pain in the right buttock and both legs, but denied any loss of consciousness or paresthesias. Physical examination showed a large area of ecchymosis and edema over the right buttock (Fig. 1), which was compressible. In addition, he had moderate tenderness over his right sacrum and buttock. The pelvis was evaluated and found to be stable. The leg compartments were soft, and there was no crepitus nor instability in his lower extremities. The neurovascular examination was normal. His hemoglobin was 8.0 g/dL. CT scan of the pelvis revealed a large right gluteal hematoma (Fig. 2). CT scan also revealed a right sacral fracture (Fig. 3) and right pubic rami fractures (Fig. 4). He was taken to the operating room where he underwent angiography and selective catheterization of the right inferior gluteal artery. There was active extravasation from several branches of the artery (Fig. 5). Coil embolization was performed using multiple microcoils (Fig. 6). Completion angiography was performed and showed no further extravasation (Fig. 7). After obtaining hemostasis, the right buttock was reexamined and found to be tense. Orthopaedic surgery confirmed the diagnosis of a gluteal compartment syndrome, and the patient underwent emergent fasciotomy through a posterior approach (Fig. 8). The gluteus maximus was incised and a large (1.5 L) hematoma was evacuated (Fig. 9). Further examination revealed healthy muscle in the buttock and hip with good hemostasis. The buttock and thigh were soft following the fasciotomy, and there was a positive wrinkle sign in the skin. The wound was therefore closed in layers over a drain, and the patient was taken to the intensive care unit for further monitoring and care. His neurovascular examination was unchanged after the surgery, and he was transferred to a higher echelon of care the following day.

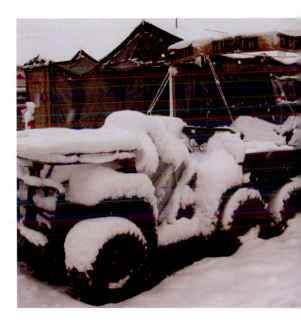

TEACHING POINTS

1. Compartment syndrome is defined as increased pressure within an enclosed osteofascial space that reduces the capillary blood perfusion below a level necessary for tissue viability. It is a clinical diagnosis and usually manifests with pain out of proportion on physical examination

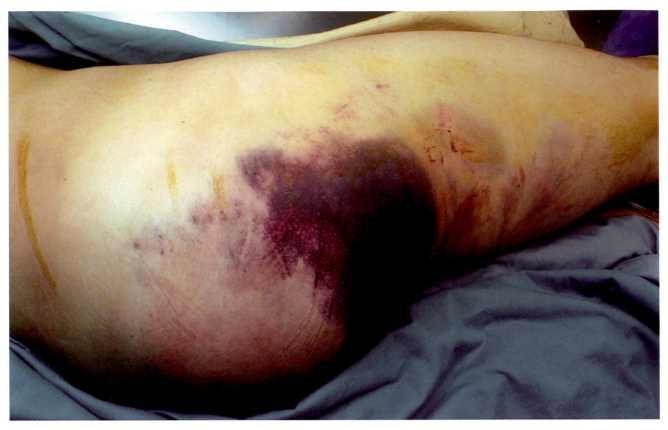

FIGURE 1. *Right buttock and thigh ecchymoses of hematoma.*

and pain that is not controlled with pain medication. In addition, patients can note paresthesias and will have pain on passive stretch of the affected extremity.

2. In patients without a reliable clinical examination (eg, an intubated or head-injured patient), compartment pressure measurements can be obtained. The diagnosis of compartment syndrome is made when either the absolute pressure is greater than 30 mm Hg or the pressure is within 30 mm Hg of the diastolic blood pressure (delta P < 30 mm Hg). Once the diagnosis is made, emergent fasciotomy is indicated. Clinical suspicion overrules pressure monitors, however, which are cumbersome and may not be available. If compartment syndrome is suspected, surgical intervention is warranted.

3. Isolated gluteal compartment syndromes are uncommon, and they are usually caused by pelvic and acetabular fractures or vascular injury. A high index of suspicion should be maintained for any patient who presents with the signs and symptoms of compartment syndrome and a plausible mechanism of injury.

4. All patients who present with pelvic fractures need a thorough physical examination of the spine, chest, pelvis, and extremities. The pelvis should be examined by applying anterior-posterior and lateral compressive forces across the iliac wings. If any instability is noted, a pelvic binder or sheet can be applied to stabilize the pelvis and prevent further bleeding.

5. Pelvic fractures are potentially complex injuries. In this instance, the pelvic fractures represented a lateral compression mechanism and were considered stable. In general, lateral compression pelvic fractures carry a high incidence of associated brain and visceral injuries; however, there is a lesser incidence of pelvic vascular injuries. Interestingly, this patient presented with a vascular injury, which may be attributed to the high-energy blast mechanism.

6. This type of lateral compression pelvic fracture is treated symptomatically with weight-bearing as tolerated using assistive devices.

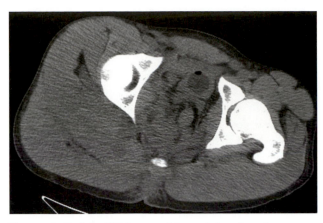

FIGURE 2. *Pelvis CT image. Note right gluteal hematoma.*

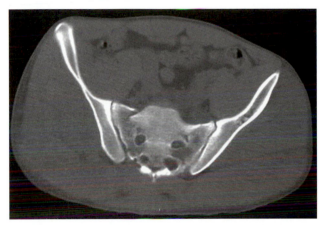

FIGURE 3. *Sacrum CT image. Note displaced fracture of the right sacrum.*

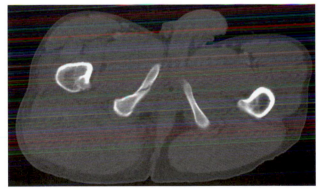

FIGURE 4. *Pelvis CT image. There is a nondisplaced fracture of the right pubic ramus. Note large right gluteal hematoma.*

CLINICAL IMPLICATIONS

Treatment of a hemodynamically unstable patient with a pelvic fracture requires a multidisciplinary approach and algorithm. Although this patient had a stable pelvic fracture, potentially life-threatening sources of hemorrhage need to be identified and controlled. Permanent muscle and nerve dysfunction can develop if a compartment syndrome is not released in a timely fashion, which makes compartment syndrome a true surgical emergency. The following treatment principles were applied in this case:

1. Control of hemorrhage can be obtained through open or endovascular techniques. Surgical ligation of the hypogastric artery can diminish pelvic blood flow and associated hemorrhage, but is nonselective and may result in ischemic complications. With this technique, persistent bleeding is also possible via collateral vascular pathways from the contralateral hypogastric artery or ipsilateral femoral artery. Direct surgical control of bleeding at the time of compartment release may also be effective, but this approach is often associated with poor exposure, and difficulties obtaining control of the artery of hemorrhage can result in significant blood loss. Finally, if the patient is stable enough to tolerate angiographic evaluation, pelvic angiography is highly sensitive and specific for determination of the source of bleeding. Embolization of the hemorrhagic artery can then be performed in a selective fashion with greater than 90% technical success in achieving thrombosis of the vessel.

2. Gluteal compartment syndromes should be released through a posterior approach to the hip, which utilizes the greater trochanter as the primary landmark. Once the greater trochanter is identified, a 15- to 20-cm incision is made that gently curves over the buttock. Because the gluteus maximus is innervated by both the superior and inferior gluteal nerves, it can be divided in line with its fibers. There are always vessels that cross the plane of dissection, so it is important to maintain good hemostasis.

3. Once the surgical plane is fully developed, the hematoma can be evacuated to relieve pressure on the surrounding tissues. After all sources of bleeding have been identified and controlled, the wound can be closed in layers over a drain.

4. It is important to monitor the patient postoperatively for improvement in symptoms and potential changes in neurovascular examination.

DAMAGE CONTROL

An unstable pelvic fracture can be temporarily stabilized with a pelvic binder or sheet. Once applied, it should not be removed until definitive stabilization can be performed. If a vascular surgeon or interventional radiologist is not available to embolize a pelvic vascular injury, emergent fasciotomy should still be performed in the face of a compartment syndrome. If the source of the bleeding cannot be identified at the time of surgery, it is prudent to pack the area in question and transport the patient to a facility with the appropriate personnel and equipment.

SUMMARY

This case demonstrates an uncommon type of compartment syndrome that was caused by high-energy blunt trauma. A team approach was used to address the vascular injury and resulting compartment syndrome. Once the inferior gluteal artery injury was embolized, the gluteal compartment was completely released to improve local tissue perfusion. Prompt diagnosis and treatment of gluteal compartment syndrome will help optimize patient recovery and long-term function.

Note: See discussion of this case on page 361.

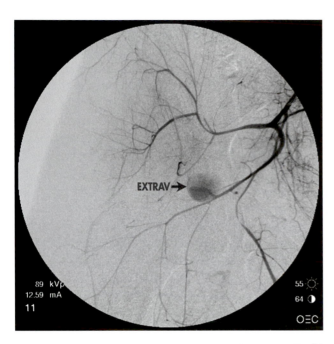

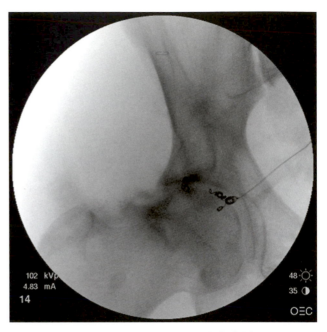

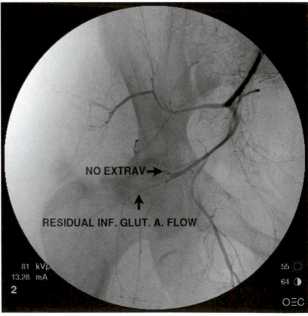

FIGURE 5. (Left) *Selective angiography of the right inferior gluteal artery. Note extravasation (EXTRAV).*

FIGURE 6. (Top Right) *Microcoil embolization of right inferior gluteal artery.*

FIGURE 7. (Bottom Right) *Completion angiogram after branch artery embolizations. No extravasation of contrast is noted. EXTRAV: extravasation; INF. GLUT. A.: inferior gluteal artery.*

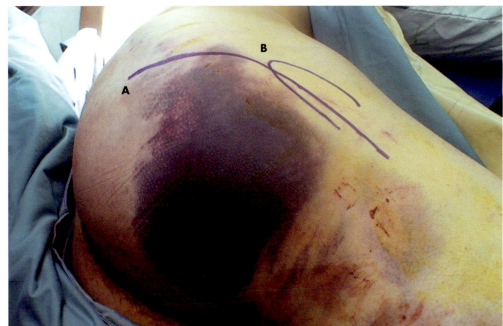

FIGURE 8. (Top) *Markings for incision to relieve right gluteal compartment syndrome (A) and to identify right greater trochanter (B).*

FIGURE 9. (Bottom) *Large gluteus hematoma exposed.*

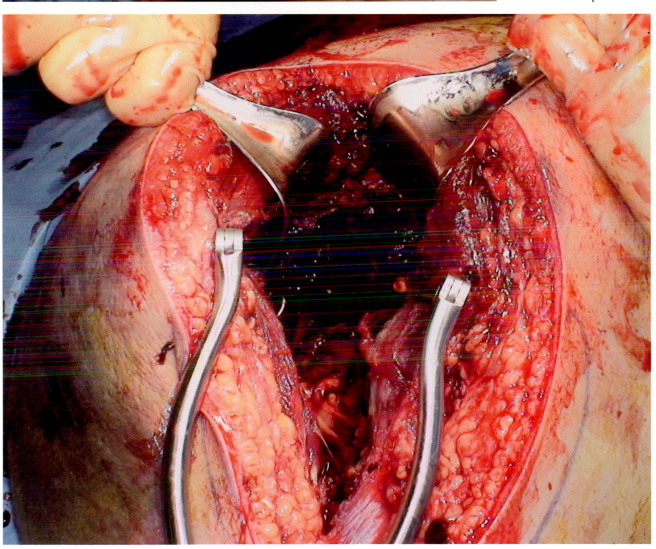

SUGGESTED READING

Browner BD, Jupiter JB, et al. *Skeletal Trauma*. 3rd ed. Philadelphia, Pa: Saunders; 2003.

Chapter 8: Vascular access. In: *Emergency War Surgery, Third United States Revision*. Washington, DC: Department of the Army, Office of The Surgeon General, Borden Institute; 2004.

Chapter 12: Damage control surgery. In: *Emergency War Surgery, Third United States Revision*. Washington, DC: Department of the Army, Office of The Surgeon General, Borden Institute; 2004.

Chapter 17: Abdominal injuries. In: *Emergency War Surgery, Third United States Revision*. Washington, DC: Department of the Army, Office of The Surgeon General, Borden Institute; 2004.

Chapter 21: Pelvic injuries. In: *Emergency War Surgery, Third United States Revision*. Washington, DC: Department of the Army, Office of The Surgeon General, Borden Institute; 2004.

Hoppenfeld S, deBoer P. *Surgical Exposures in Orthopaedics: The Anatomical Approach*. 3rd ed. Philadelphia, Pa: Lippincott Williams & Wilkins; 2003.

Vascular Trauma; Cases Review

by MAJ Niten N. Singh, MD

Numerous topics were covered in the vascular section and relevant scenarios were presented that the deploying surgeon will encounter. As a surgeon who has deployed both as a general and vascular surgeon, these collected cases can constitute a typical week in a deployed combat support hospital (CSH). The main urgency of any surgeon in theater is to transport the patient with a penetrating injury to the operating room (OR) as soon as feasible. As opposed to civilian trauma—in which blunt injury is the rule rather than the exception—the majority of combat trauma patients present after penetrating injury. Penetrating vascular injuries need to be controlled quickly. In the emergency room (ER), if a patient is found to have hard signs of arterial injury (ie, pulseless extremity, expanding hematoma, etc), then that patient should be transported to the OR for operative intervention. If the patient is hemodynamically unstable, placing a clamp or ligature on the bleeding vessel and continuing resuscitation in the OR, not the ER, is the course that should be pursued. Prolonged resuscitation should not occur in a setting where the surgeon does not have the ability to intervene surgically.

CASE VIII.1 (Innominate Vein Injury) emphasizes the importance of neck exploration in zone II injuries of the neck. There are proponents of exploration, as well as those that tout the use of endoscopy, arteriography, and bronchoscopy. I believe that, in the case of combat trauma, all zone II injuries should be explored. Resection of the clavicle to allow exposure of the subclavian vessels is a useful technique, but extending the neck incision into a median sternotomy can be the next step for venous injuries in zone I on the left. If injury of the proximal subclavian artery is suspected, a median sternotomy—along with a supraclavicular incision and fourth intercostal space anterior thoracotomy (trapdoor)—provides excellent exposure. When dealing with innominate vein injury, the surgeon may choose between repair versus ligation. Adequate control and flushing are extremely important to avoid potential air embolism.

CASE VIII.2 (External Iliac Vein Injury, Exposure and Control) provides a good example of how knowledge of various vascular exposures can be lifesaving. In this case, the patient had venous bleeding above the inguinal ligament. Using a retroperitoneal approach, they were able to identify and repair the injury. I would stress that, in these types of cases, if digital pressure is controlling the hemorrhage, the patient should be transported directly to the OR. The handholding pressure can be prepped into the field and the injury subsequently repaired or ligated. Any time spent resuscitating or attempting to clamp vessels in the ER without adequate equipment/lighting can lead to unnecessary delay in treatment.

CASE VIII.3 (Penetrating Subclavian Artery Injury) is an example of a lifesaving operation that must be performed prior to evacuation. In this case, a simple supraclavicular exposure allowed the surgeons to repair a potentially lethal injury. Given the fact that it was a minor arterial injury, debridement and repair were appropriate. If the injury were larger, proximal greater saphenous vein grafting should be used. Small size discrepancies are tolerated; otherwise, a Dacron graft soaked in rifampin is not ideal, but is a capable substitute (soak the graft in 1,200 mg of rifampin for 20 minutes).

In **CASE VIII.4** (Shunts in Vascular Injuries), the use of shunts shows the importance of shunts in level II settings. These should be removed and the artery and vein repaired expeditiously at the CSH, prior to evacuation out of theater. Remember that the proximal and distal aspects of the vessels need to be inspected because the

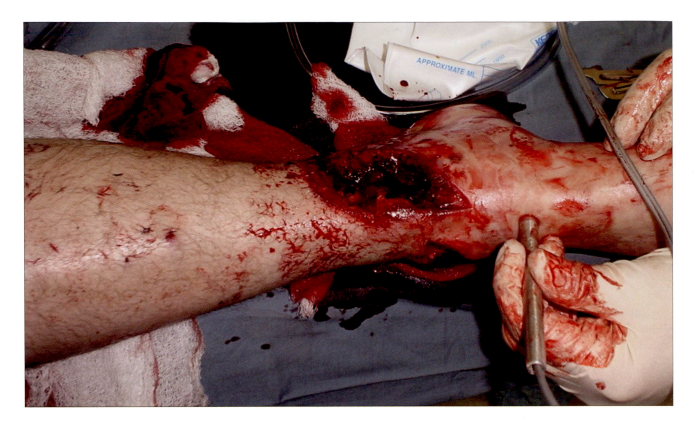

shunt and suture can injure that portion of the vessel. Up to 0.5 to 1.0 cm will need to be debrided before placing an interposition graft. If possible, which was not the case with this patient, systemic heparin should be given to all patients during vessel repair. There is no need to pass Fogarty catheters if there is good back bleeding and heparin saline flushes easily.

CASE VIII.5 (Arteriovenous Fistula)—Although not readily apparent, arteriovenous fistula and pseudo-aneurysms are fairly common in the follow-up of patients with proximity injuries. Treatment is straightforward as described. However, in difficult-to-reach areas, endovascular repair with covered stents is becoming more common practice, but is not always an option at the CSH.

CASE VIII.6 (Brachial Artery Injury, Transection) is a common one in theater. If the injury is distal to the profunda brachii and the patient is in extremis, ligation can be performed and the extremity should remain viable. Remember that the brachial artery is extremely reactive and will go into vasospasm easily. Therefore, systemic heparin, when possible, is advised. The additional use of papaverine may be necessary. The latter can be placed in heparin saline solution (5,000 units of heparin, 500 cc of normal saline, and 2 cc [60

mg] of papaverine) and injected subadventially around the artery and vein graft.

CASE VIII.7 (Femoral Vein Injury) depicts the massive blood loss that can ensue with a venous injury. With soft-tissue damage, bleeding can be worse unless the vein is repaired and venous outflow restored. If the patient is in extremis, ligation is the procedure of choice, as indicated in this case. It is unlikely that the use of activated Factor VII assisted in this case and should be avoided with vascular injuries. Once these injuries are repaired, bleeding will usually cease, and there is no need to promote potential thrombus formation in an injured vessel.

CASE VIII.8 (Brachial Artery Injury, Blunt Trauma) is another example of a brachial artery injury. It is also an example of the use of a temporizing shunt while orthopaedic procedures are performed, then performing a vein graft repair. In general, this is a good technique in the setting of major orthopaedic trauma. The greater saphenous vein can be harvested during the orthopaedic repair.

In **CASE VIII.9** (Left Subclavian Artery Gunshot Wound)—controlling hemorrhage from a penetrating thoracic wound—a Foley catheter was used to compress the bullet tract, which allowed the surgeon time to perform a thoracotomy and repair the subclavian artery. Penetrating thoracic trauma is common in theater. Wounds in proximity to the great vessels should raise a high index of suspicion for coincident injury. If the patient loses vital signs in the emergency medical treatment area, an anterolateral thoracotomy provides good exposure to the proximal subclavian artery. Combined with a median sternotomy and supraclavicular extension (trapdoor), excellent exposure to this area is obtained (see Case VIII.1). At this point, the goal is to save a life. Concern for causalgia is not warranted; many thoracotomy patients may suffer from postthoracotomy pain as well. If the patient is in extremis, the proximal subclavian artery can be ligated, as long as it is proximal to the vertebral artery. In most patients, the left vertebral artery is dominant, and flow reversal will allow for perfusion of that extremity. Reconstruction can be performed later.

In **CASE VIII.10** (Gluteal Compartment Syndrome), the use of endovascular techniques for the embolization of a gluteal compartment syndrome reveals the options available to the deployed endovascular-trained surgeon. Bleeding can be controlled in this manner if the patient is stable. However, in the face of a large gluteal hematoma, direct ligation is effective for those not trained to perform endovascular procedures and is likely more expeditious.

As stated previously, large hematomas tend to make the dissection easier. The inferior gluteal vessels are below the gluteus maximus and can be ligated relatively easily.

These cases are representative of the variety of vascular cases a surgeon will see while deployed. It might be nice to be able to perform therapeutic endovascular procedures, but a surgeon should proceed with what methods he is most comfortable performing. All of these cases call on the operating surgeon's knowledge of anatomy and exposures, which are the most important preparations I can recommend prior to deployment. Once proper exposure is obtained, repair becomes the simple part of the operation. I would highly recommend a reference text on common vascular exposures (see below) for the deploying surgeon to take along in his personal kit, because these injuries are commonly seen.

SUGGESTED READING

Rutherford RB. *Atlas of Vascular Surgery: Basic Techniques and Exposures*. Philadelphia, Pa: WB Saunders Company; 1993.

Wind GG, Valentine RJ. *Anatomic Exposure in Vascular Surgery*. 2nd ed. Baltimore, Md: Williams & Wilkins; 1991.

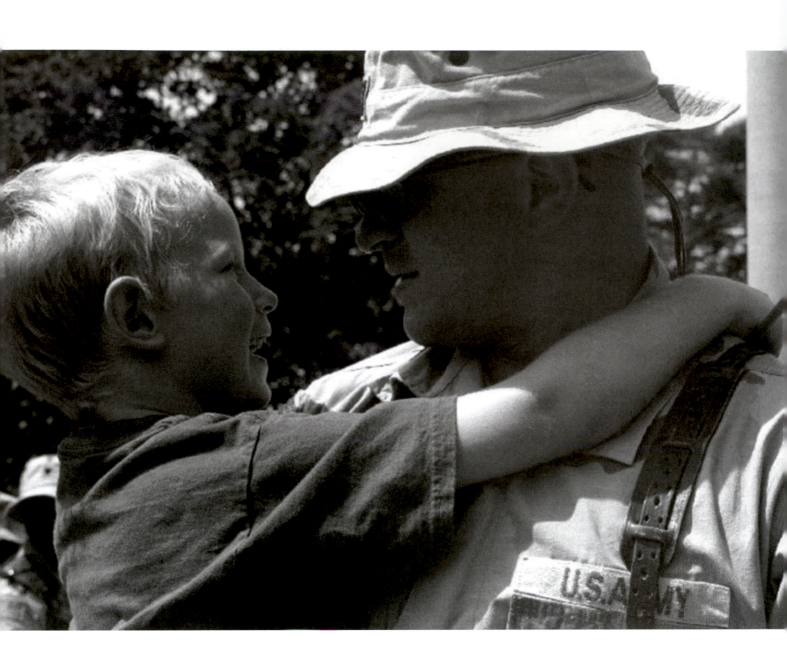

Chapter IX
SPECIAL SCENARIOS

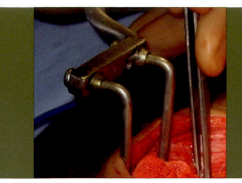

IX.1
Penetrating Pediatric Trauma, I

CASE PRESENTATION

This 5-year-old host nation male was injured by some form of exploding ordnance or improvised explosive device (IED). The patient sustained numerous penetrating fragment wounds. He presented awake, alert, and hemodynamically stable. Secondary survey revealed an open comminuted right mandibular fracture (Fig. 1), an open right nasomaxillary fracture, evisceration through a large abdominal wound to the right of the umbilicus, multiple penetrating injuries to the abdominal wall, and amputation of one digit on the right hand (Fig. 2). These injuries warranted immediate laparotomy, and the patient was taken directly to the operating room. Through a generous midline laparotomy (Fig. 3), it was discovered that he had sustained multiple intestinal perforations, including 1 hole in the gallbladder, 2 holes in the second portion of the duodenum, 8 holes in the small bowel, and 4 holes in the colon. The patient also had a large liver laceration that was bleeding minimally. His gallbladder was removed, and the common bile duct and pancreas were uninjured. There was a small bridge of duodenum connecting the two penetrating injuries that allowed debridement of the wounds, removal of the intervening bridge, and examination of the sphincter of Oddi, which was uninjured. The duodenum and portions of the small bowel and colon were repaired (with two primary anastomoses). Several other enterotomies that did not fall within reasonable resection margins were also repaired. A closed-suction drain and a Stamm gastrostomy were placed next to the duodenal repair. Postoperatively, the patient did well, although he required jaw wiring for his mandibular injury. The nasomaxillary fracture was caused by a fragment that lodged intracranially in the interhemispheric sulcus and was not removed. This condition left him with mild neurological deficits, including some gait disturbance that improved with time and therapy. A duodenal contrast study on postoperative day 7 was normal (Fig. 4), and he was allowed to eat, which resulted in a prompt and significant weight gain. The drain was removed at that time. The patient continued to do well and was eventually discharged.

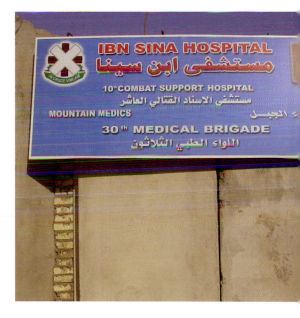

TEACHING POINTS

1. Blast and fragment injuries to children from explosive remnants of war cause enormous public health issues worldwide.

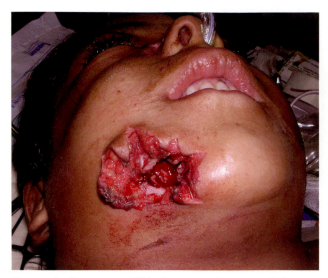

FIGURE 1. *Open mandible fracture. An open right nasomaxillary fracture is barely visible in this photograph.*

2. Children differ greatly from adults in ways that impact evaluation and management. Their vital signs vary with age and could give a false impression of physiological derangement. They have a greater ability to autoregulate perfusion than adults and are able to maintain normal blood pressures up until the last moments prior to irreversible cardiovascular collapse. Early recognition of the shock state is critical. Indicators such as tachypnea; tachycardia; ashen color; cool, clammy extremities; mottled appearance; and delayed capillary refill may be more useful than blood pressure. In children who have completely healthy hearts and lungs, the tendency should be to overtreat shock. It is unlikely that an otherwise healthy, injured child will be hydrated into congestive heart failure.

3. Airway access can be much more difficult to obtain than in adults. Even brief periods of apnea can lead to cardiac arrest. In the prehospital setting, bag-valve mask ventilation is preferred to endotracheal intubation because it is easier, quicker, and does not affect survival adversely.

4. Vascular access can be very difficult in small children. It is exacerbated by blood loss and agitation. Peripheral intravenous access should be the first choice, with a very short threshold to resort to intraosseous infusion. Insertion of an intraosseous needle is a rapid and simple procedure that may be a lifesaving bridge to more definitive venous access. Central lines should only be attempted by experienced pediatric providers and come after intraosseous infusion in order of priority.

5. Children have relatively large heads, predisposing them to head, cervical spine, and spinal cord injury. They have a larger body surface to body mass ratio, which results in a greater tendency to hypothermia. Every attempt must be made to ensure that they remain warm during resuscitation and operation.

6. Children have incompletely ossified skeletons that tend to be very elastic. Children subjected to very high-energy traumas may have relatively few fractures, but may still have sustained significant internal injuries.

7. An infant's abdomen (from birth to 12 months) is largest in the transverse direction. In this age group, a transverse incision approximately 1 fingerbreadth above the umbilicus affords maximum exposure. Above 1 year of age, midline incisions are preferable.

CLINICAL IMPLICATIONS

1. Simple duodenal injuries are best repaired primarily provided the lumen will not be reduced by more than 50%. Complex injuries may require full duodenal exposure (Kocher maneuver) and primary anastomosis or Roux-en-Y duodenojejunostomy. Pyloric exclusion should be used in all complex wounds or where repair is tenuous. This procedure can be done with absorbable pyloric sutures placed intraluminally through a distal gastrotomy or by a noncutting transverse staple line across the pylorus. Neither technique is permanent, and the lumen recanalizes in several weeks.

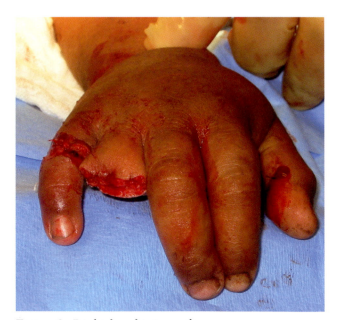

FIGURE 2. *Right-hand injury after surgery.*

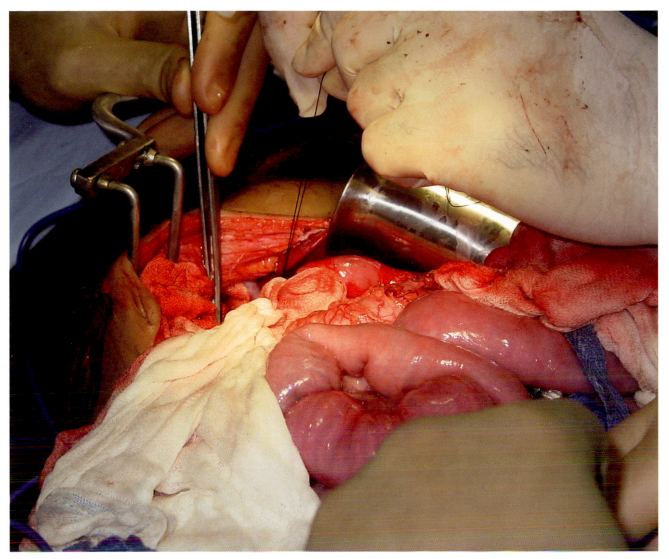

FIGURE 3. *Laparotomy in a 5-year-old male performed through a midline incision.*

2. Duodenal repairs are prone to leak, especially if complicated by shock and injuries to multiple organ systems. The patient's condition, concomitant injuries, and external factors (eg, echelon of care, total number of injured patients, and critical care assets) must be considered when deciding on treatment options.

3. Upper gastrointestinal contrast study with fluoroscopy can be performed at most level III medical treatment facilities and can be very useful prior to initiation of feeds and removal of tubes and drains.

4. Gallbladder injuries are rare and are best treated by cholecystectomy.

5. In children who have any degree of hypotension, hypoxia, hypothermia, and significant soilage or tissue destruction, primary intestinal anastomoses should be avoided. In this setting, the repair of multiple colonic perforations should be diverted proximally. The same is advisable for the small intestine, although very proximal small intestinal ostomies should be avoided because of profound postoperative derangements from intestinal fluid losses. Multiple perforations alone or combined with multiple concomitant injuries are not contraindications of primary repair. If, during such repairs, the child becomes unstable, this strategy should be switched immediately to damage control.

DAMAGE CONTROL

1. Controlling sepsis is much more important for immediate survival than intestinal continuity or definitive reconstruction.

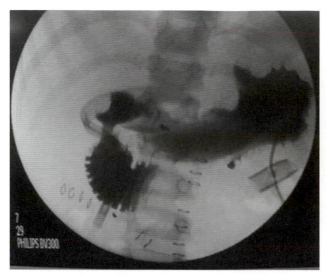

FIGURE 4. *Gastroduodenal fluoroscopy revealed no extravasation of contrast on postoperative day 7.*

2. When faced with a persistently unstable or hypothermic patient, a duodenal injury can be rapidly controlled with stapled pyloric exclusion, duodenostomy tube decompression, and multiple closed-suction drains placed around the injury. This can lead to a quick end to the operation and an opportunity to pursue aggressive rewarming and resuscitation so that the patient can survive and become stable for a second, more definitive surgery.

SUMMARY

This is an unusual case of fragment wounds in a 5-year-old boy causing multiple intestinal perforations, including gallbladder and duodenal injuries. To provide optimal care, it is important to consider anatomical and physiological differences between children and adults. Duodenal injuries vary greatly in complexity and can be highly morbid. The judicious use of adjuncts—such as gastrostomy tube, pyloric exclusion, duodenostomy tube,

and closed-suction drainage—will, hopefully, minimize the risk and sequelae of postoperative leak. In some instances, multiple intestinal and colonic perforations may be primarily repaired without diversion. Surgeons should divert proximal repairs if the patient has suffered any physiological derangement prior to or during surgery.

SUGGESTED READING

Chapter 5: Airway/breathing. In: *Emergency War Surgery, Third United States Revision*. Washington, DC: Department of the Army, Office of The Surgeon General, Borden Institute; 2004.

Chapter 8: Vascular access. In: *Emergency War Surgery, Third United States Revision*. Washington, DC: Department of the Army, Office of The Surgeon General, Borden Institute; 2004.

Chapter 13: Face and neck injuries. In: *Emergency War Surgery, Third United States Revision*. Washington, DC: Department of the Army, Office of The Surgeon General, Borden Institute; 2004.

Chapter 17: Abdominal injuries. In: *Emergency War Surgery, Third United States Revision*. Washington, DC: Department of the Army, Office of The Surgeon General, Borden Institute; 2004.

Chapter 25: Amputations. In: *Emergency War Surgery, Third United States Revision*. Washington, DC: Department of the Army, Office of The Surgeon General, Borden Institute; 2004.

Chapter 33: Pediatric care. In: *Emergency War Surgery, Third United States Revision*. Washington, DC: Department of the Army, Office of The Surgeon General, Borden Institute; 2004.

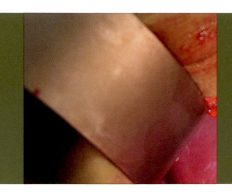

IX.2
Penetrating Pediatric Trauma, II

CASE PRESENTATION

This 5-year-old male, one of three children who presented to a combat support hospital (CSH), was wounded after triggering an unexploded ordnance (Fig. 1). His lower extremity injuries included a right femur fracture with significant associated tissue injury, as well as other soft-tissue injuries (Figs. 2 and 3). The patient had multiple wounds of the abdomen and lower extremities. After initial resuscitation, he was taken to the operating room. During surgery, colon and kidney (Fig. 4) injuries were found. The midtransverse colon injury was closed in two layers (Fig. 5), and the right kidney laceration required no further treatment after it was identified. The open femur facture was treated with external fixation after a washout. Later, the wounds were skin grafted with excellent results.

TEACHING POINTS

1. In combat zones, Forward Surgical Teams (FSTs) and CSH personnel must be prepared to treat pediatric patients. The medical rules of engagement during Operation Iraqi Freedom provided for treatment of Iraqi civilians who were injured during US Armed Forces operations. Many children were brought to US medical facilities by their parents. Treatment of medical and congenital surgical conditions was frequently authorized.

2. In a combat environment, a multispecialty team approach is normally required with all types of patients. This patient, with serious abdominal and lower extremity injuries, required general surgery and orthopaedic surgery. Pediatricians are an essential part of this team, but are typically not assigned to the CSH. Prolonged care at the CSH was necessary for this patient because civilian facilities were not available.

3. The external fixator placed on the femur fracture remained until healing was complete. Skin grafting was also performed. During his 3-month stay, the patient gained 15 pounds.

4. Family members of the patient frequently visited the hospital and interacted with staff. They were grateful for the care that the child received. Care also included hiring local, English-speaking civilians to work as translators.

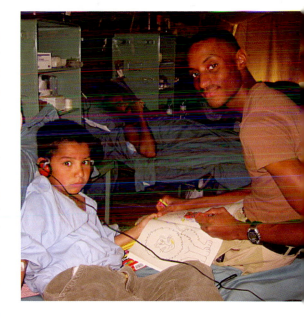

CLINICAL IMPLICATIONS

The initial, Advanced Trauma Life Support (ATLS) approach to pediatric

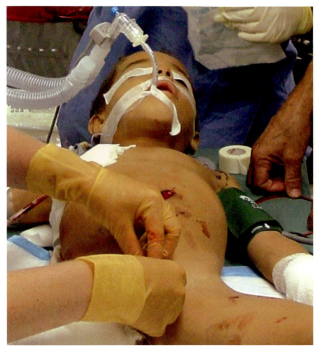

FIGURE 1. *A 5-year-old Iraqi male on admission to the CSH.*

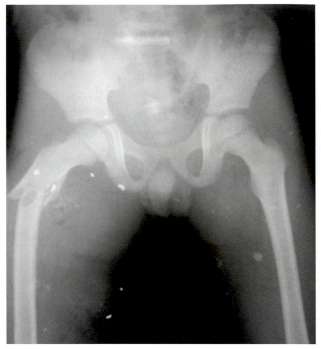

FIGURE 2. *Radiograph of the right pelvis. Note femur fracture and multiple fragments in the soft tissues.*

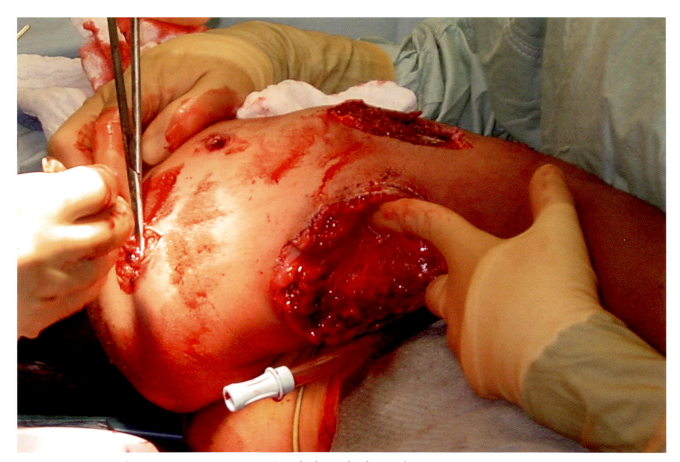

FIGURE 3. *Large soft-tissue injuries associated with the right femur fracture.*

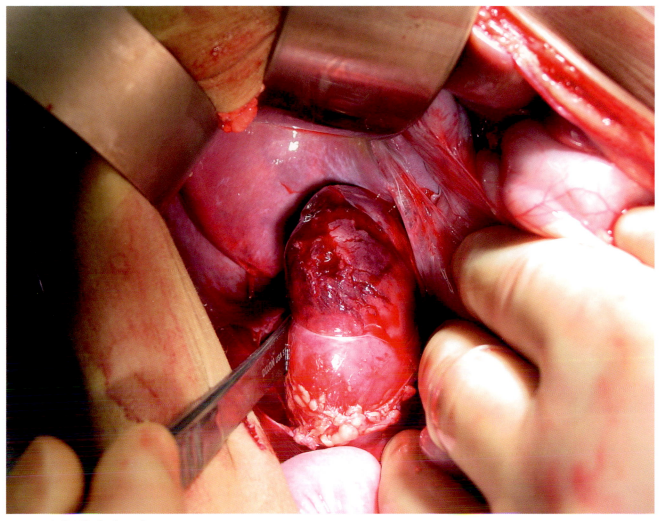

FIGURE 4. *Right kidney laceration.*

trauma patients is the same as for adults. However, there are also special considerations:

1. Infants and young children are especially prone to heat loss and must be kept warm.
2. Systolic blood pressure less than 90 mm Hg is associated with high mortality rates, and early blood transfusion is often necessary in young children with multiple wounds.
3. Children more than 3 months old have a blood volume of about 70 cc/kg. This means that a child weighing 15 kg has a total blood volume of 1,050 cc.
4. FSTs and CSHs should be equipped with the Broselow/Hinkle Pediatric Resuscitation System.
5. As a general guideline, transverse incisions should be used in infants to minimize postoperative dehiscence while still allowing adequate exposure.

DAMAGE CONTROL

If intravenous (IV) access cannot be obtained in a peripheral or femoral vein, intraosseous access is an effective alternative. The needle should be placed 2 to 3 cm below the tibial tuberosity. IV fluid, blood, and drugs (including bicarbonate, epinephrine, antibiotics, and atropine) can be infused through the intraosseous line. Fracture sites should not be used.

SUMMARY

Pediatric trauma is common in the combat environment and should be anticipated. To obtain optimum care, pediatric patients require a multispecialty team approach. Meticulous attention to postoperative care that recognizes the limited reserve of young patients is essential.

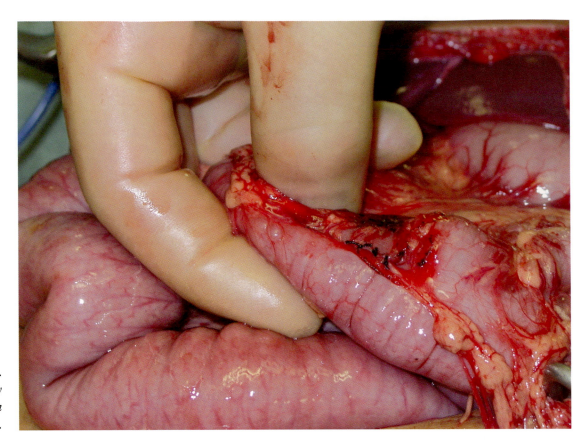

FIGURE 5.
Colon injury
repaired in
two layers.

BROSELOW/HINKLE PEDIATRIC RESUSCITATION SYSTEM

This patented system is commonly used for emergency pediatric resuscitative care. It was developed by James Broselow, MD, and Alan Hinkle, MD. This resuscitative system takes into consideration the direct correlation between the pediatric patient's body length and the proper size of emergency supplies and correct drug dosages. The Broselow/Hinkle system consists of the following items:

- Tape measure with eight color zones.
- Corresponding series of color-coded, single-patient use emergency kits.

These items are all organized and identified in a nylon organizer bag that is ready for any pediatric emergency.

SUGGESTED READING

Chapter 17: Abdominal injuries. In: *Emergency War Surgery, Third United States Revision*. Washington, DC: Department of the Army, Office of The Surgeon General, Borden Institute; 2004.

Chapter 18: Genitourinary tract injuries. In: *Emergency War Surgery, Third United States Revision*. Washington, DC: Department of the Army, Office of The Surgeon General, Borden Institute; 2004.

Chapter 22: Pediatric care. In: *Emergency War Surgery, Third United States Revision*. Washington, DC: Department of the Army, Office of The Surgeon General, Borden Institute; 2004.

Chapter 23: Extremity fractures. In: *Emergency War Surgery, Third United States Revision*. Washington, DC: Department of the Army, Office of The Surgeon General, Borden Institute; 2004.

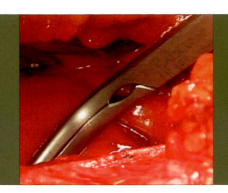

IX.3
Removal of an Unexploded Ordnance

CASE PRESENTATION

A 23-year-old male soldier was air evacuated to a Forward Surgical Team (FST) facility. The patient was described in-flight as hypotensive and having metallic fragments in the abdomen. Upon arrival, the primary survey revealed an impaled rocket. Only the tail was visible, with the majority of the rocket—and potentially the warhead—inside the patient. The rocket entered the left iliac wing, traversed the abdominal cavity, and tented the skin over the right greater trochanter (Fig. 1). The medical treatment facility was evacuated, except for the surgeon in charge of resuscitation and three medics. The explosive ordnance disposal (EOD) team was contacted. The patient's clinical condition deteriorated with worsening hypotension, marked bradycardia, and respiratory distress. Emergent intubation was performed, followed by aggressive volume resuscitation that included packed red blood cell transfusion. In addition, intravenous epinephrine was administered to reverse the bradycardia and hypotension. Epinephrine and volume resuscitation were sufficient to return the blood pressure and heart rate to within normal limits. Radiographs were used to determine the status of the suspected unexploded ordnance (UXO). No further movement of the patient was attempted because it presented an additional risk for detonation of the UXO. Radiographs revealed that the warhead was not attached to the round (Fig. 2). The patient was then moved to the operating room (OR). The decision was made to remove the UXO expediently. First, the skin was incised over the right anterior hip, where the tip of the round was protruding (Fig. 3). To gain control of the round and to remove bulky clothing that was pulled into the wound tract, a midline laparotomy was performed. While the surgeons stabilized the shaft of the rocket in the abdomen, an EOD team member sawed off the tail of the rocket at the level of the skin on the patient's left side. This allowed the UXO to be removed by pulling the round, in a left-to-right direction, across the pelvis through the abdomen (Fig. 4). Intraoperative findings included multiple, small-bowel perforations, as well as cecal and sigmoid colon perforations. These were repaired. In the original exploration, no major vascular, ureteral, or bladder injuries were identified. In addition to the intraabdominal injuries, a comminuted fracture of the left iliac crest, third-degree burns over the right proximal thigh, and extensive contamination of the lateral right thigh muscles were noted. The patient was then transferred to a level

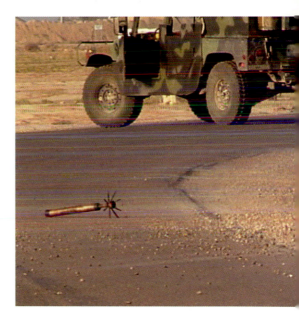

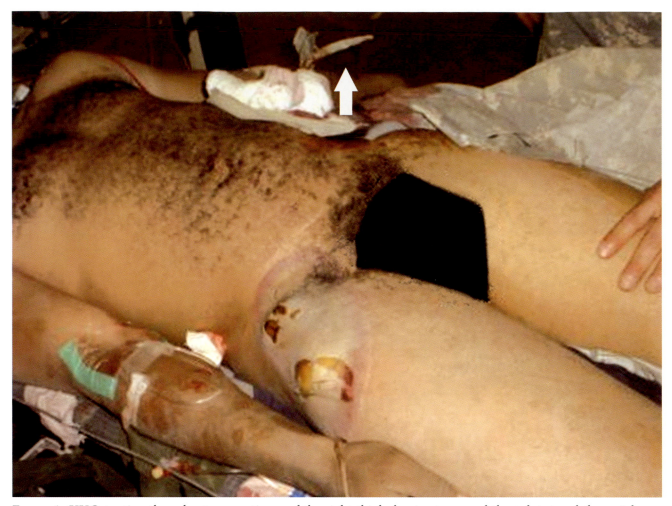

FIGURE 1. UXO *tenting the subcutaneous tissue of the right thigh, having traversed the pelvis in a left-to-right transit. The extruding tail of the rocket at the patient's left is visible in the photo* (arrow).

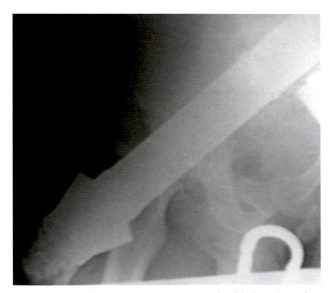

FIGURE 2. *Radiograph of the UXO embedded in the pelvis and femur. The warhead is not attached to the rocket.*

III medical treatment facility in stable condition. He survived his injuries and recovered well.

TEACHING POINTS

1. Identification of a patient with embedded UXO is critical in order to properly triage, transport, and manage the individual. Recommended management of a UXO includes triaging the patient as nonemergent and placing the patient far apart from other patients. If helicopter transport is deemed necessary, appropriate precautions include grounding the patient to the aircraft, limiting the flight crew, ensuring that the flight crew is wearing body armor, and putting other patients on a separate flight. In this case, failure to identify the UXO lead to the patient being transported by helicopter to an FST simultaneously with three routine patients, placing everyone on the aircraft at risk.

2. Proper notification of the treatment team of a patient with an embedded UXO is imperative to allow for preparation of the medical facility and expedient management of the patient. In this case, the receiving facility did not get a report indicating that the patient had a UXO. As a result, the patient was taken directly to the medical treatment facility for urgent resuscitation and damage control laparotomy, placing the entire facility and treatment personnel at risk.

3. It is necessary to isolate the patient in an area separate from the main OR and to use the minimal number of personnel required to remove the ordnance safely and treat the patient. The patient and the treatment personnel should be protected by sandbags. All personnel involved in patient treatment should wear body armor, ballistic eye protection, and helmet protection. Lein et al,[1] in a retrospective review of a 50-year military experience removing UXOs from patients, recommended that anesthesia personnel leave the OR after induction of anesthesia. From our experience, this recommended practice is situation-dependent and dictated by the type of operation planned. Further recommendations include, whenever possible, that the round be removed under spinal or local anesthesia. However, with torso injuries, positioning the patient for a spinal anesthetic would be difficult, if not impossible. It is prudent to keep the patient paralyzed during treatment to minimize physical disturbance of the ordnance. Therefore, it is simpler and quicker to intubate the patient, providing general anesthesia using a nondepolarizing paralytic agent for induction.

4. Diagnostic adjuncts must be chosen carefully. Plain radiographs have been demonstrated to be safe.[1,2] Although not substantiated, it is wise to avoid use of CT, magnetic resonance imaging (MRI), and defibrillators during the initial evaluation. During surgery, electrocautery and electromagnetic instruments should be avoided until the UXO is removed. Interestingly, Schlager et al[2] demonstrated the safety of ultrasound in identifying explosive small arms rounds seen in civilian trauma. However, it is unknown if this experience can be applied to the military, where larger munitions (eg, rocket-propelled grenades or mortars) are encountered.

CLINICAL IMPLICATIONS

1. The presence of EOD personnel is critical to the proper handling and disposal of UXO. Although resuscitation should be initiated immediately, prior to

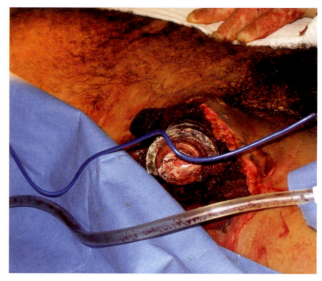

FIGURE 3. *Round protruding from the right hip.*

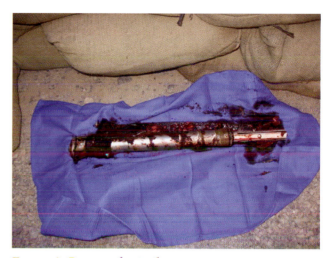

FIGURE 4. *Removed missile.*

definitive removal of the UXO the presence of EOD personnel is strongly advised.

2. In the most recent review of UXO by Lein et al,[1] 31 of 31 patients survived without further injury to the patient or medical personnel.

DAMAGE CONTROL

1. Based on the tactical situation and casualty flow, the patient with an embedded UXO may not be treatable despite apparent survivable injuries.

2. En bloc resection is the most expeditious way to minimize manipulation and risk associated with UXO removal. Manipulation of the UXO during the removal should be minimized. If embedded in an extremity, amputation should be considered.

SUMMARY

Embedded UXO is rare, but it presents many challenges to the operating surgeon. Despite previous recommendations, this clinical presentation requires constant reassessment. The type of equipment, diagnostic adjuncts, and number of personnel necessary for treatment depend on multiple factors, including the following:

1. Type of ordnance.
2. Location of the injury.
3. Condition of the patient.
4. Facilities and resources available.
5. Tactical situation/casualty flow.

We recommend that the UXO be removed in the most efficient and expedient manner possible, with minimal physical disturbance to the ordnance. To control the environment, use general versus spinal anesthesia. Having the appropriate, rather than the minimal, number of assistants in the OR to provide optimal visualization and assistance will lead to the most successful outcome.

REFERENCES

1. Lein B, et al. Removal of ordnance from patients: A 50-year military experience and current recommendations. *Mil Med*. 1999;164(3):163–165.
2. Schlager D, et al. Safety of imaging exploding bullets with ultrasound. *Ann Emerg Med*. 1996;28(2):183–187.

SUGGESTED READING

Chapter 3: Triage. In: *Emergency War Surgery, Third United States Revision*. Washington, DC: Department of the Army, Office of The Surgeon General, Borden Institute; 2004.

Chapter 12: Damage control surgery. In: *Emergency War Surgery, Third United States Revision*. Washington, DC: Department of the Army, Office of The Surgeon General, Borden Institute; 2004.

Chapter 17: Abdominal injuries. In: *Emergency War Surgery, Third United States Revision*. Washington, DC: Department of the Army, Office of The Surgeon General, Borden Institute; 2004.

Editor's Note: The use of epinephrine, as was done in this case, is not recommended in present ATLS (Advanced Trauma Life Support) protocols for the resuscitation of shock. We suspect this intervention may have been in response to the patient presenting with bradycardia. It has been noted elsewhere, however, that relative bradycardia may commonly accompany acute shock.

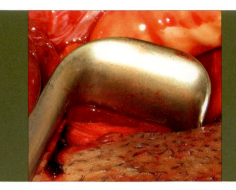

IX.4
Ectopic Pregnancy

CASE PRESENTATION

A 28-year-old female soldier presented to the combat support hospital (CSH) with complaints of unscheduled vaginal bleeding and pelvic pain. She was unsure of her last menstrual period, did not use a reliable form of contraception, and reported having unprotected intercourse 3 weeks previously while on mid-deployment leave. Physical examination revealed a tender pelvic area, old blood in the vaginal vault without active bleeding, and a closed cervical os. Laboratory results included a normal hematocrit and a positive, qualitative serum β-human chorionic gonadotropin (β-hCG) assay (quantitative titers were not available). Pelvic ultrasound revealed a cystic mass with a yolk sac in the left adenexa. The patient underwent a laparotomy. Hemoperitoneum was discovered on entry, and the left adenexa was delivered through the incision (Figs. 1 and 2) to allow a linear salpingostomy (using electrocautery) to remove the products of conception. Hemostasis was achieved, and the laparotomy incision was closed in the usual manner.

TEACHING POINTS

1. Women comprise approximately 15% of active-duty personnel in the US Armed Forces.[1] A similar proportion constitutes the forward deployed forces, therefore making the capacity to perform emergent gynecological surgery essential.
2. In a clinically stable patient suspected of having an ectopic pregnancy, laparoscopy has virtually replaced laparotomy as the standard of care within the United States. However, laparoscopic equipment is typically not available at the CSH.
3. Availability of ultrasound varies based on level of care, mobility of the unit, and the tactical situation. These conditions may make diagnosis and treatment of ectopic pregnancy difficult.

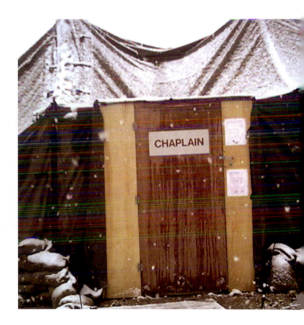

CLINICAL IMPLICATIONS

1. Surgeons skilled in the diagnosis and treatment of emergent gynecological conditions are critical to a deployed CSH.
2. Variations in available technology make the diagnosis of ectopic pregnancy more challenging and may necessitate changes in usual practice patterns.

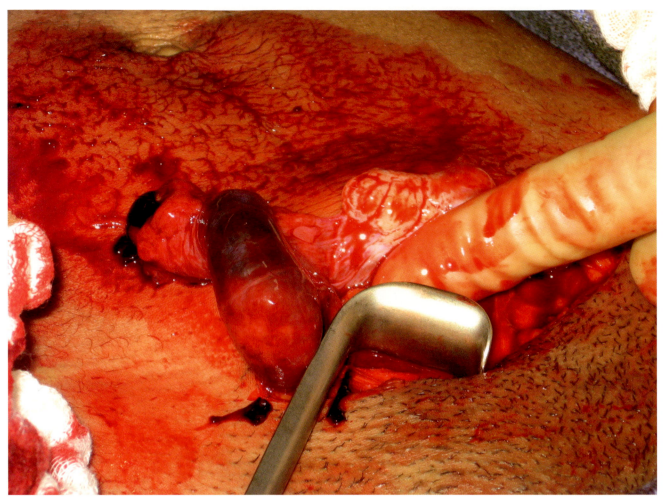

FIGURE 1. *Ectopic (left tubal) pregnancy.*

DAMAGE CONTROL

In the deployed environment, any female soldier presenting with an acute abdomen and having a positive, qualitative β-hCG should undergo an exploratory laparotomy. Choice of salpingectomy versus linear salpingostomy should be based on risk of subsequent bleeding, condition of the fallopian tube, and future fertility desires.

SUMMARY

Emergent gynecological surgery will occur in theater. Availability of diagnostic and operative tools, as well as individual skill sets, provides unique clinical challenges to the deployed clinician. Ultrasound is increasingly available, but the ability to perform and interpret these scans will vary based on tactical and clinical settings. Laparotomy replaces laparoscopy as the standard approach, if the latter is unavailable. Before deployment, female soldiers must have a negative pregnancy test. Consideration should be given to expanding this policy to include documenting a negative test before returning from leave in an effort to maintain combat power and avoid unscheduled evacuation from theater operations.

REFERENCE

1. Office of the Under Secretary of Defense, Personnel and Readiness. *Population Representation in the Military Services. Executive Summary*. Washington, DC: Department of Defense; 2004.

SUGGESTED READING

Chapter 19: Gynecologic trauma and emergencies. In: *Emergency War Surgery, Third United States Revision*. Washington, DC: Department of the Army, Office of The Surgeon General, Borden Institute; 2004.

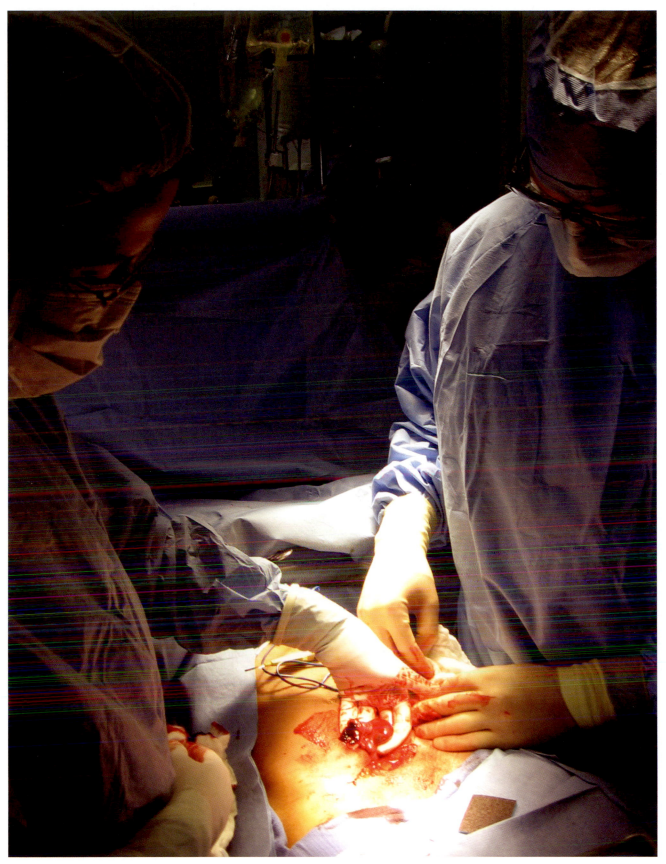

FIGURE 2. *Fallopian tube is exposed through a laparotomy incision.*

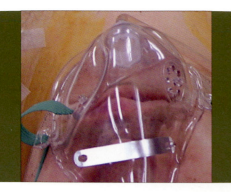

IX.5
Continuous Peripheral Nerve Block

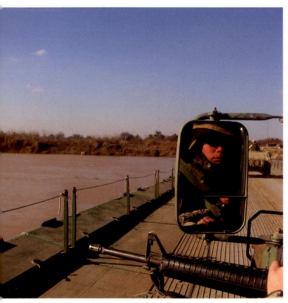

CASE PRESENTATION

A 21-year-old male sustained a rocket-propelled grenade fragment injury to his left calf. A tourniquet was applied in the field, and the patient arrived at the Combat Support Hospital (CSH) within 60 minutes of injury (Fig. 1). The soldier was in significant discomfort on arrival at the CSH despite being treated with intravenous (IV) morphine sulfate (18 mg) that was given during transport and at the CSH. His vital signs were normal, with the exception of mild tachypnea at 27 breaths/minute. His oxygen saturation was 100%, and his hematocrit was 44.4%. Neurological examination of the wounded extremity indicated loss of motor and sensory functions of the left tibial nerve. Perfusion and neurological function were otherwise intact. The patient was prepared for an emergency exploration and debridement of the wound. He was offered a left lumbar plexus and a left sciatic nerve continuous peripheral nerve block (CPNB) for surgical anesthesia and prolonged perioperative pain control. The CPNB catheters were placed by an anesthesiologist trained in advanced regional anesthesia. The patient was sedated for the block with midazolam (4 mg IV) and fentanyl (175 μg) in divided doses. He remained alert and conversant throughout the block procedure, which lasted approximately 20 minutes. He experienced complete pain relief in his left leg within 3 minutes of local anesthetic injection (30 mL of 1.5% mepivacaine with 1:400,000 epinephrine injected at each CPNB catheter site). Surgical level block was confirmed in the left extremity, with loss of hip flexion and foot dorsiflexion. The patient was lightly sedated with propofol and remained intermittently conversant throughout the 85-minute surgical procedure that included inadvertent fracture of the patient's tibia intraoperatively. Postoperatively, the patient was alert and pain free in the CSH recovery area and required minimal nursing intervention (Fig. 2). That evening, he was transported to the airport via a 40-minute helicopter flight, followed by a 5-hour flight to a level IV medical treatment facility. He remained pain free with his CPNB infusions (Fig. 3) during the flight. He required no further flight nurse interventions, allowing the nurses to focus on other patients. The patient continued using the CPNB catheters for a total of 16 days throughout dressing changes and continuous perioperative pain management during his evacuation to the United States and subsequent recovery at Walter Reed Army Medical Center. During this time, the catheters were used four additional times to reestablish a surgical level

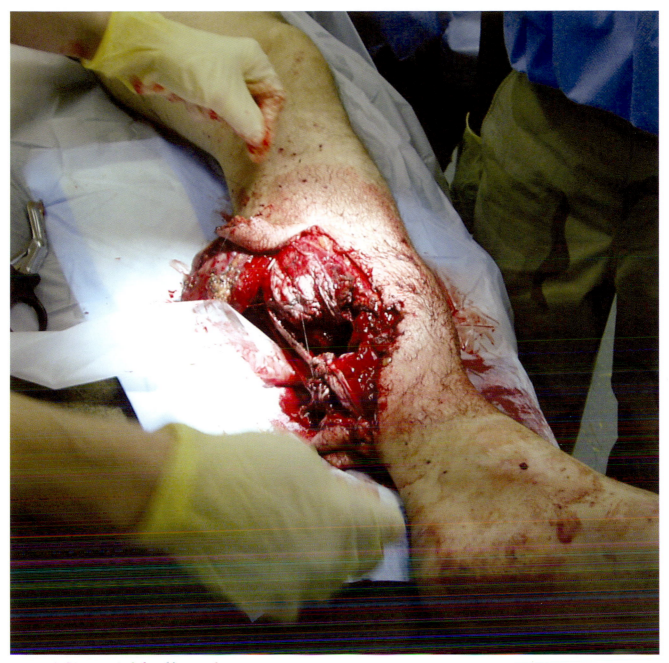

FIGURE 1. *Traumatic left calf wound.*

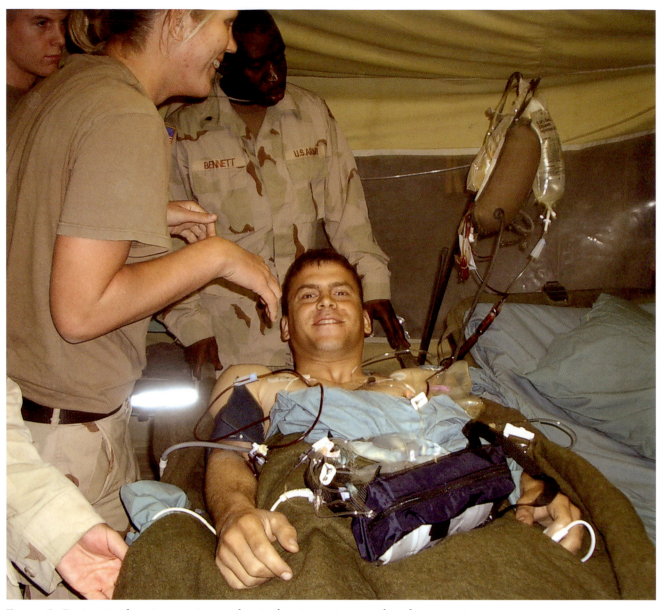

FIGURE 2. *Patient is alert, interactive, and pain free just minutes after the operation.*

nerve block. Surgical exploration revealed complete loss of the tibial nerve and deep venous system. After a prolonged course complicated by continuous ischemic pain, he elected to undergo below-the-knee amputation. The patient returned to duty with a left leg prosthesis. He remains pain free and is an active runner.

TEACHING POINTS

1. This case illustrates some of the advantages of early advanced pain control at the CSH in the management and evacuation of a seriously wounded soldier. This technique requires minimal logistics support

(compared with general anesthesia techniques), produces profound pain control during long evacuation flights (Fig. 4), and reduces the patient care burden on medical personnel during long evacuation flights. The use of CPNB in extremity wounds for surgical anesthesia promotes less anesthetic drug use, resulting in alert, pain-free patients who can participate actively in their own evacuations. The ability to reestablish surgical blocks for frequent dressing changes and surgical procedures further enhances the value of this anesthetic choice in saving medical resources. The local anesthetics

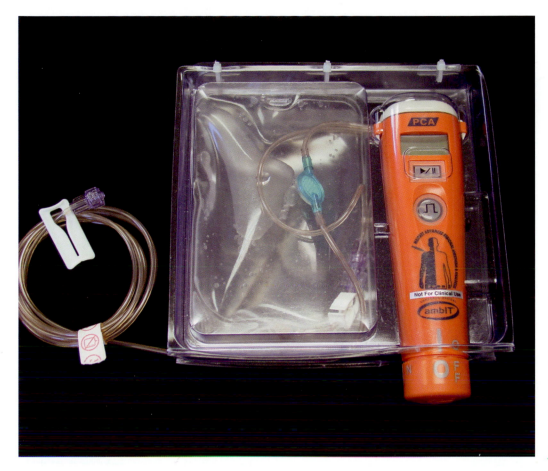

FIGURE 3. *"ambIT" pain pump currently approved for CPNB on military aircraft. (See http://www. arapmi.org for information on pain pump infusion technology currently approved for military use.) Photograph used with permission from Sorenson Medical, Inc, West Jordan, Utah.*

used in CPNB do not cause sedation or respiratory depression. These anesthetics reduce the patient's requirement for opioid pain medications that do manifest these side effects.

2. Neurological examination of the body region to be blocked is required before institution of the CPNB procedure. All CPNBs should be placed in consultation with the operative surgeon.

3. The use of advanced regional anesthesia in combat trauma patients requires significant experience and training. The level III CSH is likely the first point where advanced regional anesthesia can be practiced with consistency.

4. Specialized equipment and practice protocols are needed for safe implementation of the technology. Advanced regional anesthesia is most effective when practiced as part of a multimodal pain therapy plan instituted by the healthcare facility's acute pain service.

CLINICAL IMPLICATIONS

1. CPNB is an important battlefield anesthetic option for improved, acute pain management and evacuation.

2. Personnel trained in advanced regional anesthesia are an integral part of any deployed acute pain service.

3. It is important to note that CPNB—like other analgesic technologies—will not completely cover the pain of ischemia associated with a developing compartment syndrome. Vigilance and frequent reexamination are still required to identify this complication.

DAMAGE CONTROL

This technique is not appropriate for healthcare facilities without an acute pain service and trained personnel to manage CPNB catheter infusions.

SUMMARY

This case demonstrates the clinical advantages of CPNB in austere medical environments when appropriate resources are available for acute pain management at the CSH.

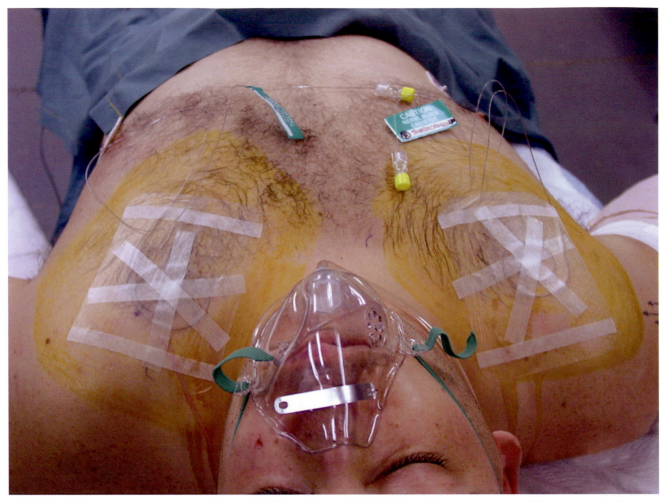

FIGURE 4. *Bilateral intraclavicular CPNB in a different patient with bilateral arm amputations following a Black Hawk tire explosion. This soldier also benefited from profound pain control during evacuation to the United States.*

SUGGESTED READING

Buckenmaier CC, Bleckner L. *The Military Advanced Regional Anesthesia and Analgesia Field Manual.* Washington, DC: Department of the Army, Office of The Surgeon General, Borden Institute. Forthcoming.

Buckenmaier CC, McKnight GM, et al. Continuous peripheral nerve block for battlefield anesthesia and evacuation. *Reg Anesth Pain Med.* 2005;30:202–205.

Chapter 9: Anesthesia. In: *Emergency War Surgery, Third United States Revision.* Washington, DC: Department of the Army, Office of The Surgeon General, Borden Institute; 2004.

Chapter 22: Soft-tissue injuries. In: *Emergency War Surgery, Third United States Revision.* Washington, DC: Department of the Army, Office of The Surgeon General, Borden Institute; 2004.

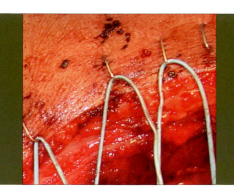

IX.6
Pediatric Popliteal Artery Trauma

CASE PRESENTATION

A 10-year-old Afghan male presented at a Forward Surgical Team (FST) facility 4 hours after being shot. The patient presented with a heart rate of 86 beats per minute, blood pressure of 120/86 mm Hg, and was awake and alert. He had an entrance wound lateral and superior to the right knee with a medial exit wound at the level of the knee (Fig. 1). A large hematoma limited the patient's range of motion at the knee joint. There were no palpable anterior tibialis or dorsalis pedis pulses. Doppler flow was also undetectable distally. The extremity was cool to the touch and appeared dusky. However, the patient was able to move his toes, and sensation was intact to light touch. No other injuries were identified. Clinical presentation in this male was consistent with popliteal artery injury. The decision was made to attempt limb salvage at the FST based on the time elapsed since injury. Per the Afghanistan culture norm, the father of the patient would only consent to an attempt to save the leg. Therefore, amputation was not considered an immediate option in this case. The patient was taken to the operating room, prepped, and draped from the nipples to the feet of both extremities. A no. 8 French Foley catheter was placed, as well as two 18-gauge intravenous catheters. The proximal femoral artery and femoral vein were exposed, and the artery was isolated with a vessel loop. The popliteal artery and vein were then approached medially (Figs. 2 and 3). On entering the hematoma, there was significant hemorrhage. Proximal control was obtained at the level of the femoral artery using the previously placed vessel loop. This maneuver allowed exposure of the popliteal artery. The artery was completely transected, and approximately 2.5 cm of the vessel had been destroyed. The proximal and distal ends of the artery were secured with vessel loops. The popliteal vein was intact. Several bridging veins were injured and secured with 3-0 silk ligatures. A no. 8 French Argyle shunt was then placed in the popliteal artery, the proximal vessel loop was loosened, and 2,500 units of heparin was administered. This did not result in acceptable distal flow determined by the absence of either palpable or Doppler flow distal to the injury. A segment of the ipsilateral greater saphenous vein was harvested and reversed. A 20-gauge angiocatheter was inserted into the reversed end of the vein and used to dilate it with normal saline. The popliteal artery was then debrided proximally, and an oblique incision was created in the artery and saphenous vein. Proximal anastomosis was made with 5-0 Prolene, and this process was repeated distally (see Fig. 2). A four-compartment fasciotomy was performed through generous medial and lateral incisions.

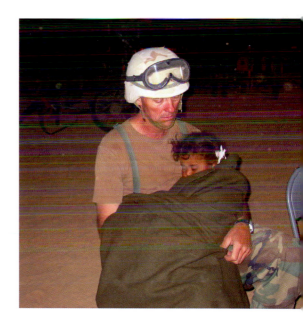

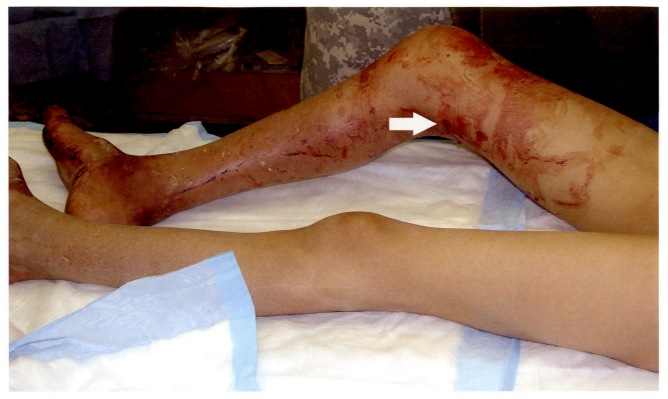

FIGURE 1. *Appearance of the extremity shortly after admission.* Arrow *indicates presumed exit wound.*

The patient had palpable distal pulses at the end of the case and a normal neurological examination.

TEACHING POINTS

1. Personnel assigned to this facility were obligated to care for this patient. There is no doubt pediatric patients will be seen by combat surgeons. Despite this fact, authorized equipment for deployed medical units is lacking in pediatric supplies. This must be corrected in the future; meanwhile, medical personnel must be proactive in obtaining required pediatric equipment and supplies.

2. Infants less than 6 months old have tremendous collateral potential even for major vessels. Control the injured vessel with bulldog clamps and see if distal perfusion is intact. If distal perfusion is adequate, then major vascular repair need not be attempted at that time, even with large vessels like the subclavian or femoral artery.

3. Because there is tremendous potential for recannulization of thrombosed vessels resulting from intimal flaps, these vessels need only be repaired if there is absence of distal flow.

4. Generally, the small shunts required in pediatric vessels are too small to provide adequate flow. This is also true of prosthetic grafts. Vein grafts or patches are usually required.

5. Unless contraindicated by other injuries, always heparinize.

6. Good technique is critical in children, and a running suture should never be used because there will be no growth potential in the injured vessel. Use interrupted sutures. As the child grows, revision of the graft may be necessary.

CLINICAL IMPLICATIONS

With the exception of the previously described teaching points, vascular injury in children is approached the same as in adults. The following points are emphasized:

1. Hard signs of vascular injury (eg, pulsatile external bleeding, enlarging hematoma, absent distal pulses, thrill/bruit, or an ischemic limb) should be explored surgically and do not require further studies.

2. External bleeding should be controlled immediately with direct pressure or a tourniquet.

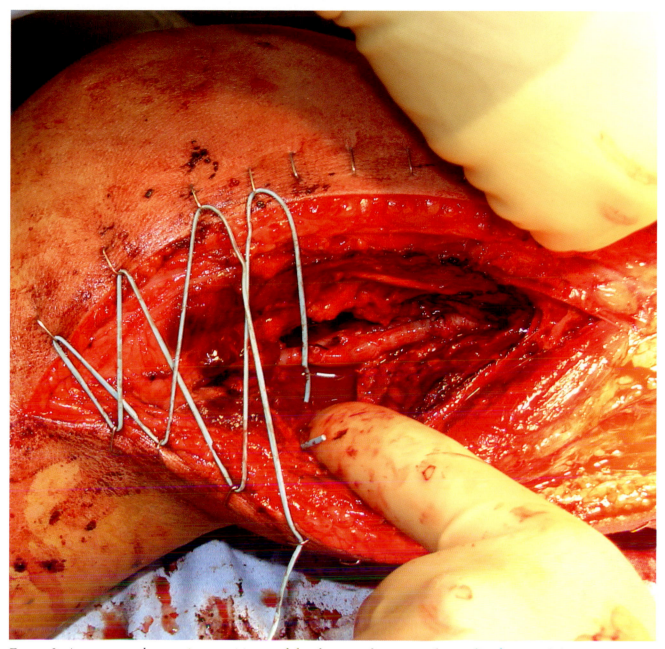

FIGURE 2. *A reverse saphenous interposition graft has been used to repair the popliteal artery defect.*

3. Combat trauma wounds are frequently caused by high-velocity missiles (> 3,000 f/s) and can cause arterial injury without major external injury. When hard signs of vascular compromise are present, thrombosis should be suspected. Soft signs of vascular injury should prompt evaluation with arteriogram, duplex ultrasound, and ankle-brachial indices.

4. Both the injured and uninjured extremities should be prepared and draped to facilitate obtaining the vein graft. If the major vein of the injured extremity is damaged, obtain the vein graft from the contralateral extremity to preserve the superficial outflow. Large injured veins should be repaired to preserve outflow.

5. The vein graft should be covered with the surrounding soft tissue at the end of the case to prevent desiccation.

6. Fasciotomy should almost always be performed in the combat setting after vascular repair.

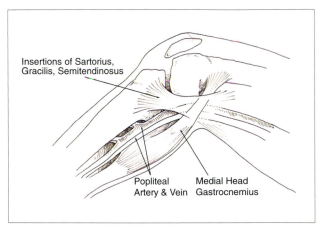

Insertions of Sartorius, Gracilis, Semitendinosus

Popliteal Artery & Vein   Medial Head Gastrocnemius

FIGURE 3. *Medial approach to popliteal vessels.*

DAMAGE CONTROL

Ligation of the injured vessel may be required if life-threatening injuries preclude repair. Shunting may be attempted; but, in pediatric vascular injuries, it may be inadequate due to the size of the shunted vessels. If shunting or collateral flow is inadequate, amputation will be required.

SUMMARY

When vascular injuries to children occur on the battlefield, combat surgeons will be required to manage these injuries. Basic tenets of vascular surgery apply, but infants and small children may not need major vascular repair due to good collateral flow. However, surgical intervention will be required if clinical evidence of distal ischemia exists.

SUGGESTED READING

Chapter 22: Soft-tissue injuries. In: *Emergency War Surgery, Third United States Revision.* Washington, DC: Department of the Army, Office of The Surgeon General, Borden Institute; 2004.

Chapter 27: Vascular injuries. In: *Emergency War Surgery, Third United States Revision.* Washington, DC: Department of the Army, Office of The Surgeon General, Borden Institute; 2004.

Chapter 33: Pediatric care. In: *Emergency War Surgery, Third United States Revision.* Washington, DC: Department of the Army, Office of The Surgeon General, Borden Institute; 2004.

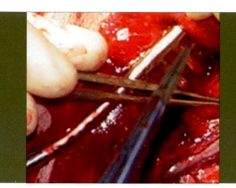

IX.7
Tetanus

CASE PRESENTATION

A 29-year-old Afghan male was brought to the combat support hospital (CSH) with a necrotic below-the-knee amputation, an inability to open his mouth fully, and spasmodic movements of the extremities. The patient reported stepping on a small landmine approximately 1 week previously and self-treating the injury with a bandage wrap. Two days prior to admission, the patient noted "stiffness" in his jaw, which had steadily worsened. He also noted involuntary muscular contractions of his arms and legs. The patient had no significant past medical history and had never received vaccinations. He was taking no medications and reported no allergies. Vital signs showed mild hypertension (150/90 mm Hg), tachycardia (pulse of 100 beats per minute), and a normal temperature. Physical examination was significant for a necrotic left below-the-knee amputation (Fig. 1) and trismus (Fig. 2). Episodic, involuntary contractions of both arms and legs were noted. An urgent amputation of the necrotic stump was performed, and the patient underwent subsequent tracheotomy for prolonged mechanical ventilation. Human tetanus immunoglobulin (hTIG) and (equine) tetanus antitoxin (TAT) were administered, at separate sites, intramuscularly. Metronidazole was infused intravenously. An intravenous infusion of midazolam was administered for sedation, but the patient required paralysis with vecuronium bromide for complete suppression of the spasms. Each day, cessation of paralysis/sedation was performed to assess the patient's clinical status, and the contractions gradually improved. After 20 days in the intensive care unit, he was finally extubated and discharged home.

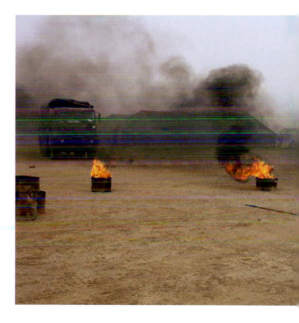

TEACHING POINTS

1. The presence of trismus and involuntary muscular contractions in the setting of a necrotic wound quickly lead clinicians to a diagnosis of tetanus in this patient.
2. Although tetanus is fairly uncommon in developed countries, lack of routine vaccination and poor access to medical care make tetanus much more prevalent in developing regions.

CLINICAL IMPLICATIONS

1. Risus sardonicus (a grimace caused by increased tone in the orbicularis oris), trismus (or lockjaw), and generalized spasm (with

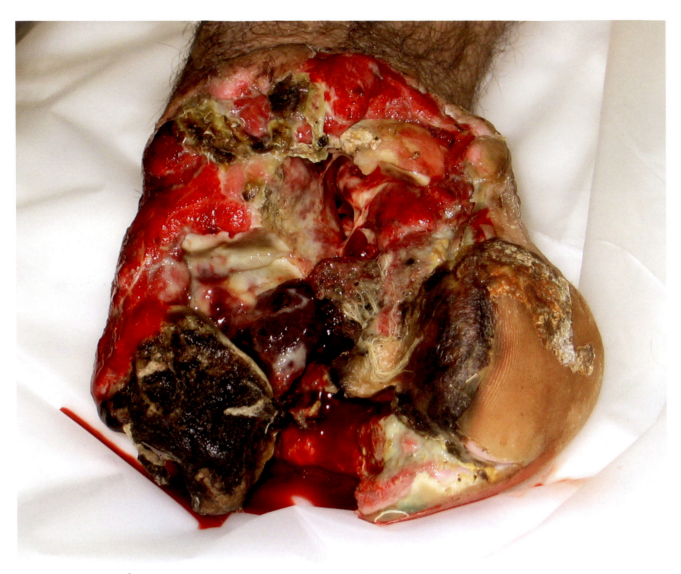

FIGURE 1. *Necrotic lower extremity, traumatic amputation site.*

flexion of the arms and extension of the legs) are the hallmarks of generalized tetanus.[1] Dysphagia follows. This neurological disorder is caused by the release of a toxin from *Clostridium tetani*. The vast majority of adult cases are associated with lacerations and punctures. The organism is found in soil worldwide, and spores may survive for years. Symptoms generally occur 3 to 10 days following inoculation. Generalized muscle spasms, induced by the slightest stimulation, may become sustained, severe, and compromise respiratory effort. Diagnosis is secured by clinical observation. Culture of suspected wounds is not useful because cultures are frequently negative, and a positive culture may be present without disease in patients with adequate immunity.

2. Treatment is supportive and relies on providing a secure airway, as well as maintaining nutrition and having good nursing care. Benzodiazepines are used for control of spasms, although occasionally neuromuscular junction blockade is required. Passive immunization with hTIG shortens the course of tetanus, and active immunization should also be initiated. Antimicrobial therapy with metronidazole is recommended. Autonomic dysfunction may occur as hypertension and/or hypotension.

DAMAGE CONTROL

Tetanus is a preventable disease by using vaccination. A series of three monthly intramuscular injections of tetanus toxoid provides protection for at least 5 years,

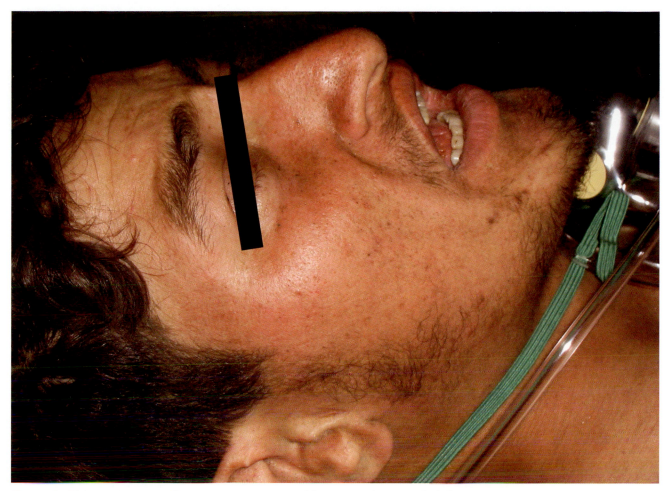

FIGURE 2. *Trismus (risus sardonicus). Patient is unable to open his mouth fully on command.*

with booster vaccinations recommended every 10 years. Patients suffering from tetanus-prone wounds (puncture wounds, dirty wounds, etc) who have not received adequate vaccination within the past 5 years should receive passive immunization with hTIG, in addition to active immunization.

SUMMARY

Most physicians having received medical training in the United States will be unfamiliar with diseases afflicting patients who have not benefited from modern medical care. Tetanus is one such disease. Clinical presentation of a patient with a wound and muscular spasms should prompt the diagnosis. Although the mortality for severe tetanus is reportedly as high as 60%, many patients who receive intensive medical support, not always available in a forward medical facility, will survive.[2]

REFERENCES

1. Bleck T. *Clostridium tetani* (tetanus). In: Mandell G, Bennett J, Dolin R, eds. *Mandell, Douglas, and Bennett's Principles and Practice of Infectious Diseases*. Philadelphia, Pa: Elsevier; 2005: 2817–2822.

2. Nolla-Salas M, Garces-Bruses J. Severity of tetanus in patients older than 80 years: Comparative study with younger patients. *Clin Infect Dis.* 1993;16:591–592.

SUGGESTED READING

Chapter 10: Infections. In: *Emergency War Surgery, Third United States Revision*. Washington, DC: Department of the Army, Office of The Surgeon General, Borden Institute; 2004.

Chapter 25: Amputations. In: *Emergency War Surgery, Third United States Revision*. Washington, DC: Department of the Army, Office of The Surgeon General, Borden Institute; 2004.

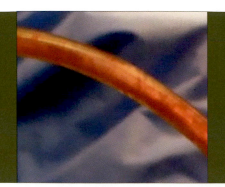

IX.8
Penetrating Abdominal Trauma in the Pregnant Patient

CASE PRESENTATION

This 30-year-old female sustained a single gunshot wound to the abdomen from an AK-47 rifle. She was approximately 34 to 38 weeks pregnant. The bullet entered the abdomen just left of the umbilicus and exited the left side of the abdominal wall, leaving a substantial exit wound and obvious evisceration of the small bowel. Despite being 2 hours postinjury on arrival, the patient was alert, awake, and hemodynamically stable, with a heart rate of 122 beats per minute and blood pressure of 124/88 mm Hg. Fetal heart tones could not be assessed. Large-bore intravenous access was obtained, as well as initial laboratory values. The patient was then taken to the operating room for exploratory laparotomy. A midline incision was used to deliver the gravid uterus into the operative field and also to provide exposure for obvious bowel injuries. On initial inspection, a through-and-through wound from the uterine fundus to the left lateral aspect of the uterus was seen. The exit wound was large, and the fetus was presumed to be in distress. Therefore, the vesicouterine fold was mobilized and an emergency cesarean section was performed using a standard low transverse incision (Fig. 1). Once delivered and the cord controlled, the baby boy was aggressively suctioned and stimulated (Figs. 2 and 3). The initial Apgar score was 2, but with continued efforts the child began to breathe spontaneously, his color improved, and he began to move all extremities (Fig. 4). The child was passed off the operative field, and attention was turned back to the mother. The placenta was delivered without incident, and the uterus was massaged vigorously to cause contraction and achieve hemostasis. At initial surgery, there were no agents available to produce uterine contraction; therefore, uterine massage and selective ligation of several large bleeding sites were used to achieve hemostasis. The uterus was closed using a running locking 0 VICRYL suture, and the two bullet wounds were debrided and closed in a similar fashion. With the uterus contracted, the remainder of the patient's abdomen was evaluated for injuries. The only significant injuries found were four small bowel enterotomies located in the mid-jejunum. Resection and primary anastomosis were performed. During rescusitation and surgery, the mother received 5 units of packed red blood cells, 4 units of fresh frozen plasma, 1 dose of recombinant Factor VIIa, 2 units of whole blood, and 3 L of crystalloid. The abdomen was thoroughly irrigated, and the bowel and colon were reinspected.

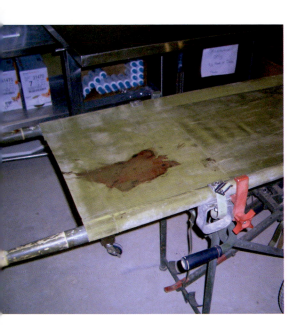

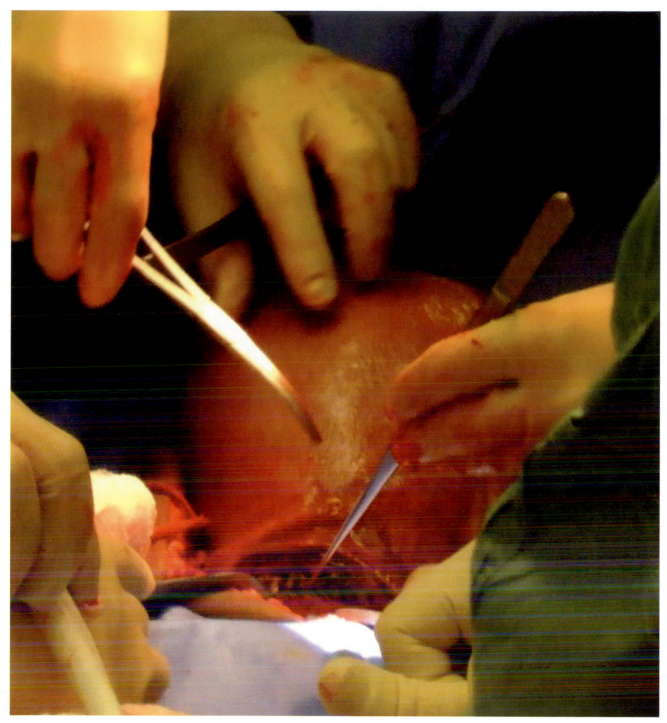

FIGURE 1. *The abdomen is opened with a vertical midline incision, and a low transverse incision has been made on the uterus.*

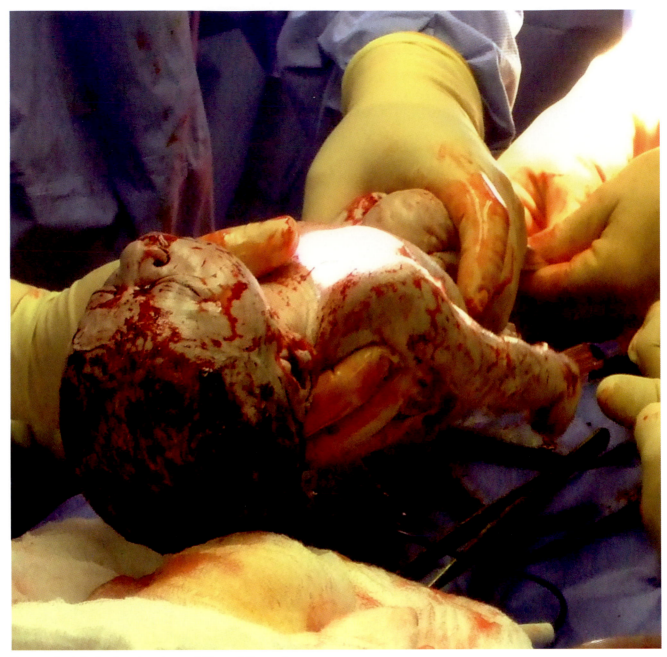

FIGURE 2. *A baby boy has been delivered from the uterus.*

The lateral abdominal wall defect (exit wound) was closed by approximating the peritoneum and the fascia. Laxity of the lateral abdominal wall allowed a tension-free fascial closure. The abdomen was closed using a no. 1 looped PDS suture (polydioxanone suture) in a running fashion. The lateral wound was packed open using Kerlix sponges, and the patient was transferred in stable condition to a postoperative holding area. Following the mother's surgery, the baby was evaluated and found to have a minor tangential wound from the bullet. This wound was dressed, and both patients were transferred to a level III medical treatment facility for continued care.

TEACHING POINTS

Penetrating abdominal trauma in pregnant females is likely to include injury to the uterus and fetus. The incidence of injury increases in proportion to the size of the uterus as the pregnancy progresses. The upward displacement of abdominal organs in late pregnancy

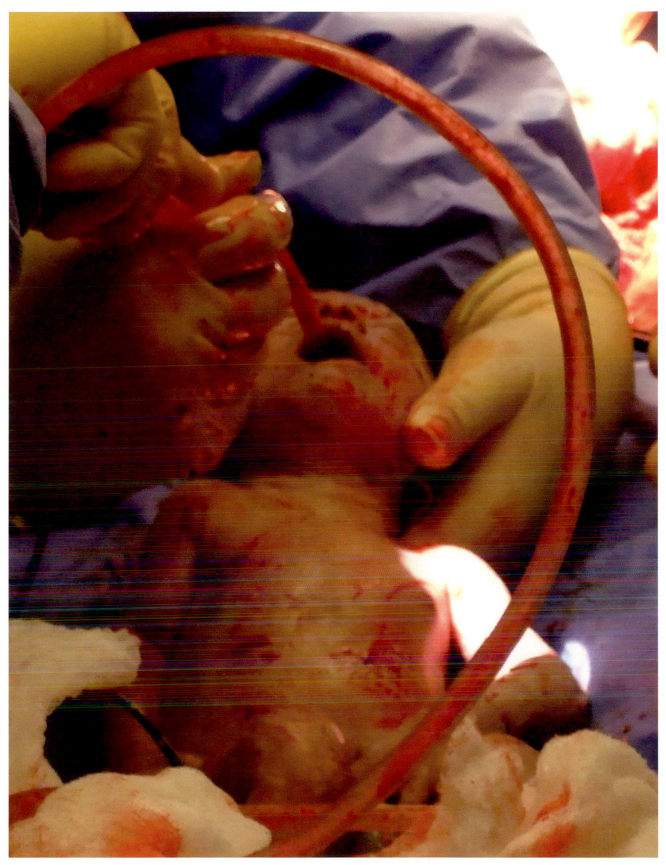

FIGURE 3. *The neonate is suctioned in the operative field and given an initial Apgar score of 2.*

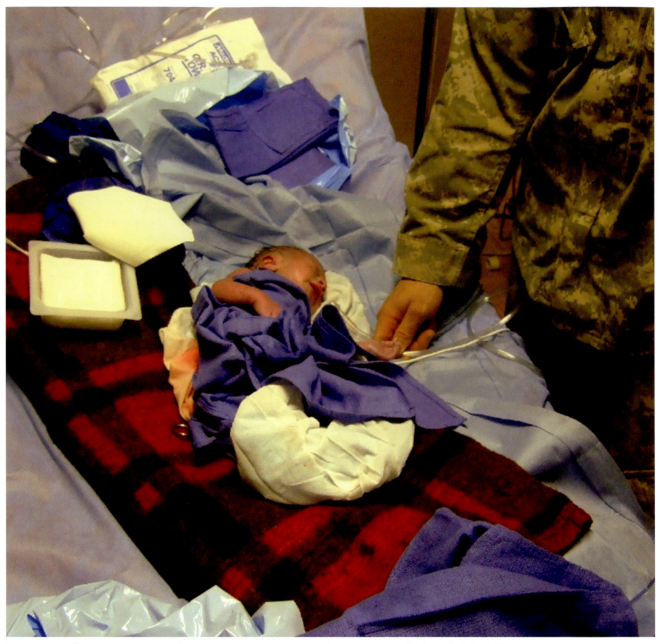

FIGURE 4. *After resuscitation, the neonate was given an Apgar score of 10 and did well.*

SUPINE HYPOTENSIVE SYNDROME OF PREGNANCY

In late pregnancy, the large gravid uterus can compress the inferior vena cava resulting in decreased return of blood to the heart. This may result in tachycardia, hypotension, sweating, nausea, and dizziness. It is also possible for the uterus to compress the aorta, thus decreasing blood flow to the uterus and placing the fetus in jeopardy. Both of these conditions can be prevented by placing the patient on the left side or, if the spine is not cleared, by slanting the patient on the backboard to the left.

can result in multiple organs damaged in wounds that involve the upper abdomen. Resuscitation and surgical intervention of the pregnant patient have several unique aspects.

1. The most common cause of fetal death in the traumatized pregnant patient is maternal death. The priority in resuscitation is the mother, and the primary ATLS (Advanced Trauma Life Support) survey is completely focused on the mother.
2. As soon as feasible, place the mother on her left side to shift the weight of the uterus off the inferior vena cava and prevent supine hypotensive syndrome of pregnancy (see box on page 396).
3. Evidence of shock during pregnancy suggests massive blood loss. Signs of shock in the pregnant patient will manifest late when the patient has lost as much as 35% of circulating blood volume.
4. Mild hypoxia in the mother results in severe hypoxia for the fetus. Start all pregnant patients on supplemental oxygen and maintain their saturation at 95% to 100%, if possible.
5. X-ray examination of the patient should be carefully planned, but needed radiographs should be obtained. When possible, shield the abdomen with a lead apron. Ultrasound is an excellent modality and may be used to assess both the mother and fetus.
6. The secondary survey includes assessment of the reproductive organs and the fetus. Consultation with an obstetrician is highly desirable, if possible at this point.

    a. The presence of any blood in the vagina is suggestive of injury to the uterus in penetrating trauma or of placental abruption in blunt trauma.
    b. Initial assessment should include fetal heart tones. Normal fetal heart rate is 120 to 160 beats per minute. A fetal heart rate of less than 120 indicates fetal hypoxia. If available, a cardiotocographic device will allow continuous assessment of the fetus and detect uterine contractions that may indicate preterm labor.
    c. If available, ultrasound and CT can be used to further assess the fetus, uterus, and placenta.
    d. Measuring fundal height will give an estimation of fetal age. When the fundus is at the level

of the umbilicus, the fetal age is roughly 20 weeks. When the fundus is palpated midway between the umbilicus and the xiphoid, fetal age is approximately 26 weeks. At this age, when a neonatal intensive care unit is available, the fetus is considered viable in a normal hospital setting. This level of sophistication will rarely be encountered in the combat setting, and viability of the prematurely delivered neonate will depend largely on its physiological maturity.

7. Almost all patients with penetrating abdominal injuries in the combat setting will require surgical exploration. This includes pregnant patients.

    a. The patient should be approached just like any other trauma patient and damage control performed as needed.
    b. The uterus should be carefully examined and, if injured and the fetus is in good condition, it may be repaired using 0 VICRYL suture.
    c. If injury to the uterus causes fetal distress and the fetus is mature enough for delivery, perform a cesarean section (Fig. 5).

8. In the event the baby is delivered, it may require resuscitation and other necessary equipment, including warm towels, a bulb syringe, a stethoscope, oxygen, and a suction catheter. Airway management instruments should be available immediately.
9. Injury to the uterus can be controlled usually with suture ligation. After the cesarean section, uterine atony may result in uncontrollable hemorrhage. In this case, if tocolytic agents are available, they should be given and uterine massage performed. If this fails to arrest the bleeding, ligation of the uterine arteries or hysterectomy may be required.

CLINICAL IMPLICATIONS

The physiological changes that occur during pregnancy impact the patient's ability to respond to trauma and should be remembered when caring for the injured pregnant patient. Some of these changes are reviewed here briefly.

1. Pregnant patients retain sodium and total body water resulting in a 30% to 40% increase in plasma volume. There is a concurrent increase in red blood cell mass of about 15%. This results in a

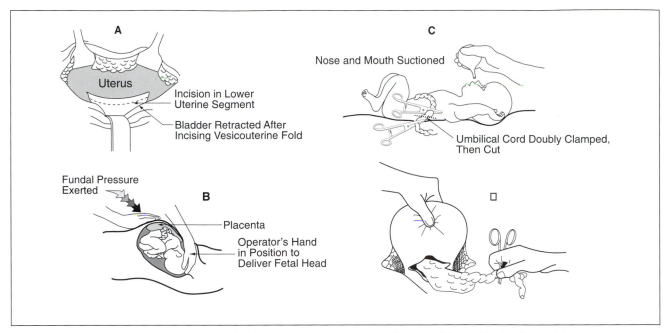

FIGURE 5. *Emergency cesarean section.* (A) *Uterine incision.* (B) *Delivery of fetus.* (C) *Delivered infant on abdomen.* (D) *Uterine fundus exteriorized.*

normal hematacrit of 30% to 36%. A moderate leukocytosis is also common.

2. Cardiac output and resting heart rate increase in pregnancy. Heart rate will typically increase 10 to 20 beats per minute for a given patient. Peripheral vascular resistance is slightly decreased, and average blood pressure is also decreased 10 to 15 mm Hg.

3. Significant changes occur in the pregnant patient's respiratory system. Anatomical changes occur that result in an increased subcostal angle and increased chest circumference. As the pregnancy progresses, the diaphragm is increasingly elevated. The result of all these changes is an increase in tidal volume and minute ventilation. However, functional residual capacity is decreased. The P_{CO_2} is also decreased, and the body compensates for this by decreasing bicarbonate. This results in a compensated respiratory alkalosis during pregnancy.

4. Hormonal and anatomical changes in the pregnant patient lead to decreased intestinal mobility and decreased lower esophageal sphincter competency. They are particularly susceptible to aspiration. Nasogastric decompression should be considered early.

5. Trauma patients are hypercoaguable with increased levels of Factor VII, VIII, IX, X, XII, and fibrinogen and decreased fibrinolysis. Heparin does not cross the placenta and can be used in pregnant patients.

DAMAGE CONTROL

The damage control approach to the pregnant patient is the same as any patient. However, the uterus can be a source of rapidly fatal hemorrhage. If bleeding from the uterus cannot be controlled, then cesarean section—followed by emergency hysterectomy—may be required and can be lifesaving. If the fetus is dead, it should be delivered either vaginally or by cesarean section as soon as practicable. This may be delayed if damage control is required.

SUMMARY

This case demonstrates that civilians injured in combat zones inevitably will include the pregnant female. In this case, a Forward Surgical Team (FST) operating in an austere environment was able to safely deliver a viable infant and salvage the gravely wounded mother and her reproductive organs. The physiological maturity of the fetus, appropriate resuscitation of the mother, and the professional knowledge of the team all contributed to the successful outcome in this case.

SUGGESTED READING

Chapter 19: Gynecologic trauma and emergencies. In: *Emergency War Surgery, Third United States Revision.* Washington, DC: Department of the Army, Office of The Surgeon General, Borden Institute; 2004: 19.15.

Management of Pediatric Trauma

by COL Kenneth S. Azarow, MD

When dealing with children in wartime situations, two principles need to be understood. The first principle is to be prepared. Soldiers will be dealing with children. American history demonstrates that the US Army Medical Department has taken care of children in every conflict that our nation has been involved in. Generally, the American soldier will try to help a child immediately, regardless of whether that child has been injured as a result of "collateral damage" or if that child is part of the enemy force. In addition, the soldier will bring a child to his own medical facility rather than to the local medical facility.

The second principle is that children are not small adults, and infants are not small children. Given the same mechanism of injury, both infants and children are usually more physiologically forgiving than adults. Management principles of trauma are the same in all age groups. However, the means to achieve those goals are different. In the cases presented in this chapter, the surgeons should be complimented on their pediatric trauma management skills, and a few practical points should be emphasized: IV access, resuscitation, and operative decision making.

IV ACCESS

Given a severe traumatic injury and no identifiable peripheral veins, the first choice for peripheral access is the external jugular vein for all age groups. It is reliably present in the vast majority of patients when they are positioned in a small degree of Trendelenburg. If central access is required, the first choice is the femoral vein in all age groups. The femoral vein has reliable landmarks. If the vein is missed while attempting access, very little harm is done relative to the alternative choices for access. Unless the provider has significant experience in placing subclavian lines in pediatric patients, cannulization is not recommended in almost any circumstance. If these sites are unavailable, access in children under the age of 6 can be an intraosseous line (and is described in the case comments). The caveat is that your unit has to have intraosseous lines in stock. You can use a 16-gauge or an 18-gauge spinal needle for that purpose. However, these are harder to place, and most deployed units do not have spinal needles of that size readily available.

RESUSCITATION

After the first few months of life, blood volume drops from 80 cc/kg to 70 cc/kg. For practical purposes, think of all children as having a blood volume of 80 cc/kg. This is important because we think of giving fluid and blood products in terms of 20 cc/kg boluses. Think of this as one-quarter blood volume boluses. Just as in adults, children—undergoing massive transfusions—need 1:1 packed red blood cells to fresh frozen plasma, unless they are receiving whole blood. Although the definition of a massive transfusion in adults is 10 units, in children it should be 1.5 blood volumes (ie, 120 cc/kg). Airway management is simple: obtain one and secure it without performing a cricothyroidotomy. Remember, the formula for tube size is as follows: (age + 16)/4. Also, remember that children have an intense vagal response and a profound bradycardia when their vocal cords are manipulated; pretreat when possible.

OPERATIVE DECISION MAKING

When in a deployed combat environment, there is a much higher percentage of penetrating trauma than when working in a nonhostile environment. However, blunt trauma still occurs. The usual nonoperative management of most blunt traumatic injury can only be followed if adequate blood products are available. When the decision is made to operate, all subsequent decisions with regard to vascular control, damage control, and resuscitative surgery apply. To make these decisions easier, the following guidelines are useful. In the setting of severe abdominal and thoracic trauma, always operate on the abdomen first (even more so for children than for adults). In general, patients will triage themselves out of the immediate hemorrhagic catastrophe in the chest if they have survived transport. The incision of choice is a midline incision, unless the child is less than 18 months of age. For those patients, a transverse supraumbilical incision can give better exposure to retroperitoneal structures. When deciding what operation to perform, know what the local resources are for postoperative rehabilitation and nutrition. For example, it serves no purpose to insert a jejunal feeding tube if there are no replacement tubes available and no jejunal feeds available. However, a major challenge is to have the proper size tube available in the operating room (OR). Although Broselow kits are popular and most resuscitative bays have appropriately sized instruments and tubes for resuscitation, once in the OR there is a void of pediatric equipment unless prior planning included it. A few helpful items include the following:

- Size 10 French nasogastric tubes,
- Size 14-gauge and 16-gauge Malecot catheters,
- Size 12 French red rubber catheters,
- Size 12 French t-tubes, and
- Size 6 and 8 French Foley catheters.

Colostomies should be used if indicated; however, keep in mind that bags may be an issue. Thus, if given the choice between a colostomy and an ileostomy—although an ileostomy is preferred in the United States—a colostomy is easier to take care of and is preferable when deployed.

One of the most emotional challenges the OR staff will face is a decision to amputate a child's extremity. It is well known that prosthetics, wheelchairs, and even crutches are not available in most theater ORs. Thus, an amputation is not only a life-changing event, but also it may be a life-ending event over time. This fact is not new to deployed surgeons. For adults, Argyle shunts can be placed to preserve blood flow when in damage control mode, and delayed vascular reconstruction can save some limbs that have sufficient muscle mass and neurological function remaining. Because of blood vessel size, if shunts are placed in children, they must be fully heparinized immediately. Therefore, do not place a shunt as the first step to damage control. Clamp the vessels, stop all bleeding, then heparinize, place shunts, and perform fasciotomies. Unfortunately, amputations to save lives are a gruesome reality of war, especially where children are concerned.

When an individual is injured and needs to undergo operation, postinjury and postoperative pain will be an unavoidable consequence. Use of continuous peripheral and continuous regional anesthetic techniques has been a major advance that has been used by deployed anesthesia providers (see Case IX.5). Although there have been concerns about transportation of the electrically driven pump to provide continuous local or regional anesthetic, the principle is sound and has many advantages. The most obvious advantage is decreased use of narcotics. For abdominal and thoracic procedures, a continuous epidural has been a major advance in postoperative pain relief. Caution should be taken not to place an epidural when a neurosurgeon is more than 8 hours away for fear of the inability to decompress an epidural hematoma. However, when an epidural is utilized, it is the optimal method of pain relief to avoid all complications associated with postoperative narcotic usage. For both regional and peripheral techniques, if pump compatibility with electronic configuration of the aircraft is of concern, the catheter can be simply left in place, and intermittent injections by a flight medic or nurse can be administered.

The unborn fetus represents an infrequent patient to a deployed surgeon. The unborn fetus can present to a deployed surgical team in two ways. First, a patient with an ectopic pregnancy can appear (see Case IX.4). This is not a diagnosis that can be easily made at a Forward Surgical Team (FST) facility without a laboratory or an ultrasound unit. Transportation to a level III medical treatment facility should be triaged as urgent (surgical) when the diagnosis is suspected. However, in the case of a ruptured ectopic pregnancy with a significant hemoperitoneum, the diagnosis can be made on a FAST examination. On diagnosis, treatment is a relatively straightforward surgical intervention to remove the tube, ovary, and ectopic fetus.

Second, the fetus may also present as a maternal traumatic injury. Successful treatment of the mother will be the optimal treatment for the fetus. Even if the mother's outcome is poor, there have been many reports of successful, traumatic cesarean sections (or C-sections). Neonatal ventilators are not available for deployed units. Thus, traumatic C-sections will have a chance at being successful when the newborn is mature enough to breathe without support (a minimum of 34–36 weeks gestation). After ventilation, temperature control and heat loss are the next immediate challenges. Dry the infant and use plastic wrap (especially covering the head) if incubators are not available. Intravenous access, if required, is easily obtained via the hands/wrist/scalp/or external jugular vein. If the mother survives, breast milk is the only acceptable choice. If the mother does not survive, look to the family or local village for nursemaids because it will be very unusual for infant formula or total parenteral nutrition to be available for this age group. The best advice for a forward or rear echelon surgical unit in this scenario, in which a fetus is recovered and resuscitated, is to gain access to a pediatric specialist as soon as possible. Physiological changes that occur during the transition out of the uterus vary, depending on the maturity of the infant. Pediatric subspecialty expertise can be very helpful.

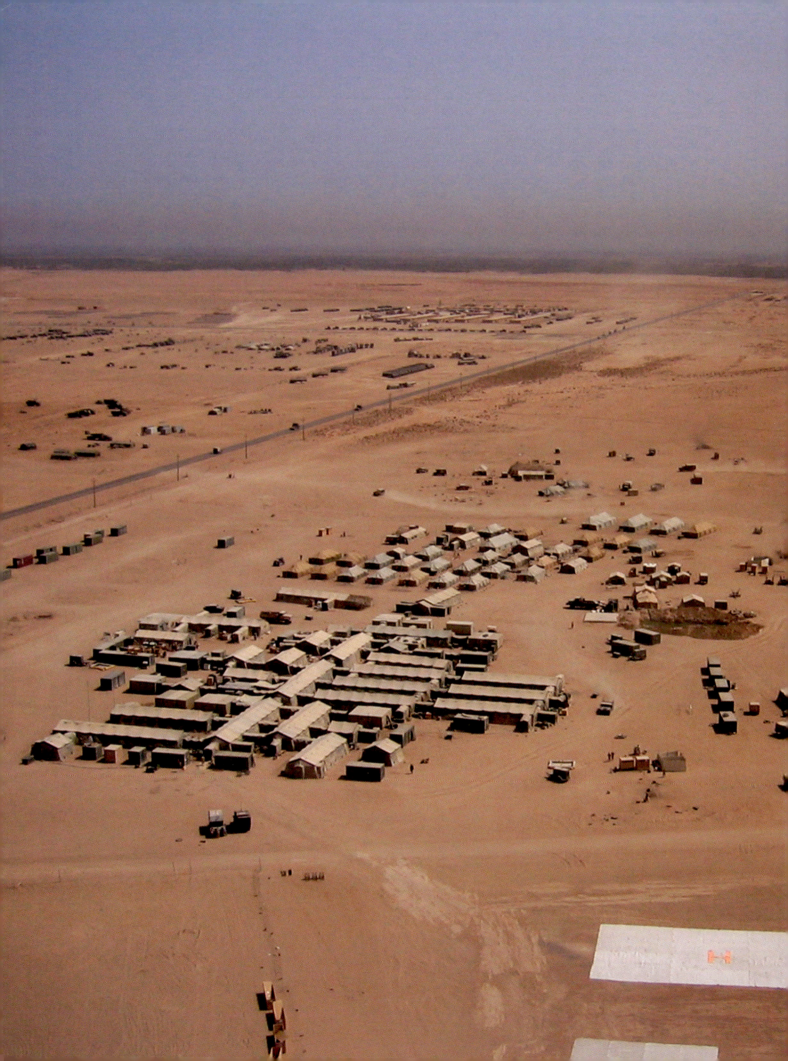

AFTERWORD

Sunt lacrimae rerum et mentem mortalia tangunt.

—Virgil

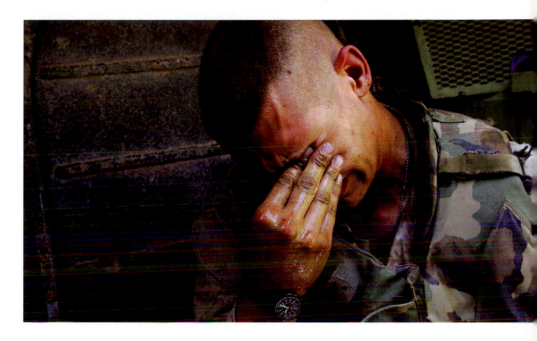

. . . Though nothing can bring back the hour
Of splendour in the grass, of glory in the flower,
We will grieve not, rather find
Strength in what remains behind;
In the primal sympathy
Which having been must ever be;
In the soothing thoughts that spring
Out of human suffering;
In the faith that looks through death,
In years that bring the philosophic mind.

. . . Thanks to the human heart by which we live,
Thanks to its tenderness, its joys, and fears,
To me the meanest flower that blows can give
Thoughts that do often lie too deep for tears.

—William Wordsworth, 1807

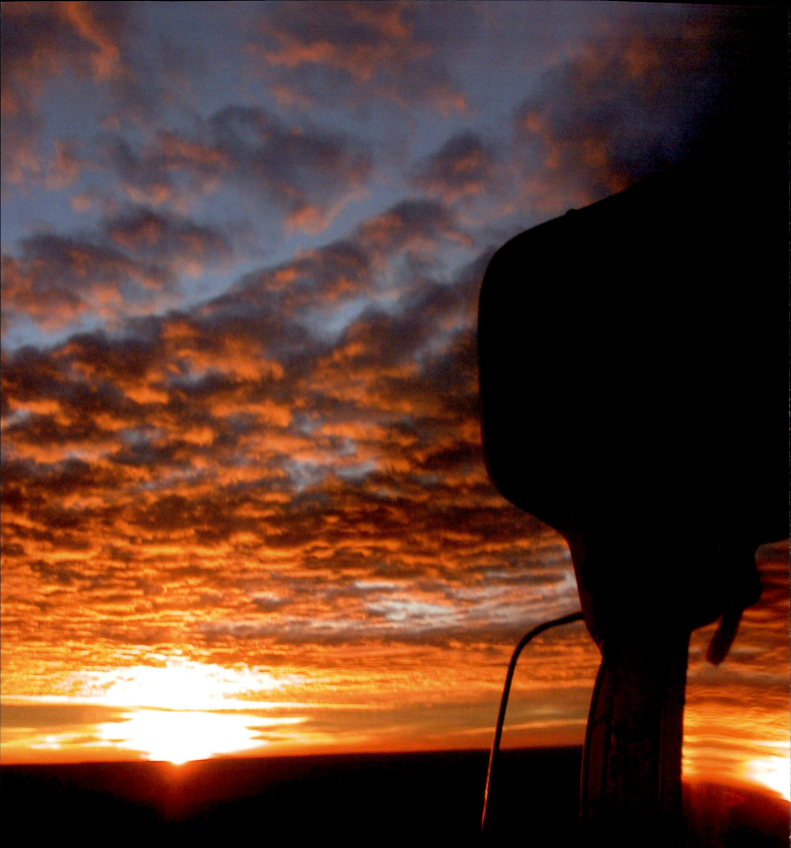

APPENDIX A   Abbreviations and Acronyms

A

ABC: *Acinetobacter baumannii-calcoaceticus* complex
ABN: airborne
ACS: American College of Surgeons
AP: anteroposterior
APC: Armored Personal Carrier
aPLTs: apheresis platelets
ATLS: Advanced Trauma Life Support

B

BAMC: Brooke Army Medical Center (Fort Sam Houston, TX)
β-hCG: β-human chorionic gonadotropin
BVM: bag valve mask

C

CAT: Combat Application Tourniquet
CATS: Combat Application Tourniquet System
CBC: complete blood count
CBF: cerebral blood flow
CCATT: Critical Care Air Transport Team
CEEG: continuous electroencephalogram
CENTCOM: Central Command
coag: coagulopathy
CONUS: continental United States
COT: Committee on Trauma
CPDA: citrate, phosphate, dextrose, adenine (solution)
CPGs: Clinical Practice Guidelines
CPNB: continuous peripheral nerve block
CRNA: certified registered nurse anesthetist
CSF: cerebrospinal fluid
CSH: combat support hospital
CT: computed tomography
CXR: chest X-ray

D

DCCS: Deputy Commander for Clinical Services
DOW: died of wounds
DPL: diagnostic peritoneal lavage
DVBIC: Defense and Veterans Brain Injury Center

E

EBL: estimated blood loss
ED: emergency department
EDTA: ethylenediamine tetraacetic acid
EMEDS: Expeditionary Medical Squadron
EMS: emergency medical system (or service)
EMT: Emergency Medical Treatment (area/section)
EOD: explosive ordnance disposal
EPW: enemy prisoner of war
ETT: endotracheal tube
evac: evacuation
EWS: *Emergency War Surgery, Third United States Revision* (2004 manual)

F

FAST: Focused Abdominal Sonography for Trauma
FDA: Food and Drug Administration
FFP: fresh frozen plasma
FRSS: Fast Response Survey System
FST: Forward Surgical Team
FWB: fresh whole blood

G

GCS: Glasgow Coma Scale
GI: gastrointestinal
GIA: gastrointestinal anastomosis
GU: genitourinary

H

HBV: hepatitis B virus
HCV: hepatitis C virus
HIPAA: Health Insurance Portability and Accountability Act
HIV: human immunodeficiency virus
HMMWV: High-Mobility Multipurpose Wheeled Vehicle ("Humvee")
HPMK: Hypothermia Prevention and Management Kit
HPPL: high-pressure pulsatile lavage
HTIG: human tetanus immunoglobulin

I

IBA: Individual Body Armor
ICH: intracranial hemorrhage
ICP: intracranial pressure
ICU: intensive care unit
IED: improvised explosive device
IFAK: Individual First-Aid Kit
INR: international normalized ratio
ISO: International Organization for Standardization
(also called International Standards Organization)
ISR: (US Army) Institute of Surgical Research
IV: intravenous
IVC: inferior vena cava

J

JTTS: Joint Theater Trauma System

K

KIA: killed in action

L

LRMC: Landstuhl Regional Medical Center
(Landstuhl, Germany)

M

MASH: Mobile Army Surgical Hospital
MEDCOM: Medical Command
MEDEVAC: medical evacuation
MFST: Mobile Field Surgical Team
MNC-I: Multi-National Corps-Iraq
MRE: Meal, Ready-to-Eat
MRI: magnetic resonance imaging
MRSA: methicillin-resistant *Staphylococcus aureus*
MT: massive transfusion

N

NATO: North Atlantic Treaty Organization
NG: nasogastric
NNMC: National Naval Medical Center (Bethesda, MD)
NPA: nasopharyngeal airway
NSAID: nonsteroidal anti-inflammatory drug

O

OEF: Operation Enduring Freedom (Afghanistan)
OIF: Operation Iraqi Freedom
OMF: oral and maxillofacial
OMFS: oral and maxillofacial surgeon
OR: operating room
OSD-HA: Office of the Assistant Secretary of Defense for
Health Affairs

P

PA: posteroanterior
PCO_2: partial pressure of carbon dioxide
PDS: polydioxanone
PEEK: polyetheretherketone
PFA: profunda femoris artery
PLTs/plts: platelets
PRBCs: packed red blood cells (also pRBCs)
PT: prothrombin time
PTFE: polytetrafluoroethylene
PTT: partial thromboplastin time

R

RBC: red blood cell
RCT: randomized controlled trial
rFVIIa: recombinant Factor VIIa (also hrFVIIa)
R/O: rule out
RPG: rocket-propelled grenade

S

SFA: superficial femoral artery
SFV: superficial femoral vein
SG: Surgeon General
SOFTT: Special Operations Forces Tactical Tourniquet
s/p: status post (Latin for "after condition")
STP: Shock Trauma Platoon
STSG: split-thickness skin graft

T

TAT: tetanus antitoxin
TCD: transcranial Doppler
THAM: tris-hydroxymethyl aminomethane (or tromethamine)
t.i.d.: three times a day
TOA: total obligation authority
TRAC: Therapeutic Regulated Accurate Care
Tx: treatment

U

UXO: unexploded ordnance

V

VA: Veterans Administration
VAC: vacuum-assisted closure
VP: ventriculoperitoneal

W

WHMC: Wilford Hall Medical Center
WRAMC: Walter Reed Army Medical Center

APPENDIX B Product Manufacturers

Argentum Medical LLC, Willowbrook, Illinois (Silverlon)

Arizant Healthcare, Inc, Eden Prairie, Minnesota (Bair Hugger)

AstraZeneca Pharmaceuticals LP, Wilmington, Delaware (Diprivan [propofol])

Bausch & Lomb, Rochester, New York (Optima FW Trial)

Bayer Corporation, Pittsburgh, Pennsylvania (ciprofloxacin)

Belmont Instrument Corporation, Billerica, Massachusetts (rapid fluid infuser, blood and fluid warmer)

BlackHawk Products Group, Norfolk, Virginia (military outdoor gear)

Cloward Instruments Corporation, Honolulu, Hawaii (Hudson brace)

Derma Sciences, Inc, Princeton, New Jersey (Silverseal burn contact dressings)

DeRoyal Industries, Inc, Powell, Tennessee (Dermanet Wound Contact Layer)

Edward Weck Company, Research Triangle Park, North Carolina (Weck cell sponge)

E. I. du Pont de Nemours and Company, Wilmington, Delaware (Kevlar and Tyvek products/equipment)

Ethicon, Inc, Somerville, New Jersey (DERMABOND, VICRYL suture, Prolene suture)

GlaxoSmithKline, Research Triangle Park, North Carolina (Ancef [cephazolin])

Hospira, Inc, Lake Forest, Illinois (Hextend)

Integra LifeSciences Corporation, Plainsboro, New Jersey (DuraGen)

Integra NeuroSciences, Plainsboro, New Jersey (NeuroGen nerve guide, Mayfield pins, Sundt shunt)

Kendall Healthcare Products Company, Mansfield, Massachusetts (Kerlix rolls and sponges)

Kinetic Concepts, Inc/KCI Licensing, Inc, San Antonio, Texas (wound VAC [therapy system], VAC Abdominal Dressing System, TRAC Pad)

Kontur Kontac Lens Company, Richmond, California (Kontur[55])

LifeCell, Branchburg, New Jersey (AlloDerm)

Mallinckrodt, Hazelwood, Missouri (Shiley tracheostomy tube)

McNeil Consumer Healthcare, Guelph, Ontario, Canada (Tylenol)

MEDICON, Tuttlingen, Germany (Javid shunt)

Medisave Services, Inc, Markham, Ontario, Canada (butyl cyanoacrylate [corneal glue])

Miltex, Inc, York, Pennsylvania (Penfield dissector)

Mopec, Oak Park, Michigan (Gigli saw)

North American Rescue Products, Inc, Greenville, South Carolina (Hypothermia Prevention and Management Kit [HPMK])

Novartis International AG, Basel, Switzerland (Sandostatin)

Parks Medical Electronics, Inc, Aloha, Oregon (Doppler ultrasound)

Pfizer, Inc–US Pharmaceuticals Group, New York, New York (Dilantin [phenytoin])

Phil Durango, LLC, Golden, Colorado (Combat Application Tourniquet System [CATS])

Polymed Chirurgical, Inc, St. Laurent, Quebec, Canada (MSI-EpiDermGlu)

Procter & Gamble Pharmaceuticals, Inc, Cincinnati, Ohio (Didronel [etidronate])

Rocky National, Eau Claire, Wisconsin (Gerber "Seal 'n Go" sterile bag)

Sanofi-aventis U.S. LLC, Bridgewater, New Jersey (Lovenox)

Sherwood Medical Company, Norfolk, Nebraska (Argyle shunt)

SonoSite, Inc, Bothell, Washington (SonoSite duplex ultrasound device)

Sorenson Medical, Inc, West Jordan, Utah (ambIT pain pump)

Synthes, Inc, West Chester, New York (Synthes compression plate)

Velcro USA, Inc, Manchester, New Hampshire (Velcro strap)

Welch Allyn, Inc, Skaneateles Falls, New York (Propaq monitor)

W. L. Gore & Associates, Inc, Flagstaff, Arizona (GORE-TEX)

Z-Medica Corporation, Wallingford, Connecticut (QuikClot)

APPENDIX C Glasgow Coma Scale

Component	Response	Score
Motor response (best extremity)	Obeys verbal command	6
	Localizes pain	5
	Flexion (withdrawal)	4
	Flexion (decortication)	3
	Extension (decerebration)	2
	No response (flaccid)	1
	Subtotal	(1–6)
Eye opening	Spontaneously	4
	To verbal command	3
	To pain	2
	None	1
	Subtotal	(1–4)
Best verbal response	Oriented and converses	5
	Disoriented and converses	4
	Inappropriate words	3
	Incomprehensible sounds	2
	No verbal response	1
	Subtotal	(1–5)
	Total	(3–15)

APPENDIX D Clinical Practice Guidelines*

BURN CARE

The large number of burn casualties treated by coalition forces in the Iraq theatre has prompted a reevaluation of the optimal treatment plan. Many lessons have been learned and relearned during the last 4 years of treating casualties during OIF/OEF. Burn patients are very labor intensive and consume significant personnel and class VIII (medical logistic supply materials) resources. Despite the best efforts of providers at every level of care, the mortality for burn casualties who cannot be evacuated out of the theater of operations is significantly higher than that experienced in US facilities (Table 1). Experience among US treatment facilities in the past 3-4 years reveals no survivors among host nation casualties sustaining full thickness burns to 50% or greater total body surface area (TBSA). The spread of infection in large open wards is a real concern, which can threaten the outcome of non-burn patients. Furthermore the average burn patient in Accredited Burn Centers in the US stays 1-2 days for each percent burn. The factors have prompted a reevaluation of the optimal treatment plan based on severity of injury, treatment facility capabilities and potential for evacuation. The following recommendations are provided to assist the physician in making patient management decisions unique to the deployment environment. Chapter 28 of the 2004 edition of the *Emergency War Surgery* handbook is an excellent general reference for burn care.

In every case, use of the Burn Patient Admission Orders (Appendix A) and the JTTS Burn Resuscitation Flow Sheet (Appendix B) is highly recommended, especially if the patient may transfer to another facility.

1. **Coalition Casualties Who Can Be Evacuated Out of Country**
   a. Protect airway early, using a large-sized endotracheal tube (ETT) as possible (i.e., 8 mm) is strongly preferred, especially if inhalation injury is noted on bronchoscopy. A large ETT tube ensures ease of bronchoscopy and facilitates pulmonary suction, which are critical with inhalation injuries.
   b. Calculate burn size using a Lund and Browder chart (Appendix C).
   c. Initiate resuscitation using a standard burn formula (1-2 mL/kg/%BSA—see Burn Resuscitation Flow Sheet) and avoid boluses if possible; uptitrate the rate of intravenous fluids to maintain adequate urine output (UOP) as described below.
   d. Monitor UOP closely and decrease or increase the LR infusion 20% per hour to maintain a UOP of 30-50 mL/hour.
      1) Overresuscitation is as harmful as underresuscitation; patients who receive over 6 mL/kg/%BSA burn are susceptible to severe complications.
      2) Hour-to-hour fluid management is critical, especially during the first 24 hours.
      3) Use of the Burn Resuscitation Flow Sheet to record fluid intake and UOP is mandatory. Refer to Appendix D for the Burn Resuscitation Flow Sheet Protocol.
   e. Keep the patient warm.
   f. Debride in the operating room (OR) with hibiclens, removing all blistered or sloughing skin (do not perform excision).
   g. Perform escharotomy and/or fasciotomies early if pulses are not palpable and circumferential burns are present.

*Reprinted from CENTCOM's Clinical Practice Guidelines.

h. Wrap burns on scalp, trunk, neck, and extremities in 5% Sulfamylon solution soaked dressings TID and as needed to keep dressings moist:
  1) There is less mess as opposed to Sulfamylon or Silvadene cream
  2) Easier for receiving institution to clean and evaluate on arrival
i. Measure abdominal compartment pressure for casualties with large burns and those who receive a large resuscitation. Pressures > 25 mm Hg warrant intervention.
j. Shave and debride face and scalp.
k. Apply Sulfamylon cream to ear burns BID.
l. Apply Bacitracin to face burns QID.
m. If available, consult ophthalmology for all patients with deep facial burns or corneal injury by Wood's lamp exam.
  1) Apply Bacitracin ophthalmic ointment to eye lids QID.
  2) Apply Erythromycin ophthalmic ointment QID in the eyes.
n. Change dressings every day until evacuated.
o. Consult the Army Burn Center at the USAISR at DSN 312-429-2876 or burntrauma.consult@us.army.mil.

2. Host Nation Burn Casualties
a. Triage casualties with full thickness burns of 50% or greater TBSA as expectant and provide adequate comfort measures. This requires careful and accurate calculation of burn size using a Lund and Browder chart (Appendix C).
b. Remember that inhalation injury, comorbidities, and extremes of age, in addition to the burn, increase mortality. Take these factors into consideration as treatment plans are initiated.
c. For patients with combined partial and full thickness burns of 50% TBSA or greater, with less than half of the burn being full thickness, initially treat the patient as above (section 1) and allow the partial thickness component to declare itself after 2 days. It is initially sometimes difficult to determine the full extent of the full thickness burn. After 48 hours, reassess the percentage of full thickness burn.
d. For patients with a less than 50% TBSA burn, attempts at early excision and grafting are recommend.
e. Presently, no allograft (cadaveric skin) or xenograft (Pig skin) are available in theater; therefore, the extent of excision should be guided by amount of autograft donor skin available, meshing no wider than 3:1.
f. Consider using a Negative Pressure Wound Dressing

(NPWD) over fresh graft with intervening non-adherent layer (i.e. Dermanet, Silverlon) and leave in place for 3-5 days.
g. Following NPWD removal, use Sulfamylon moistened gauze dressings for next 5-7 days before transitioning to Bacitracin.
h. Initially excise only as much as donor skin is available to cover.
  1) Do not excise wounds and leave open. If patients arrive in this state, re-excise and apply a NPWD until granulation tissue is present.
  2) Rarely need to mesh skin wider than 2:1.
i. Take the patient to the OR for staged excisions and grafting of the full thickness burns with a goal of complete excision within 1 week of injury.
j. Once grafts are healed, continue to keep patient clean using showers, when available.
k. Early ambulation and physical therapy, with range of motion of all affected joints, is critical to the long-term functioning of these casualties.
l. Early and continuous nutrition are key to wound healing. Use a nasoenteric feeding tube and supplement with high protein, low fat tube enteral feedings, even when patient is able to eat. Utilize nutritionist whenever available. Supplement diet with a daily multivitamin.
m. Questions about burn care in theater can be answered by the in-theater burn consultant who can be reached at DSN 318-239-7664.

3. Pitfalls
a. Excising uninfected full thickness burns before having donor skin to cover the wound.
b. Pseudomonas infections:
  1) High rate of graft loss.
  2) Ominous sign.
  3) Liberal use of Dakin's solution.
  4) Delay subsequent grafting until topical pseudomonas is well-treated.
c. Transition from aggressive care to comfort care:
  1) Difficult decision.
  2) Initial burn may appear survivable but graft loss, topical infections, or donor site conversion may convert a potentially survivable situation into a nonsurvivable injury.
  3) Be aware of this possibility and the need for potential change to an expectant category.
  4) Elicit opinions from medical leaders, partners, and nurses, as this is a decision that should not be made solely by the treating physician.

d. Consider inhalational injury in relationship to the TBSA burned when deciding whether to treat the patient or deem the patient expectant. (i.e., a patient with a 40% TBSA burn and an inhalational injury will likely not do well as a patient with a 40% TBSA burn and no inhalational burn)

e. Perform large dressing changes in the OR (not ICU or ICW), especially early in the treatment process:
   1) Better evaluation.
   2) Improved ability to clean wounds.
   3) Improved pain control.

f. Initial burn may appear survivable but graft loss, topical infections, or donor site conversion may lead to transition from a potentially survivable situation into a nonsurvivable injury. Be aware of this possibility and the need for potential change to an expectant category.

g. The decision to do less than everything possible should not be viewed as failure, but rather part of reality in a combat zone. The attending physician should not feel isolated about making the decision to decrease the level of care but should seek the opinions of leaders, partners, and nurses. Consult the Chaplain and, if needed, an interpreter to counsel the patient's family about the prognosis and plans.

4. Recommendations for Complicated Burn Care

a. Recommendations for the difficult fluid resuscitation:
   1) At 12-18 hours post-burn, calculate the PROJECTED 24-hour resuscitation if fluid rates are kept constant. If the projected 24-hour resuscitation requirement exceeds **6 mL/kg/% TBSA**, the following steps are recommended:
      a) Initiate 5% albumin early as described previously in the *Emergency War Surgery* handbook.
      b) Check bladder pressures every 4 hours.
      c) If available, strongly consider placing a pulmonary artery (PA) catheter to guide resuscitation with specific PCWP and SvO_2 goals (Goal PCWP 10-12 mm Hg, SvO_2 65-70%). If PA catheter placement is not practical, consider monitoring central venous pressures from a subclavian or IJ catheter along with central venous O_2 saturations (Goal CVP 8-10 cm H_2O, $ScvO_2$ 60-65%).
         • If CVP or PCWP is not at goal, increase fluid rate.
         • If CVP or PCWP is at goal, consider vasopressin 0.02-0.04 units/min to augment MAP (and thus UOP) or

dobutamine 5 mcg/kg/min IV (titrate until SvO_2 or $ScvO_2$ at goal). The maximum dose of dobutamine is 20 mcg/kg/min.
         • If both CVP or PCWP and SvO_2 or $ScvO_2$ are at GOAL, stop increasing fluids (EVEN if UOP < 30 mL/hr). Consider the patient hemodynamically optimized and that the oliguria is likely a result of an established renal insult. Tolerate and expect some degree of renal failure. **Continued increases in fluid administration despite optimal hemodynamic parameters will only result in "resuscitation morbidity" that is often times more detrimental than renal failure.**
      d) If the patient becomes hypotensive and oliguric (UOP < 30 mL/hr), then follow the **hypotension guidelines.**
      e) Every attempt should be made to minimize fluid administration while maintaining organ perfusion. If UOP > 50 mL/hr, then decrease the fluid rate by 20%.
   2) After 24 hours, titrate LR infusion down to maintenance levels and continue albumin until the 48-hour mark.
   3) War burn patients have exhibited multisystem injury to include soft tissue injury secondary to blunt/penetrating injury/blast and inhalational injury, which all affect resuscitation amounts and may result in marked increased fluid needs above and beyond standard burn resuscitation formulas. The air evacuation environment may also increase fluid requirements and wound edema.

b. Recommendations for hypotension:
   1) The optimal minimum blood pressure for burn patient must be individualized. Some patients will maintain adequate organ perfusion (and thus have adequate UOP) at MAPs lower than 70 mm Hg. True hypotension must be correlated with UOP. If a MAP is not adequate (generally < 55 mm Hg) to maintain the UOP goal of at least 30 mL/hr, the following steps are recommended.
      a) Vasopressin 0.02-0.04 units/min IV drip (DO NOT TITRATE).
      b) Monitor CVP (Goal 8-10 cm H_2O).
      c) If CVP not at goal, increase fluid rate.
      d) If CVP at goal, add Levophed (norepinephrine) 2-20 mcg/min IV.
      e) If additional pressors are needed, consider inserting a PA catheter to guide resuscitation with specific PCWP and SvO_2 goals (goal

PCWP 10-12 mm Hg, SvO_2 65-70%). These patients may be volume depleted, but also suspect a missed injury.

- If PCWP at goal, consider a dobutamine drip at 5 mcg/kg/min IV (titrate until SvO_2 at goal). The maximum dose of dobutamine is 20 mcg/kg/min.
- If hypotension persists, look for a missed injury.
- Consider adding epinephrine or neo-synephrine as a last resort.

f) If the patient exhibits catecholamine-resistant shock, consider the following diagnoses:

- Missed injury and on-going blood loss.
- Acidemia. If pH < 7.20, adjust ventilator settings to optimize ventilation (target PCO_2 30-35 mm Hg). If despite optimal ventilation, patient still has a pH < 7.2, consider bicarb administration.
- Adrenal insufficiency. Check a random cortisol and start hydrocortisone 100 mg every 8 hours.
- Hypocalcemia. Maintain ionized calcium > 1.1 mmol/L.

c. Recommendations for inhalational injury:

1) Inhalation injury is further exacerbated by retained soot and chemicals. Remember, inhalation injury is mostly a chemical injury that will benefit from removing the chemical.

2) Upon arrival, if patients are found to have visible soot in the airways, make every attempt to debride through bronchoscopic suction as much soot as possible. In addition, keep in mind that irrigation may actually make the injury worse by transporting injurious substances to new, uninjured parts of the lung, so irrigate judiciously.

3) If a diagnosis of inhalation injury is made, use aerosolized heparin 5,000 units every 4 hours. Mix heparin with albuterol as heparin can induce bronchospasm.

d. Recommendations for abdominal compartment syndrome:

1) Massive fluid replacement (> 6 mL/kg/% burn) has led to abdominal compartment syndrome (increased bladder pressure, increased airway pressures, decreased UOP, hypotension) and extremity compartment syndromes (beyond standard escharotomy treatment).

2) If the patient requires a decompressive laparotomy, do a full midline incision (NOT a small mini-laparotomy incision) followed by a temporary abdominal closure. If the abdominal wall skin is burned, Ioban dressing will not adhere to burnt skin. Use a traditional Bogotá bag or 3 L NS IV bag sewn to the skin (keep loose).

e. Recommendations for escharotomy/fasciotomy:

1) The requirement for escharotomy or fasciotomy usually presents in the first few hours following injury. If the need for either procedure has not presented in the first 24 hours, then circulation is likely to remain adequate without surgical intervention. For this reason, it would be unusual for a patient to require a new escharotomy or fasciotomy by the time of arrival at an Level IV facility.

2) More likely, a patient with previous escharotomy or fasciotomy performed in the field might require extension of the incision or placement of a second incision on the other side of an extremity to restore circulation. This can occur if significant volumes of intravenous fluid are given in transit between the time of initial escharotomy and patient arrival at a rear medical facility.

3) On arrival, assess distal circulation of all extremities by palpating the radial, dorsalis pedis and posterior tibial arteries. If a pulse is palpable in one or more arteries in each extremity, neither escharotomy nor fasciotomy is indicated, and serial assessments are appropriate. Elevate injured extremities 30-45°. Use Doppler ultrasound to assess distal circulation in the absence of palpable pulses. Absent Doppler signals or pulses that are diminishing on serial exam 30 minutes to one hour apart should prompt consideration of escharotomy.

4) Escharotomy is normally performed when an extremity has a circumferential full thickness burn. If the burn is superficial or not circumferential and pulses are absent, consider inadequate circulation from other causes such as hypovolemia, hypotension, or occult traumatic injury.

5) Extend escharotomy incisions the entire length of the full-thickness burn and carry across the joint when the burn extends across the joint. In the lower extremity, make a mid-lateral or mid-axial incision with a knife or electrocautery through

the dermis to the level of fat. It is not necessary to carry the incision to the level of fascia. Although full-thickness burn is insensate, the patient will often require intravenous narcotics and benzodiazepines during this procedure. Give morphine 2-5 mg IV and midazolam 1-2 mg IV at 5- to 10-minute intervals as needed. On completion of midlateral or midmedial escharotomy, reassess the pulses. If circulation is restored, bleeding should be controlled with electrocautery and the extremity dressed and elevated at a 30-45° angle. Assess pulses hourly for at least 12-24 hours. If circulation is not restored, perform a second incision on the opposite side of the extremity.

6) For upper extremities, place the hand in the anatomic position (palm facing forward) and make an incision in the midradial or mid ulnar line. Ulnar incisions should stay anterior (volar) to the elbow joint to avoid the ulnar nerve, which is superficial at the elbow. If pulses are not restored, a second incision may be necessary on the opposite side of the extremity. If both the hand and arm are burned, continue the incision across the mid ulnar or midradial wrist and onto the mid ulnar side of the hand or to the base of the thumb and then the thumb webspace.

7) Finger escharotomies are controversial. Before performing finger escharotomies, consider that there is little other than bone and tendon in the fingers and that fingers burned badly enough to require escharotomy frequently end up as amputations. If finger escharotomies are performed, avoid functional surfaces (radial surface of the index and ulnar surface of the little finger). Place the fingers in a clenched position and note the finger creases at DIP and PIP joints. Escharotomy incisions should be just dorsal to a line drawn between the tops of these creases.

8) If bilateral extremity incisions do not restore circulation, re-evaluate the adequacy of the patient's overall circulation. A well-resuscitated adult burn patient should have a clear sensorium, a heart rate in the range of 110-130 beats per minute, and a UOP of 30 mL/hr or more.

9) In unusual cases, following escharotomy, fasciotomy may be necessary to restore circulation. This is more common in electrical injuries and in crush or other traumatic injuries. Leg fasciotomies should release all four compartments. Forearm fasciotomies should decompress all three compartments. The dorsal compartment may be accessed via a 3 inch longitudinal mid dorsal forearm incision. Dissect to the fascia, enter the fascia and then slide a Metzenbaum scissor distal to the level of the wrist and proximal to the upper forearm. The volar compartment is approached via a lazy-S curved incision from the elbow to wrist. Avoid straight incisions on the volar surface as these may lead to later contractures. Also use the volar incision to access the mobile compartment, which is the fascia overlying the brachioradialis muscle. If escharotomies have already been performed, it may be possible to access the dorsal, volar, and mobile compartments by dissection between the dermis and fascia from the escharotomy site to the desired areas. Circulation should not be compromised by a desire to avoid additional incisions; however, the burned tissue will be excised later during burn surgery. When performing an arm fasciotomy, some hand surgeons prefer to also decompress the median nerve at the carpal tunnel and/or the ulnar nerve at the Canal of Guyon.

10) Following escharotomy or fasciotomy, late bleeding may occur as pressure is decompressed and circulation restored. Examine the surgical site every few minutes for up to 30 minutes for signs of new bleeding, which is usually easily controlled with electrocautery.

For use of this form, see MEDCOM Circular 40-5

DIRECTIONS: The provider will SIGN, DATE, and TIME each order or set of orders recorded. Only one order is allowed per line. Orders completed during the shift in which they are written will be signed off adjacent to the order and do not require recopying on other ITR forms.

DATE / TIME ORDERS

(SIGNATURE REQUIRED FOR EACH ORDER/SET OF ORDERS. SIGNATURE MUST BE LEGIBLE; PROVIDER WILL USE SIGNATURE STAMP OR PRINT NAME).

BURN PATIENT ADMISSION ORDERS   (Page 1 of 5)

1. Admit/Transfer to ICU (1 / 2 / 3), SDU, ICW (1 / 2 / 3) to Physician _____

2. Diagnosis:

3. Condition: VSI   SI   NSI   **Category:** Nation/Service (e.g., US/USA, HN/IA)_____

4. Allergies: Unknown   NKDA   Other:

5. Monitoring

5.1 Vital signs: Q _____ hrs

5.2 Urine output: Q _____ hrs

5.3 Transduce bladder pressure Q _____ hrs

5.4 Neurovascular/Doppler pulse checks Q _____ hrs

5.5 Transduce: _____ CVP _____ A-line _____ Ventriculostomy

5.6 Neuro checks: Q _____ hrs

5.7 Cardiac monitor: Yes / No

6. Activity

6.1 _____ Bedrest _____ Chair Q shift _____ Ad lib _____ Roll Q 2 hrs

6.2 _____ Passive ROM to UE and LE Q shift

6.3 Spine precautions: _____ C-Collar/C-Spine _____ TLS spine

7. Wound Care

7.1 _____ NS wet to dry BID to: _____

7.2 _____ Dakin's wet to dry BID to: _____

7.3 _____ VAC dressing to: _____ 75 mm Hg _____ 125 mm Hg

7.4 _____ Abdominal closure drains to LWS

7.5 _____ Other: _____

8. Tubes/Drains

8.1 _____ NGT to LCWS or _____ OGT to LCWS

8.2 _____ Place DHT _____ Nasal _____ Oral and confirm via KUB

8.3 _____ Foley to gravity

8.4 _____ Flush feeding tube Q shift with 30 mL water

8.5 _____ JP(s) to bulb suction; strip tubing Q 4 hrs and PRN

8.6 _____ Chest tube to: _____ 20 cm H_2O suction (circle: R   L   Both) or _____ Water seal (circle: R   L   Both)

Physician Signature _____   **Date/Time** _____

| MEDCOM FORM 688-RB (TEST) (MCHO) JUL 07 | PREVIOUS EDITIONS ARE OBSOLETE | MC V2.00 |

PATIENT IDENTIFICATION *(For typed or written entries note: Name – last, first, middle initial; grade; DOB; hospital or medical facility)*	Nursing Unit	Room No.	Bed No.	Page No.
	Complete the following information on page 1 of provided orders only. Note any changes on subsequent pages.			
	Diagnosis:			
	Allergies and reaction:			
	Height: _____			
	Weight (Kg): _____			
	Diet: _____			

DIRECTIONS: The provider will SIGN, DATE, and TIME each order or set of orders recorded. Only one order is allowed per line. Orders completed during the shift in which they are written will be signed off adjacent to the order and do not require recopying on other ITR forms.

DATE / TIME ORDERS

(SIGNATURE REQUIRED FOR EACH ORDER/SET OF ORDERS. SIGNATURE MUST BE LEGIBLE; PROVIDER WILL USE SIGNATURE STAMP OR PRINT NAME).

BURN PATIENT ADMISSION ORDERS   (Page 2 of 5)

9. Nursing

9.1 Strict I & O and document on the JTTS Burn Resuscitation Flow Sheet Q 1hr for burns > 20% TBSA

9.2 _____ Clear dressing to Art Line/CVC, change Q 7D and prn

9.3 _____ Bair Hugger until temperature > 36° C

9.4 _____ Lacrilube OU Q 6hrs while sedated

9.5 _____ Oral care Q 4hrs; with toothbrush Q 12 hrs

9.6 _____ Maintain HOB elevated 45°

9.7 _____ Fingerstick glucose Q _____ hrs

9.8 _____ Routine ostomy care

9.9 _____ Ext fix pin site care

9.10 _____ Trach site care Q shift

9.11 _____ Incentive spirometry Q 1 hr while awake; cough & deep breath Q 1 hr while awake

10. Diet

10.1 _____ NPO

10.2 _____ PO Diet: _____

10.3 _____ TPN per Nutrition orders

10.4 _____ Tube Feeding: _____ @ _____ mL/hr OR _____ Advance per protocol

11. Burn Resuscitation (%TBSA > 20%)

11.1 Post Burn 1-8 hrs: LR at _____ mL/hr IV (0.13 mL x Wt in kg x %TBSA)

11.2 Post Burn 8-24 hrs: LR at _____ mL/hr IV (0.06 mL x Wt in kg x %TBSA)

11.3 Titrate resuscitation IVF as follows to maintain target UOP (Adult: 35-50 mL/hr; Children: 1.0 mL/kg/hr)

-   Decrease rate of LR by 20% if UOP is greater than 50 mL/hr for 2 consecutive hrs

-   Increase rate of LR by 20% if UOP is less than 30 mL/hr (adults) or pediatric target UOP for 2 consecutive hrs

11.4 If CVP > 10 cm H_2O and patient still hypotensive (SBP < 90 mm Hg), begin vasopressin gtt at 0.02 – 0.04 Units/min

11.5 Post burn day #2 (Check all that apply)

_____ Continue LR at _____ mL/hr IV

_____ Begin _____ at _____ mL/hr IV for insensible losses

_____ Start Albumin 5% at _____ mL/hr IV ((0.3 – 0.5 x %TBSA x wt in kg) / 24) for 24 hrs

Physician Signature _____   Date/Time _____

| MEDCOM FORM 688-RB (TEST) (MCHO) JUL 07 | PREVIOUS EDITIONS ARE OBSOLETE | MC V2.00 |

PATIENT IDENTIFICATION (For typed or written entries note: Name – last, first, middle initial; grade; DOB; hospital or medical facility)	Nursing Unit Room No. Bed No. Page No.
	Complete the following information on page 1 of provided orders only. Note any changes on subsequent pages.
	Diagnosis:
	Allergies and reaction:
	Height: _____
	Weight (Kg): _____
	Diet: _____

DIRECTIONS: The provider will SIGN, DATE, and TIME each order or set of orders recorded. Only one order is allowed per line. Orders completed during the shift in which they are written will be signed off adjacent to the order and do not require recopying on other ITR forms.

DATE / TIME ORDERS

(SIGNATURE REQUIRED FOR EACH ORDER/SET OF ORDERS. SIGNATURE MUST BE LEGIBLE; PROVIDER WILL USE SIGNATURE STAMP OR PRINT NAME).

BURN PATIENT ADMISSION ORDERS   (Page 3 of 5)

12. IVF (% TBSA $\leq$ 20%): ___ LR ___ NS ___ D5NS ___ D5LR ___ D5 .45NS ___ + KCl 20 meq/L @ ____ mL/hr

13. Laboratory Studies & Radiology

13.1 ____ CBC, Chem-7, Ca/Mg/Phos: _____ ON ADMIT _____ DAILY @ 0300

13.2 ____ PT/INR ____ TEG ____ Lactate: _____ ON ADMIT _____ DAILY @ 0300

13.3 ____ LFTs ____ Amylase ____ Lipase: _____ ON ADMIT _____ DAILY @ 0300

13.4 ____ ABG: ____ ON ADMIT _____ 30 mins after ventilator change ____ Q AM (while on ventilator)

13.5 ____ Triglyceride levels after 48 hours on Propofol

13.6 ____ Portable AP CXR on admission

13.7 ____ Portable AP CXR Q AM

14. Prophylaxis

14.1 ____ Protonix 40 mg IV Q day

14.2 ____ Lovenox 30 mg SQ BID OR ____ Heparin 5000 U SQ BID starting _____

14.3 ____ Pneumatic compression boots

15. Ventilator Settings

15.1 Mode: ____ SIMV ____ CMV ____ AC ____ CPAP

15.2 FiO$_2$: _____ %

15.3 Rate: _____

15.4 Tidal Volume: _____ cc

15.5 PEEP: _____

15.6 Pressure Support: ____

15.7 Insp Pressure: _____

15.8 I/E Ratio: _____

15.9 ____ APRV: Phi ____ Plow ____ Thi ____ Tlow ____ FiO$_2$: ____ %

15.10 ____ Maintain patient in soft restraints while on ventilator

15.11 ____ Wean FiO$_2$ to keep SpO$_2$ > 92% or PaO$_2$ > 70 mm Hg

15.12 ____ Nebulizer/MDIs: ____ Albuterol ____ Atrovent ____ Xopenex Unit Dose Q 4 hrs

Physician Signature _____ **Date/Time** _____

MEDCOM FORM 688-RB (TEST) (MCHO) JUL 07   PREVIOUS EDITIONS ARE OBSOLETE   MC V2.00

PATIENT IDENTIFICATION (For typed or written entries note: Name – last, first, middle initial; grade; DOB; hospital or medical facility)	Nursing Unit	Room No.	Bed No.	Page No.
	Complete the following information on page 1 of provided orders only. Note any changes on subsequent pages.			
	Diagnosis:			
	Allergies and reaction:			
	Height: _____			
	Weight (Kg): _____			
	Diet: _____			

DIRECTIONS: The provider will SIGN, DATE, and TIME each order or set of orders recorded. Only one order is allowed per line. Orders completed during the shift in which they are written will be signed off adjacent to the order and do not require recopying on other ITR forms.

DATE / TIME ORDERS

(SIGNATURE REQUIRED FOR EACH ORDER/SET OF ORDERS. SIGNATURE MUST BE LEGIBLE; PROVIDER WILL USE SIGNATURE STAMP OR PRINT NAME).

BURN PATIENT ADMISSION ORDERS   (Page 4 of 5)

16. Analgesia/Sedation/PRN Medications

16.1 _____ Propofol gtt at _____ mcg/kg/min, titrate up to 80 mcg/kg/min for SAS 3-4.

16.2 _____ Versed gtt at _____ mg/hr, titrate up to 10 mg/hr for SAS 3-4; may give 2-5 mg IVP Q 15 minutes for acute agitation or burn wound care.

16.3 _____ Ativan gtt at _____ mg/hr, titrate up to 15 mg/hr for SAS 3-4; may give 1-4 mg IVP Q 2-4 hours for acute agitation.

16.4 _____ Fentanyl gtt at _____ mcg/kg/hr, titrate up to 250 mcg/kg/hr; for analgesia may give 25-100 mcg IVP Q 15 minutes for acute pain or burn wound care.

16.5 _____ Morphine gtt at _____ mg/hr, titrate up to 10 mg/hr, for analgesia may give 2-10 mg IVP Q 15 minutes for pain or burn wound care

16.6 Important: Hold continuous IV analgesia/sedation at 0600 hrs for a SAS ≥ 4. If further analgesia/sedation is indicated, start medications at ½ of previous dose and titrate for a SAS 3-4.

16.7 _____ Morphine 1-5 mg IV Q 15 minutes prn pain

16.8 _____ Fentanyl 25-100 mcg IV Q 15 minutes prn pain

16.9 _____ Ativan 1-5 mg IV Q 2-4 hrs prn agitation

16.10 _____ Percocet 1-2 tablets po Q 4 hrs prn pain

16.11 _____ Motrin 800 mg po TID prn pain

16.12 _____ Toradol 30 mg IV loading dose, then 15 mg IV Q 8 hrs for 48 hours

16.13 _____ Tylenol _____ mg / Gm PO / NGT / PR Q _____ hrs PRN for fever or pain

16.14 _____ Morphine PCA: Program (circle one): 1   2   3   4

16.15 _____ Zofran 4-8 mg IVP Q 4 hrs PRN for nausea/vomiting

16.16 _____ Dulcolax 5 mg PO / PR Q day PRN for constipation

17. Specific Burn Wound Care

17.1 Cleanse and debride facial burn wounds with Sterile Water or (0.9% NaCl) Normal Saline Q 12 hrs, use a washcloth or 4x4s to remove drainage/eschar

17.2 Cleanse and debride trunk and extremities with chlorhexidine gluconate 4% solution (Hibiclens) and Sterile Water or Normal Saline, before prescribed dressing changes

17.3 Change fasciotomy dressings and outer gauze dressings daily and as needed; moisten with sterile water Q 6 hours and as needed to keep damp, not soaking wet

Physician Signature _____   Date/Time _____

MEDCOM FORM 688-RB (TEST) (MCHO) JUL 07   PREVIOUS EDITIONS ARE OBSOLETE   MC V2.00

PATIENT IDENTIFICATION (For typed or written entries note: Name – last, first, middle initial; grade; DOB; hospital or medical facility)	Nursing Unit	Room No.	Bed No.	Page No.
	Complete the following information on page 1 of provided orders only. Note any changes on subsequent pages.			
	Diagnosis:			
	Allergies and reaction:			
	Height: _____			
	Weight (Kg): _____			
	Diet: _____			

DIRECTIONS: The provider will SIGN, DATE, and TIME each order or set of orders recorded. Only one order is allowed per line. Orders completed during the shift in which they are written will be signed off adjacent to the order and do not require recopying on other ITR forms.

DATE/ TIME ORDERS

(SIGNATURE REQUIRED FOR EACH ORDER/SET OF ORDERS. SIGNATURE MUST BE LEGIBLE; PROVIDER WILL USE SIGNATURE STAMP OR PRINT NAME).

BURN PATIENT ADMISSION ORDERS   (Page 5 of 5)

17. Specific Burn Wound Care (continued)

Face & Ears

_____ Bacitracin ointment BID & PRN

_____ Sulfamylon cream to ears BID & PRN

_____ 5% Sulfamylon solution dressing changes Q AM & wet downs Q 6 hrs

_____ Bacitracin ophth ointment: apply OU Q 6 hrs

BUEs & Hands, BLEs, Chest, Abdomen & Perineum

_____ Silvadine cream Q AM & PRN (*deep partial & full thickness*)

_____ Sulfamylon cream Q PM & PRN (*deep partial & full thickness*)

_____ 5% Sulfamylon solution - change Q AM & wet downs Q 6 hrs (*superficial partial thickness, perineal burn wounds, or Pt O/C to OR/AE*)

_____ Silverlon dressing & Sterile Water wet downs Q 6 hrs (apply dressing and DO NOT remove for 72 hrs)

Back

_____ Silvadine cream Q AM & PRN (*deep partial & full thickness*)

_____ Sulfamylon cream Q PM & PRN (*deep partial & full thickness*)

_____ 5% Sulfamylon powder dressing changes Q AM & wet downs Q 6 hrs (*superficial partial thickness, Pt O/C to OR/AE*)

18. Other Orders

18.1 _____

18.2 _____

18.3 _____

19. Notifiy Physician if: SBP < _____ , MAP < _____ , HR < _____ or > _____ ,
SaO_2 < _____% , T > _____, UOP < 30 mL for 2 consecutive hours

Physician Signature _____   **Date/Time** _____

MEDCOM FORM 688-RB (TEST) (MCHO) JUL 07	PREVIOUS EDITIONS ARE OBSOLETE	MC V2.00

PATIENT IDENTIFICATION (*For typed or written entries note: Name – last, first, middle initial; grade; DOB; hospital or medical facility*)	Nursing Unit Room No. Bed No. Page No.
	Complete the following information on page 1 of provided orders only. Note any changes on subsequent pages.
	Diagnosis:
	Allergies and reaction:
	Height: _____
	Weight (Kg): _____
	Diet:

BURN ESTIMATE AND DIAGRAM

Total Area front/back (circumferential)		one side-- anterior	one side-- posterior				
	Adult	adult	adult	1st	2nd	3rd	TBSA
Head	7	3.5	3.5				0
Neck	2	1	1				0
Anterior trunk*	13	13	0				0
Posterior trunk*	13	0	13				0
Right buttock	2.5	na	2.5				0
Left buttock	2.5	na	2.5				0
Genitalia	1	1	na				0
Right upper arm	4	2	2				0
Left upper arm	4	2	2				0
Right lower arm	3	1.5	1.5				0
Left lower arm	3	1.5	1.5				0
Right hand	2.5	1.25	1.25				0
Left hand	2.5	1.25	1.25				0
Right thigh	9.5	4.75	4.75				0
Left thigh	9.5	4.75	4.75				0
Right leg	7	3.5	3.5				0
Left leg	7	3.5	3.5				0
Right foot	3.5	1.75	1.75				0
Left foot	3.5	1.75	1.75				0
	100	48	52	0	0	0	0

Age: _____
Sex: _____
Weight: _____

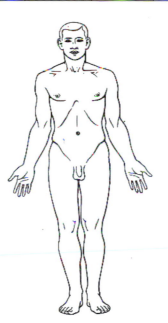

DIAGRAM A

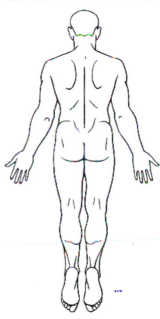

Figure 25 (17)

BABY BURN ESTIMATE AND DIAGRAM

Total Area front/back (circumferenti	Birth to1 year	1st	2nd	3rd	TBSA
Head	19				0
Neck	2				0
Anterior trunk*	13				0
Posterior trunk	13				0
Right buttock	2.5				0
Left buttock	2.5				0
Genitalia	1				0
Right upper ar	4				0
Left upper arm	4				0
Right lower arr	3				0
Left lower arm	3				0
Right hand	2.5				0
Left hand	2.5				0
Right thigh	5.5				0
Left thigh	5.5				0
Right leg	5				0
Left leg	5				0
Right foot	3.5				0
Left foot	3.5				0

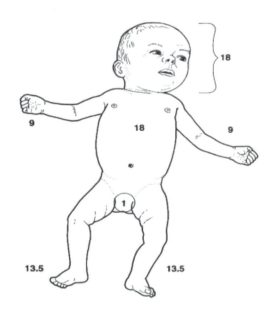

CHILD BURN ESTIMATE AND DIAGRAM

Total Area front/back (circumferential)	1 to 4 years	5 to 9 years	10 to14 years	15 years	1st	2nd	3rd	TBSA
Head	17	13	11	9				0
Neck	2	2	2	2				0
Anterior trunk*	13	13	13	13				0
Posterior trunk*	13	13	13	13				0
Right buttock	2.5	2.5	2.5	2.5				0
Left buttock	2.5	2.5	2.5	2.5				0
Genitalia	1	1	1	1				0
Right upper arm	4	4	4	4				0
Left upper arm	4	4	4	4				0
Right lower arm	3	3	3	3				0
Left lower arm	3	3	3	3				0
Right hand	2.5	2.5	2.5	2.5				0
Left hand	2.5	2.5	2.5	2.5				0
Right thigh	6.5	8	8.5	9				0
Left thigh	6.5	8	8.5	9				0
Right leg	5	5.5	6	6.5				0
Left leg	5	5.5	6	6.5				0
Right foot	3.5	3.5	3.5	3.5				0
Left foot	3.5	3.5	3.5	3.5				0

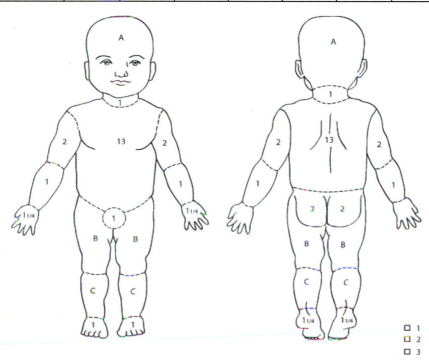

JTTS Burn Resuscitation Flow Sheet Protocol

Purpose: The JTTS Burn Resuscitation Flow Sheet provides clinicians with a tool to track burn resuscitation over a 72-hour period. Conceptually, the flow sheet creates a continuum between clinicians during the resuscitation phase. This format allows clinicians to accurately trend intake and output, hemodynamics and vasoactive medications, and promotes optimal outcomes through precise patient management.

I. The clinicians at the first medical facility where the patient receives treatment will initiate the JTTS Burn Resuscitation Flow Sheet. This treatment facility will be listed in the "Initial Treatment Facility" block. Clinicians at any level of care may initiate the flow sheet.

II. Record today's date in the "Date" block according to the current date where the recorder is located (do not adjust this date based on the patient's origin or destination; use the local date).

III. Record the patient's full name and social security number in the "Name" and "SSN" blocks. Document name and SSN on all three pages of the flow sheet.

IV. Record the patient's weight in the "Pre-burn est. wt (kg)" block. In theater, record the estimated weight based on the patient's weight prior to injury or "dry weight." If a patient presents prior to initiating resuscitation and an accurate weight can be easily obtained without delaying care, providers are urged to weigh the patient and record the result.

V. Record the total body surface area burned in the "% TBSA" block. Clinicians will assess the burn size and use this value to determine fluid resuscitation requirements. Following the patient's transfer to another facility, the receiving clinicians are required to "re-map" the burn, considering that burn wound may "convert" between assessments at one facility or during transport between two facilities.

VI. Burn Fluid Resuscitation Calculations: Use the ABLS guidelines to determine fluid requirements for the first 24 hours post-burn. At 8-12 hours post-burn, reevaluate resuscitation efforts and recalculate fluid resuscitation needs. If fluid resuscitation needs exceed ABLS formula calculations,

consider the guidelines established in the *Emergency War Surgery* handbook and the addendum to the handbook, "Recommendations for Level IV Burn Care." [*LRMC specific: USAISR/BAMC Burn Unit Guidelines can also be found in the LRMC Burn Care Guide*]

a. Clinicians at the first medical facility to treat the patient will calculate the fluid requirements for the first 24 hours post-burn and record the amount in the block on page 1 labeled "Estimated fluid vol. pt should receive."

b. Clinicians will record the "fluid volume ACTUALLY received" during the first 24 hours of resuscitation in the block labeled as such at the top of page 2. This amount will equal the actual volume delivered during the first 24 hours (as recorded on page 1).

c. Clinicians will transcribe the 24-hour fluid volume totals recorded on pages 1 and 2 of the flow sheet onto page 3 in the block labeled "fluid volume ACTUALLY received." This allows clinicians to see the first 48-hour totals as the patient enters into the last 24 hours of the 72-hour period.

VII. Record the local date and time that the patient was injured in the "Date & Time of Injury" block. This date and time IS NOT the time that the patient arrived at the medical facility, but rather the date and time of INJURY.

VIII. Record the facility name and/or treatment team in the "Tx Site/Team" block. The facility name/team name is the team of clinicians who managed the patient during each specified hour on the flow sheet. This team may reside within a facility, in which case the facility name is recorded, or be a transport team (e.g., Medevac, CCATT, Aerovac).

IX. "Hr from burn" is defined as the number of hours after the burn injury occurred. If a patient does not arrive at a medical facility until 3 hours after the burn occurred, clinicians do not record hourly values for hours 1-3 but begin recording in the row marked "4th" hour post-burn. To the extent possible, clinicians should confer with level I and II clinicians to determine fluid intake and urine output. These totals may be recorded in the 3rd hour row.

X. Record the current local time of the recorder in the "Local Time" block, be it Baghdad Time, Berlin Time, ZULU, or CST. As with date, do not adjust this time based on the patient's origin or destination; use the local time.

XI. Record the total volume of crystalloids and colloids administered in the "crystalloid/colloid" column, not the specific fluids delivered. Clinicians should refer to the critical care flow sheet to determine the fluid types and volumes. This burn flow sheet is designed to track total volumes. Examples of crystalloid solutions are LR, 0.45% NS, 0.9% NS, D5W, and D5LR. Examples of colloids are Albumin (5% or 25%), blood products, and other volume expanders such as dextran, hespan, or hextend.

XII. Document the name, dosage, and rate of vasoactive agents in the "Pressors" block. Patients who receive vasoactive agents may also have invasive pressure monitoring devices (e.g., arterial line, central venous line, pulmonary artery catheter), in which case significant values should be recorded in the "BP" and "MAP (>55)/CVP" columns

XIII. For additional burn resuscitation guidelines refer to the *Emergency War Surgery* handbook and the "Recommendations for Level IV Burn Care."

Burn Flow Sheet Documentation

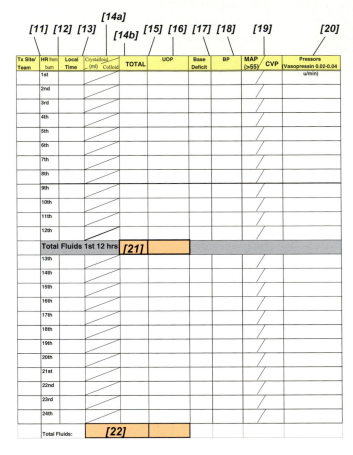

JTTS Burn Resuscitation Flow Sheet								Page 1
Date: **[1]**		Initial Treatment Facility:			**[2]**			
Name		SSN	Pre-burn est. wt (kg)		Estimated fluid vol. pt should receive			
				% TBSA	1st 8 hrs	2nd 16th hrs	Est. Total 24 hrs	
[3]		**[4]**	**[5]**	**[6]**	**[7]**	**[8]**	**[9]**	
Date & Time of Injury		**[10]**			BAMC/ISR Burn Team DSN 312-429-2876			

Tx Site/ Team [11]	HR from burn [12]	Local Time [13]	Crystalloid (ml) [14a] / Colloid [14b]	TOTAL [15]	UOP [16]	Base Deficit [17]	BP [18]	MAP (>55) / CVP [19]	Pressors (Vasopressin 0.02-0.04) [20] u/min
	1st								
	2nd								
	3rd								
	4th								
	5th								
	6th								
	7th								
	8th								
	9th								
	10th								
	11th								
	12th								
Total Fluids 1st 12 hrs				**[21]**					
	13th								
	14th								
	15th								
	16th								
	17th								
	18th								
	19th								
	20th								
	21st								
	22nd								
	23rd								
	24th								
Total Fluids:				**[22]**					

[1] **Date**: Today's date

[2] **Initial Treatment Facility**: Where this form is initiated

[3] **Name**: Patient's name

[4] **SSN**: Patient's social security number

[5] **Weight (Kg)**: Estimated weight PRE-BURN "dry weight"

[6] **% TBSA**: Total body surface area burned

[7] **1st 8 Hrs**: ½ total calculated fluids per burn resuscitation formula (ABLS), given over 1st 8 hrs post-burn

[8] **2nd 16 Hrs**: Remaining ½ of the calculated fluids over the next 16 hrs

[9] **Estimated Total Fluids**: Total fluids calculated for the first 24 hrs post-burn injury

[10] **Time of Injury**: Time the patient burned, **NOT** the time patient arrived at the facility

[11] **Treatment (Tx) Site/Team**: Facility, CCATT or care team providing care at specified hour

[12] **Hour From Burn**: "1st" hour is the first hour post burn. For example: pt arrives @ facility 3 hrs post-burn. Clinicians will start their charting for the "4th" hour. Enter IVF & UOP totals from level I & II care, prior to arrival at the current facility, in the "3rd" hour row.

[13] **Local Time**: Current time being used by recorder

[14a] **Crystalloid (mL)**: Total crystalloid volume given over last hour (LR, NS, etc.)

[14b] **Colloid (mL)**: Total colloid volume given over the last hour (Albumin 5%-25%, blood products, Hespan, etc.) **Note when using Albumin**: With large resuscitations, start 5% Albumin at the 12 hour mark; with normal resuscitations, start at the 24 hour mark.

[15] **Total**: Total volume (crystalloid + colloid) for the hour

[16] **UOP**: Urine output for last hour

[17] **Base Deficit**: enter lab value, if avail. (indicates acidemia)

[18] **BP**: Systolic BP / Diastolic BP

[19] **MAP/CVP**: MAP and/or CVP if available.

[20] **Pressors**: Vasopressin, Levophed, etc., and rate/dose

[21] **12-hr Total**: Total IVF & UOP for 1st 12 hours post-burn

[22] **24-hr Total**: Total IVF & UOP for 1st 24 hours post-burn

Pre-burn Est. Wt (kg)	%TBSA	Fluid Volume ACTUALLY received		
		1st 8 hrs	2nd 16th hrs	24 hr Total
		[a]	**[b]**	**[c]**

Page 2 (24-48 hrs)

The guidelines for page 2 remain the same as for page 1, with the exception of the calculation table. On page 2, the values in [a] and [c] are the **actual** volumes delivered and recorded from page 1, blocks 21 & 22. [b] is the **actual** volume delivered from the 9th hour through the 24th hour. These values allow caregivers to re-calculate the mL/kg/% TBSA, and evaluate for over-resuscitation

Pre-burn Est. Wt (kg)	%TBSA	Fluid Volume ACTUALLY received		
		1st 24 hrs	2nd 24 hrs	48 hr Total
		[d]	**[e]**	**[f]**

Page 3 (48-72 hrs)

The guidelines for page 3 remain the same as for pages 1 & 2, with the exception of the calculation table. On page 3, the values in [d] and [e] are the **actual** 24 hour fluid totals recorded from pages 1 & 2. [f] is the **total** volume delivered over the first 48 hrs ([d] + [e]). Once again, these values allow caregivers to re-calculate the mL/kg/% TBSA, and evaluate for over-resuscitation

MANAGEMENT OF PATIENTS WITH SEVERE HEAD TRAUMA

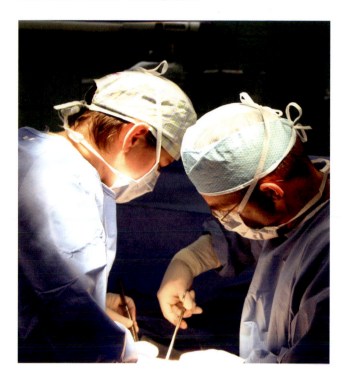

Severely head injured patients are those comatose patients with Glasgow Coma Scores (GCS) of 3 to 8. The current Coalition referral center for patients with severe head injuries is the 332nd EMDG in Balad. All severely head injured Coalition and civilian patients are referred to Balad for definitive neurosurgical care. Several trends have been observed since 2003, warranting the standardization of care for these patients. The mortality of American service members with severe head injuries is 30% for GCS 3–5 and 10% for GCS 6–8. Of these survivors, progression to independent living in the United States is 30% for GCS 3–5 and 60% for GCS 6–8. These excellent outcomes are achieved through rapid evacuation from the battlefield, timely neurosurgical intervention, meticulous critical care, and team rehabilitation that often continues for months. On the contrary, many Iraqi patients cannot be afforded even basic critical care and rehabilitation. During the past four years, approximately 90% of severely head injured patients treated in Balad are Iraqi Nationals. After resuscitative surgery and initial critical care, all comatose Iraqi patients are transported to Baghdad. Those with isolated head injures are treated at the "CNS" hospital. Those with multi-system injuries are treated at "Medical City." Personal communication with staff neurosurgeons at

these facilities confirms that patients who fail to quickly recover to independent or minimally-assisted living will not be aggressively treated. Given this standard of care, all Coalition patients with GCS 3–8 and Iraqi patients with GCS 6–8 should be referred to Balad for definitive neurosurgical care. Transfer of Iraqi patients with GCS 3–5 is optional, as these patients are likely to be treated expectantly.

RECOMMENDATIONS

1. Always address immediate life-threatening injuries and begin resuscitation using ATLS protocols.
   a. Normal saline is the preferred crystalloid solution.
   b. Blood products are preferred over albumin and hespan if colloids are necessary.
   c. Consider recombinant Factor VIIa for life threatening intracranial bleeding.
   d. Consider hyperventilation (goal $PaCO_2$ 30–35 mm Hg) to decrease ICP.
   e. Antibiotics are unnecessary for isolated closed head injuries. Patients with open head injuries should receive 2 grams (child 50 mg/kg) cefazolin (Ancef) IV on admission and every 8 hours until wounds are closed.
   f. Steroids provide no benefit to head injured patients.

2. Two most important factors to manage:
   a. Hypotension: keep SBP > 90 mm Hg.
   b. Hypoxemia: keep SpO_2 Sat > 93%.

3. Document neurological examinations. These should include:
   a. Glasgow Coma Score (GCS).
   b. Size and reactivity of pupils.
   c. Presence of gross unilateral weakness, paraplegia, or quadriplegia.
   d. Interval changes while at your facility.

4. Neurosurgeons in Balad prefer to examine patients when they arrive. Avoid medications which cause long lasting sedation or paralysis.

Note: at no time should these preferences override the need for safe transport

   a. Vecuronium (Norcuron) 5–10 mg (child 0.1 mg/kg) IV is preferred for paralysis. Avoid redosing within one hour of arrival in Balad.

MONITORING & LAB EVALUATION	INDICATIONS & GUIDELINES
INTRACRANIAL PRESSURE (ICP)	Glasgow Coma Score 8 or less.
ARTERIAL LINE	Any head trauma that requires tracheal intubation or other definitive airway.
CENTRAL VENOUS PRESSURE	When ICP or CPP management requires mannitol (Osmitrol) or hypertonic saline.
NEUROIMAGING	Non-contrast head CT upon admission then at 6-24 hours after admission.
EEG	Continuously when barbiturates are employed to manage ICP.
LABS	ABG, CBC, Chem 10, PT, PTT, and INR *at least* q12 hrs during the first 48 hours of care.
GENERAL MANAGEMENT PRINCIPLES	
PHILOSOPHY	• Maintain continuous communication between the care teams. • Aggressively avoid hypotension, hypoxemia, fever, and hyponatremia. • Remember, the longer the ICP is elevated and the MAP/CPP are low, the worse the outcome.
RESUSCITATION FLUID	Prefer Normal Saline. (Beware of iatrogenic, hyperchloremic acidosis)
MAINTENANCE FLUID	Prefer Normal Saline 1 cc/kg/hr. (Child use 4/2/1 rule X 80%)
SEDATION	• Prefer propofol (Diprivan) 10-50 mcg/kg/min IV. • Consider other short-acting agents such as fentanyl (Sublimaze) 1 mcg/kg/hr IV or midazolam (Versed) 1-2 mg/hr IV.
ULCER PROPHYLAXIS	• All patients should receive pantoprazole (Protonix) 40 mg QD. • Child dosing for pantoprazole (Protonix) is 1 mg/kg to maximum of 40 mg QD.
DVT PROPHYLAXIS	• Pneumatic stockings for all adults. • Consider enoxaparin (Lovenox) 30 mg SC bid 24 hours after injury. • DVT Prophylaxis is not indicated in children (age < 16 yrs).
SEIZURE PROPHYLAXIS	• For all patients with injuries penetrating the cortex or blunt injuries with abnormal CT. • Minimum treatment 7 days. • Fosphenytoin (Cerebyx) loading dose: 18 mg/kg IV over 10 minutes. Adult maintenance: 100 mg q8h (child 2 mg/kg q8h). Therapeutic level: 10-20 μg/ml: [Phy corrected] = [Phy measured]/(0.2 x [albumin]) + 0.1. • Phenytoin (Dilantin) causes irritation of peripheral veins; run IV bolus over 20 minutes.
ANTIBIOTICS	Cefazolin (Ancef) 1 gm IV (child 25 mg/kg) q8h X 5 days for all open injuries.
NURSING	Assess neurologic status hourly; document ICP/CPP ventriculostomy output.
STEROIDS	• Steroids are *not* recommended for head trauma. • High dose methylprednisolone (Solu-Medrol) is contraindicated in penetrating injuries. • Consider methylprednisolone (Solu-Medrol) in blunt trauma with incomplete cervical spinal cord injuries. This protocol is not recommended for thoracic and lumbar trauma. • The protocol for methylprednisolone (Solu-Medrol) is 30 mg/kg bolus IV, then 5.4 mg/kg/hr.
NUTRITION	≈140% of basal energy expenditure by seventh day post injury. Give 15% of calories as protein.

GENERAL MEDICAL MANAGEMENT GOALS			
NEUROLOGIC	Intracranial Pressure (ICP)	**< 20 mm Hg**	See page 2
	Cerebral Perfusion Pressure (CPP)	**> 60 mm Hg**	

HEMODYNAMIC	Mean arterial pressure (MAP)	**Maintain CPP**	• Hypotension (SBP < 90 mm Hg) worsens mortality and outcome • Provide a rapid physiologic resuscitation utilizing Normal Saline, Hypertonic Saline, or colloids.
	Central venous pressure (CVP)	**> 5 mm Hg**	
	Cardiac index (CI)	**> 2.5L/m/m²**	
PULMONARY	Oxygen saturation (Sp0₂%)	**> 93%**	Aggressively avoid hypoxemia
	PaC0₂	**30-35 mm Hg**	First 24-48 hours of care
HEMATOLOGIC Consider titrating components using thromboelastography (TEG)	INR	**< 1.5**	Transfuse fresh frozen plasma
	Platelets	**> 100,000/mm³**	Transfuse platelets
	Hemoglobin	**> 10 g/dL**	Transfuse packed red blood cells
METABOLIC	Glucose	**> 80 & < 150 mg/dl**	Have low threshold for insulin drip
RENAL	Serum osmolarity	**> 280 & < 320 mOsm**	• sOsm = (2 x Na) + (Glucose/18) + (BUN/2.8) • See sodium disorders on page 2
	Serum sodium	**> 135 & < 150 mEq/L**	

INTRACRANIAL PRESSURE MANAGEMENT

GENERAL MEASURES	Keep head in neutral position, avoid of tight cervical collars and circumferential ETT ties, elevate the head of the bed to 30-60 degrees.
SEDATION	• Propofol (Diprivan) preferred during first 72 hours (see above for dosing). • Confirm level of sedation when intracranial pressure increases.
TEMPERATURE	Consider cooling measures (Tylenol, cooling blanket) even for *modest* temperature elevations (100-101° F).
INTRACRANIAL HYPERTENSION MANAGEMENT	• Treat elevations ≥ 20 mm Hg sustained for > 5 minutes. • Always consider repeat CT scan with ICP elevations refractory to medical therapy.

TITRATE TO EFFECT GOAL: ICP < 20 mmHg

1. Deep sedation/analgesia	Propofol/fentanyl/midazolam (see above for dosing).
2. Chemical paralysis	Cisatracurium (Vecuronium): Loading dose 0.2 mg/kg IV. Maintenance infusion 1-3 mcg/kg/hr IV.
3. Modest hyperventilation	• PaC0₂ 30-35 mmHg during evaluation or evacuation. • Discontinue after 24-48 hours.
4. Hypertonic saline	• Recommended during the first 24-48 hours. • 3% NS 250-500 cc bolus over 15 minutes (child 5 cc/kg). • 3% NS infusion 40 cc/hr (child 0.5 cc/kg/hr).
5. Mannitol	• Avoid in dehydration and hypotension. • 1 gm/kg IV fast push, then 0.25 gm/kg push q4h.
6. Ventricular drainage	When open, ventriculostomy may drain as much as 10-20 cc/hr.
7. Decompressive craniectomy	Discuss indications with neurosurgeon on call.

CEREBRAL PERFUSION PRESSURE MANAGEMENT (CPP = MAP – ICP)

GOAL > 60 mm Hg	1. Ensure euvolemia	Utilize endpoints of resuscitation (exam, vital signs, urine output, CVP, PCWP, CI).
	2. Control the ICP	Beware of mannitol use in hypovolemic patients.
	3. Consider pressors	Dopamine preferred, 0.5 mcg/kg/min IV.

ACUTE CLINICAL DETERIORATION
(e.g. Mental status change, unilateral dilated pupil, new focal neurological deficit, progressive or refractory ICP elevation)

1. Confirm level of sedation	**UNCAL HERNIATION SYNDROME** (Commonly seen in head trauma)
2. Verify oxygenation and ventilation	• Unilateral dilating pupil → progression to fixed and dilated
3. Hyperventilate bag with 100% O₂; goal PaC0₂ 20-30 mmHg	• Altered mental status → progression to comatose • Contralateral babinski → contralateral weakness → bilateral flexor or extensor posturing • Tachycardia/hypertension → bradycardia/hypertension → bradycardia/hypotension
4. Re-bolus 3% saline or mannitol	
5. Repeat CT/call neurosurgery	
6. Consider damage control crani	

GLASGOW COMA SCORE	Eye Opening	Best Verbal Effort	Best Motor Effort
1	None	None	No response to pain
2	To Pain	Nonspecific sounds	Extensor posturing
3	To verbal stimuli	Inappropriate words	Flexor posturing
4	Spontaneously	Confused	Withdraws to pain
5	-	Oriented	Localizes pain
6	-	-	Follows commands

COMMON SODIUM DISORDERS SEEN IN HEAD TRAUMA			
Disorder	Na+	Diagnostic Clues	Treatment
SIADH	↓	Low Sosm, usually euvolemic, ↑ Uosm	Restrict free water, administer hypertonic saline if severe
Cerebral salt wasting	↓	Sosm may be normal, ↑ UOP, signs of volume depletion & hemoconcentration, very high U Na	Replace volume with Normal Saline or hypertonic saline. Administer oral sodium. Beware of rapid sodium correction.
Mannitol use	↑	Polyuria, ↑ [Na+] & Sosm	Hold mannitol if Sosm > 320.
Diabetes Insipidus	↑	Polyuria (> 250 cc/hr), ↑ [Na+] & Sosm, U Sp Gr <1.005	DDAVP ≈ 2-4 μg SQ bid.

BRAIN DEATH DETERMINATION – Adhere to separate "Guidelines for Diagnosing Brain Death."

b. Propofol (Diprivan) 5–10 mcg/kg/min IV is preferred for sedation.

c. Intermittent administration of narcotics is preferred over continuous intravenous drips for pain control.

5. If therapy for intracranial hypertension is needed prior to transfer:

a. Consider 23% NS 30 cc one time bolus IV over 15 minutes (child 0.5 cc/kg).

b. If 23% sodium chloride is unavailable, consider 3% NS 250-500 cc IV bolus (child 5 cc/kg) followed by continuous infusion 40 cc/h (child 5 cc/kg/hr).

c. If signs of herniation or severe edema are present, consider Mannitol 1 g/kg bolus IV, followed by 0.5 g/kg rapid IV push q4h.

Note: do not use mannitol in hypotensive or under-resuscitated patients

6. Antiepileptic medications for seizure prophylaxis:

a. Consider for all patients with intracranial hemorrhage, penetrating brain injury, seizure following the injury, or GCS 3–8.

b. Fosphenytoin (Cerebyx) is the preferred parenteral (IV or IM) medication:

   i. Adults: load 1 gram IV over 10 minutes, followed by 100 mg IV q8h.

   ii. Children: load 20 mg/kg over 10 minutes, followed by 2 mg/kg IV q8h.

c. Discontinue after 7 days if no penetrating brain injury, no prior seizure history, and no development of seizures since the injury.

DAMAGE CONTROL RESUSCITATION AT LEVELS IIb AND III

The leading cause of potentially preventable death on the battlefield is noncompressible hemorrhage. Following Tactical Combat Casualty Care (TCCC) guidelines, tourniquets and hemostatic dressings are being used by medics to treat compressible hemorrhage, thus truncal bleeding is the unmet problem. At the FST and CSH level many physicians use the standard ATLS guidelines, starting resuscitation with crystalloid, then moving to PRBC and only after liters of these fluids adding plasma. For the severely injured a new method of resuscitation utilizes objective criteria outlined below to initiate rFVIIa, thawed plasma and RBC use in the ED, within minutes of arrival. Crystalloid infusion is extremely limited. rFVIIa has recently shown improved hemostasis (decreasing blood loss by 23%) in combat casualties. Likewise increased use of plasma has recently been shown to improve mortality rates in combat casualties. These products are very safe in trauma patients and are currently in widespread use, both in military and civilian trauma patients. Conversely, excessive crystalloid has resulted in a greater incidence of abdominal compartment syndrome (16% vs 8%), multiple organ failure (22% vs 9%), and death (27% vs 11%) in a large series of civilian trauma patients. Administration of rFVIIa, PRBC, thawed plasma, platelets and cryoprecipitate and fresh whole blood at the FST and CSH, within the confines of the tactical situation, may decrease hemorrhagic morbidity and mortality of casualties with truncal hemorrhage.

ED/EMT RESUSCITATION

rFVIIa and plasma and PRBC (1:1 ratio) are indicated for any one of the following findings:

1. Truncal/axillary/neck or groin bleeding not controlled with tourniquets, HemCon dressings or QuikClot
2. Large soft tissue injuries not controlled with tourniquets, HemCon dressings or QuikClot
3. A proximal amputation or mangled extremity
4. > 1000 cc blood out of a chest tube, or > 200 cc/hr for 4 consecutive hours
5. Physical exam findings:

    a. decreased mental status from injury and shock
    b. severe head injury
    c. clinically coagulopathic
6. Objective physical exam or laboratory findings:

    a. an INR ≥ 1.5
    b. a base deficit ≥ 6
    c. a Hgb ≤ 12
    d. hypothermic from blood loss (T < 96°F)
    e. hypotensive from blood loss (SBP < 90 mm Hg) or a weak/absent radial pulse
7. Need for fresh whole blood transfusion:

    a. bilateral proximal amputations
    b. large hemoperitoneum and significant shock

Casualties with any one of these parameters have > 25% mortality and should be given rFVIIa and RBC:thawed plasma in a 1:1 ratio as soon as possible.

OR RESUSCITATION

Most of the seriously injured casualties that receive hemostatic resuscitation in the ED will require the massive transfusion protocol, outlined in another CPG. In general this calls for coolers of products from the blood bank containing 6 units of PRBC, 6 units of plasma, 6 units of platelets and 10 packs of cryoprecipitate. Again crystalloid resuscitation is minimized, and rFVIIa is given when the INR is > 1.0. THAM is administered to keep the pH > 7.2 and Ca++ is given after every 4 units of PRBC, and/or to keep ionized Ca++ > 1.0 (on the ISTAT). The goal of OR resuscitation is to normalize all laboratory parameters, patient temperature, INR and base deficit. The operating room must be kept as warm as possible, usually 108°F. Major resuscitations in the OR (20–40 units) frequently only receive 3–4,000 cc of crystalloid.

ICU RESUSCITATION

Patients treated in the above fashion frequently arrive in the ICU warm (98), a base deficit of −3 and an INR of 1. This is after receiving an average of 17 PRBC, 13 plasma, 20 cryoprecipitate, 18 platelets, 7.2 mg rFVIIa and 4 liters crystalloid. Occasionally the patients require ongoing plasma and rFVIIa resuscitation, for an elevated INR and volume deficit. These patients are put on 50 cc/hr of crystalloid and because they are much less edematous than after traditional resuscitation regimens are able to extubate within 10 hours on average.

Dose of rVIIa:
1. The usual trauma dose is 100 mcg/kg rFVIIa IV push
   a. this dose can be safely repeated as many as 3–4 times in 20 minute intervals or greater

Route:
1. rFVIIa can be given through an IV or an intra-osseous line.

Contraindications:
1. patient with active cardiac disease

Storage of rFVIIa:
1. Keep rVIIa refrigerated at 2–8 degrees C/36-46 degrees F prior to reconstitution with sterile H_2O.
2. May store rFVIIa for up to 3 hours at room temperature (15–30 degrees C/59–86 degrees F) after reconstitution. If not maintained at these temperatures, the rVIIa is rendered inactive.

Plasma:
See separate guidance on use of plasma from Joint Theater Blood Program USCENTCOM/CCSG.

Thawed plasma not used under the precise conditions listed here may cause serious harm to the patient (infection or transfusion reactions); thus, it should be administered only by those trained to do so.

Infuse 250 cc plasma IV or IO after the rFVIIa; this can be by drip or by IV/IO push. No more than two units of un-typed plasma should be administered under these conditions; thus, immediately send blood to lab for typing, as all subsequent transfusions should be done with type-specific plasma where possible.

Storage of Thawed Plasma (see separate guidance on use of plasma from Joint Theater Blood Program USCENTCOM/CCSG)

Plasma not stored under the precise conditions listed here may cause serious harm to the patient (infection or transfusion reactions) and should be properly discarded immediately.

1. FFP can stay thawed (Thawed Plasma) for up to 5 days but it must be relabeled as "Thawed Plasma" complete with a new expiration annotated and stored at 1–6 degrees C.
2. Thawed plasma for emergency use should be type AB or A; **DO NOT** allow more than 2 emergency plasma units to be administered until an ABO forward type or complete ABO type has been performed.
3. Administer plasma through standard blood administration set.
4. Use the HemaCool® Mobile Blood Storage Refrigerator/Freezer* or other refrigeration device to safely store these products (see further information as noted* below).

*HemaCool® Mobile Blood Storage Refrigerator/Freezer Model: HMC-MIL-1. NSN: 4110-01-506-0895
Helmer Rapid Plasma Thawer has a 4 plasma unit model (DH4) and an 8 plasma unit model (DH8). NSN for the DH4 is 6640-01-510-3136. There is no NSN currently for the 8-unit model.

MILITARY ACUTE CONCUSSION EVALUATION (MACE)

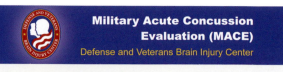

Military Acute Concussion Evaluation (MACE)
Defense and Veterans Brain Injury Center

Patient Name: _____

SS#: _____-_____-_____ Unit: _____

Date of Injury: ____/____/____ Time of Injury: _____

Examiner: _____

Date of Evaluation: ____/____/____ Time of Evaluation: _____

History: (I – VIII)

I. Description of Incident
Ask:
a) What happened?
b) Tell me what you remember.
c) Were you dazed, confused, "saw stars"? ☐ Yes ☐ No
d) Did you hit your head? ☐ Yes ☐ No

II. Cause of Injury (Circle all that apply):
1) Explosion/Blast   4) Fragment
2) Blunt object   5) Fall
3) Motor Vehicle Crash 6) Gunshot wound
7) Other _____

III. Was a helmet worn? ☐ Yes ☐ No   Type _____

IV. Amnesia Before: Are there any events just BEFORE the injury that are not remembered? (Assess for continuous memory prior to injury)
☐ Yes ☐ No If yes, how long _____

V. Amnesia After: Are there any events just AFTER the injuries that are not remembered? (Assess time until continuous memory after the injury)
☐ Yes ☐ No If yes, how long _____

VI. Does the individual report **loss of consciousness** or **"blacking out"**? ☐ Yes ☐ No If yes, how long _____

VII. Did anyone observe a period of **loss of consciousness** or **unresponsiveness**? ☐ Yes ☐ No If yes, how long _____

VIII. Symptoms (circle all that apply)
1) Headache   2) Dizziness
3) Memory Problems   4) Balance problems
5) Nausea/Vomiting   6) Difficulty Concentrating
7) Irritability   8) Visual Disturbances
9) Ringing in the ears 10) Other _____

08/2006   DVBIC.org   800-870-9244
This form may be copied for clinical use.
Page 1 of 6

Military Acute Concussion Evaluation (MACE)
Defense and Veterans Brain Injury Center

Examination: (IX – XIII)

Evaluate each domain. Total possible score is 30.

IX. Orientation: (1 point each)

Month:	0	1
Date:	0	1
Day of Week:	0	1
Year:	0	1
Time:	0	1

Orientation Total Score _____/5

X. Immediate Memory:
Read all 5 words and ask the patient to recall them in any order. Repeat two more times for a total of three trials. (1 point for each correct, total over 3 trials)

List	Trial 1	Trial 2	Trial 3
Elbow	0 1	0 1	0 1
Apple	0 1	0 1	0 1
Carpet	0 1	0 1	0 1
Saddle	0 1	0 1	0 1
Bubble	0 1	0 1	0 1
Trial Score			

Immediate Memory Total Score _____/15

XI. Neurological Screening
As the clinical condition permits, check
Eyes: pupillary response and tracking
Verbal: speech fluency and word finding
Motor: pronator drift, gait/coordination
Record any abnormalities. **No points are given for this.**

08/2006   DVBIC.org   800-870-9244
This form may be copied for clinical use.
Page 2 of 6

Reprinted courtesy of the Defense and Veterans Brain Injury Center (DVBIC), Walter Reed Army Medical Center, Washington, DC.

XII. <u>Concentration</u>

Reverse Digits: (go to next string length if correct on first trial. Stop if incorrect on both trials.) 1 pt. for each string length.

4-9-3	6-2-9	0	1
3-8-1-4	3-2-7-9	0	1
6-2-9-7-1	1-5-2-8-5	0	1
7-1-8-4-6-2	5-3-9-1-4-8	0	1

Months in reverse order: (1 pt. for entire sequence correct)
Dec-Nov-Oct-Sep-Aug-Jul-Jun-May-Apr-Mar-Feb-Jan
0   1

Concentration Total Score _____/5

XIII. <u>Delayed Recall</u> **(1 pt. each)**

Ask the patient to recall the 5 words from the earlier memory test (Do NOT reread the word list.)

Elbow	0	1
Apple	0	1
Carpet	0	1
Saddle	0	1
Bubble	0	1

Delayed Recall Total Score _____/5
TOTAL SCORE _____/30

Notes: _____

_____

Diagnosis: (circle one or write in diagnoses)

No concussion
850.0 Concussion without Loss of Consciousness (LOC)
850.1 Concussion with Loss of Consciousness (LOC)

Other diagnoses _____

_____

Defense & Veterans Brain Injury Center
1-800-870-9244 or DSN: 662-6345

Instruction Sheet

Purpose and Use of the MACE
A concussion is a mild traumatic brain injury (TBI). The purpose of the MACE is to evaluate a person in whom a concussion is suspected. The MACE is used to confirm the diagnosis and assess the current clinical status.

Tool Development
The MACE has been extensively reviewed by leading civilian and military experts in the field of concussion assessment and management. While the MACE is not, yet, a validated tool, the examination section is derived from the *Standardized Assessment of Concussion* (SAC) (McCrea, M., Kelly, J. & Randolph, C. (2000). *Standardized Assessment of Concussion (SAC): Manual for Administration, Scoring, and Interpretation.* (2nd ed.) Waukesa,WI: Authors.) which is a validated, widely used tool in sports medicine. Abnormalities on the SAC correlate with formal comprehensive neuropsychological testing during the first 48 hours following a concussion.

Who to Evaluate
Any one who was dazed, confused, "saw stars" or lost consciousness, even momentarily, as a result of an explosion/blast, fall, motor vehicle crash, or other event involving abrupt head movement, a direct blow to the head, or other head injury is an appropriate person for evaluation using the MACE.

Evaluation of Concussion
History: (I – VIII)
I.   Ask for a description of the incident that resulted in the injury; how the injury occurred, type of force. Ask questions A – D.
II.   Indicate the cause of injury
III.   Assess for helmet use. Military: Kevlar or ACH (Advanced Combat Helmet). Sports helmet, motorcycle helmet, etc.
IV – V   Determine whether and length of time that the person wasn't registering continuous memory both **prior** to injury and **after** the injury. Approximate the amount of time in seconds, minutes or hours, whichever time increment is most appropriate. For example, if the assessment of the patient yields a possible time of 20 minutes, then 20 minutes should be documented in the "how long?" section.
VI – VII   Determine whether and length of time of **self reported** loss of consciousness (LOC) or **witnessed/observed** LOC. Again, approximate the amount of time in second, minutes or hours, whichever time increment is most appropriate.
VIII   Ask the person to report their experience of each specific symptom since injury.

Examination: (IX – XIII)

Standardized Assessment of Concussion (SAC):

Total possible score = 30
Orientation = 5
Immediate Memory = 15
Concentration = 5
Memory Recall= 5

IX Orientation: Assess patients awareness of the accurate time
Ask: WHAT MONTH IS THIS?
WHAT IS THE DATE OR DAY OF THE MONTH?
WHAT DAY OF THE WEEK IS IT?
WHAT YEAR IS IT?
WHAT TIME DO YOU THINK IT IS?
One point for each correct response for a total of 5 possible points. It should be noted that a correct response on time of day must be within 1 hour of the actual time.

X Immediate memory is assessed using a brief repeated list learning test. Read the patient the list of 5 words once and then ask them to repeat it back to you, as many as they can recall in any order. Repeat this procedure 2 more times for a total of 3 trials, even if the patient scores perfectly on the first trial.
Trial 1: I'M GOING TO TEST YOUR MEMORY, I WILL READ YOU A LIST OF WORDS AND WHEN I AM DONE, REPEAT BACK AS MANY WORDS AS YOU CAN REMEMBER, IN ANY ORDER.
Trial 2 &3: I AM GOING TO REPEAT THAT LIST AGAIN. AGAIN, REPEAT BACK AS MANY AS YOU CAN REMEMBER IN ANY ORDER, EVEN IF YOU SAID THEM BEFORE.
One point is given for each correct answer for a total of 15 possible points.

XI Neurological screening
Eyes; check pupil size and reactivity.
Verbal: notice speech fluency and word finding
Motor: pronator drift- ask patient to lift arms with palms up, ask patient to then close their eyes, assess for either arm to "drift" down. Assess gait and coordination if possible. Document any abnormalities.
No points are given for this section.

XII Concentration: Inform the patient:
I'M GOING TO READ YOU A STRING OF NUMBERS AND WHEN I AM FINISHED, REPEAT THEM BACK TO ME BACK-WARDS, THAT IS, IN REVERSE ORDER OF HOW I READ THEM TO YOU. FOR EXAMPLE, IF I SAY 7-1-9, YOU WOULD SAY 9-1-7.
If the patient is correct on the first trial of each string length, proceed to the next string length. If incorrect, administer the 2nd trial of the same string length. Proceed to the next string length if correct on the second trial. Discontinue after failure on both trials of the same string length. Total of 4 different string lengths; **1** point for each string length for a total of **4** points.
NOW TELL ME THE MONTHS IN REVERSE ORDER, THAT IS, START WITH DECEMBER AND END IN JANUARY.
1 point if able to recite ALL months in reverse order.
0 points if not able to recite ALL of them in reverse order.
Total possible score for concentration portion: **5.**

XIII Delayed Recall
Assess the patient's ability to retain previously learned information by asking he/she to recall as many words as possible from the initial word list, without having the word list read again for this trial.
DO YOU REMEMBER THAT LIST OF WORDS I READ A FEW MINUTES EARLIER? I WANT YOU TO TELL ME AS MANY WORDS FROM THE LIST AS YOU CAN REMEMBER IN ANY ORDER.
One point for each word remembered for a total of 5 possible points.
Total score= Add up from the 4 assessed domains: immediate memory, orientation, concentration and memory recall.

Significance of Scoring

In studies of non-concussed patients, the mean total score was 28. Therefore, a score less than 30 does not imply that a concussion has occurred. Definitive normative data for a "cut-off" score are not available. However, scores below 25 may represent clinically relevant neurocognitive impairment and require further evaluation for the possibility of a more serious brain injury. The scoring system also takes on particular clinical significance during serial assessment where it can be used to document either a decline or an improvement in cognitive functioning.

Diagnosis

Circle the ICD-9 code that corresponds to the evaluation. If loss of consciousness was present, then circle 850.1. If no LOC, then document 850.0. If another diagnosis is made, write it in.

08/2006   DVBIC.org   800-870-9244
This form may be copied for clinical use.
Page 5 of 6

08/2006   DVBIC.org   800-870-9244
This form may be copied for clinical use.
Page 6 of 6

APPENDICES | **433**

JTTS CLINICAL PRACTICE GUIDELINES FOR UROLOGIC TRAUMA

MONITORING & LAB EVALUATION	INDICATIONS & GUIDELINES
HEMATURIA	• During trauma evaluation, place foley catheter unless contra-indicated. Perform RUG first if blood at the meatus, high riding prostate or other evidence urethral injury **RUG- Obtain a KUB plain film first, then 14-16 fr foley, primed with contrast to rid air, is placed in the urethra past the balloon. 1-2 cc saline to fill the balloon snugly in the fossa navicularis. A pelvic film in a semi-lateral position is obtained after injecting approximately 30cc of straight contrast (con-ray) under steady, gentle pressure. Study is considered normal only if contrast enters the bladder without any extravastaion.** • If anterior urethral injury, plan to repair in OR. If posterior urethral injury, attempt to gently place a foley catheter. If unable, then place supra-pubic tube in EMT or in OR. • If catheter passes, and gross hematuria noted, proceed with GU diagnostic evaluation for bladder injury or a renal/ureteral source. CT scan with delayed images ± a CT cystogram is ideal imaging study (see technique description following).
LABS	• CBC, Chem 10, PT, PTT, UA. Type and Screen or Type and Cross x 4 units.
GENERAL MANAGEMENT PRINCIPLES	
RENAL INJURY Penetrating renal injury = Abdominal exploration	• Blunt trauma with gross hematuria or microscopic hematuria in a patient with a SBP <90, should be imaged with contrast enhanced CT. • Renal Injury Grading Grade 1: Sub-capsular hematoma Grade 2: Small parenchymal laceration Grade 3: Deeper parenchymal laceration without entry into collecting system Grade 4: Laceration into collecting system with extravasation; vascular injury with contained hemorrhage Grade 5: Shattered kidney or renal pedicle avulsion • Hemodynamically stable patients can usually be managed without operation. • Vascular repair is indicated for salvageable kidneys with renal artery or vein injury. • Ureteral stent may need to be placed for persistent urinary extravasation.
RENAL EXPLORATION DURING ABDOMINAL OPERATION	• Absolute indications: persistent bleeding or expanding/pulsatile hematoma • Relative indications: urinary extravasation, nonviable tissue (> 20%), and segmental arterial injury on pre-op study. • Urinary extravasation from a grade IV parenchymal laceration or forniceal rupture can be managed nonoperatively in most patients.
RENAL REPAIR AND PARTIAL NEPHRECTOMY PRINCIPLES	• Complete renal exposure, débridement of nonviable tissue, hemostasis by individual suture ligation of bleeding vessels, watertight closure (absorbable suture), drainage of the collecting system, and coverage/approximation of the parenchymal defect. Perform partial nephrectomy if reconstruction not possible: the collecting system must be closed and the parenchyma covered with omentum. • Place ureteral stent for persistent urinary extravasation
NEPHRECTOMY	• Total nephrectomy is immediately indicated in extensive renal injuries when the patient's life would be threatened by attempted renal repair: **vascular control of renal pedicle prior to exploration is paramount.** • Damage control by packing the wound to control bleeding and attempting to correct metabolic and coagulation abnormalities, with a plan to return for corrective surgery within 24 hours **is an option.**

JTTS CLINICAL PRACTICE GUIDELINES FOR UROLOGIC TRAUMA

URETERAL INJURIES	• Hematuria not universal: a high index of suspicion must be maintained. • Can be diagnosed with IV contrast and a delayed KUB or CT • Middle and upper 1/3 ureteral contusion is treated by excision and ureteroureterostomy: mobilize injured ureter, sparing adventitia widely to prevent devascularization; débride ureter liberally until edges bleed; repair ureter (absorbable suture) under magnification with spatulated, tension-free, stented, watertight anastomosis, and drain. Consider omental interposition to isolate repair. • UPJ avulsion injuries should undergo re-anastamosis of the ureter to the renal pelvis. A stent and drains need to be placed. • Lower 1/3 ureteral injuries should be reimplanted into the bladder. Use a psoas hitch or Boari flap if required.
BLADDER INJURIES	• Most patients will present with gross hematuria. If CT is planned for other injuries, a CT cystogram (*use DILUTED conray*) should be performed. If no CT, obtain a plain film cystogram. *(need minimum 300cc to be adequate study)* • **Cystogram:** Obtain scout film. Fill bladder via foley by gravity with at least 350cc contrast (7 cc/kg for pedi). Obtain AP image $\pm$ Oblique view. Drain bladder completely and obtain AP image. Many bladder injuries are detected only on the post-drainage film. • **Extraperitoneal** extravasation of contrast can be managed with foley catheterization alone, unless: bone fragment projecting into the bladder, open pelvic fracture, or rectal perforation. Open repair is indicated in these cases (see below). • **Intraperitoneal** ruptures require open repair, two-layer closure with absorbable suture and perivesical drain placement. Last, place a large-bore suprapubic catheter and a urethral catheter to maximize bladder drainage of blood and clots.
POSTERIOR URETHRAL INJURIES	• Initial Management- Surgeon to attempt foley placement, consider urethroscopic-assisted stenting of the injury with a urethral catheter. • If unable to pass a urethral foley catheter, operatively place an open suprapubic tube. At the time of open s-p tube placement, inspect the bladder to rule out injury.
ANTERIOR URETHRAL INJNURIES	• Diagnosis- As with posterior urethral injury, a high index of suspicion must be maintained in all patients with blunt or penetrating trauma in the urogenital region, and a RUG should be performed in any case of suspected urethral injury. • Anterior urethral injuries may also be associated with large hematoma or swelling from extravasated urine. In severe trauma, Buck's fascia may be disrupted, resulting in blood and urinary extravasation into the scrotum. • Management- Initial suprapubic urinary diversion is recommended after high-velocity gunshot wounds to the urethra, followed by delayed reconstruction.
EXTERNAL GENITALIA INJURIES	• **Penis**- superficial wounds can be irrigated and closed primarily. Corporal injures are repaired by approximation of the tunical margins with absorbable sutures. Associated anterior urethral injuries should be closed primarily with a watertight, spatulated, catheter-stented technique and absorbable suture; posterior urethral injuries should be managed in staged fashion with suprapubic catheterization. • **Scrotum/Testicle**- Diagnosis by physical exam and ultrasound. Equivocal cases should be explored. Explore all testicles with overlying shrapnel on pelvic film or if there is a scrotal laceration and any abnormality on exam. Necrotic testicular tissue should be débrided and the capsule closed with running absorbable suture. In some cases, loss of capsule requires removal of intratesticular tissue to allow closure.

INDEX

ABOUT THE EDITORS

Shawn Christian Nessen, DO, FACS
LTC, MC, US Army

Dr Nessen is a graduate of Idaho State University in Pocatello and the College of Osteopathic Medicine at Des Moines University in Des Moines, Iowa. He did his general surgery residency at William Beaumont Army Medical Center in El Paso, Texas. In 2003, he served as a staff surgeon with the 10th and 28th Combat Support Hospitals in Iraq. As this book went to press, LTC Nessen was completing a 15-month deployment as Commander of the 541st FST (ABN) in Afghanistan.

Dave Edmond Lounsbury, MD, FACP
COL, MC, US Army (Ret.)

Dr Lounsbury is a graduate of Bates College in Lewiston, Maine, and the University of Vermont College of Medicine in Burlington, Vermont. He did his residency training in medicine and neurology at Letterman Army Medical Center in San Francisco. He was assigned to the 300th Field Hospital (EPW) in the first Gulf War (1991) and served as Brigade Surgeon in the Balkans (UNPREDEP) in the winter of 1995–1996. In 2003, Colonel Lounsbury was Deputy Commander of the 10th Combat Support Hospital in Kuwait. He retired from the US Army Medical Department in 2005. Dr Lounsbury is presently Developmental/Consulting Editor at the Borden Institute at Walter Reed Army Medical Center in Washington, DC.

Stephen P. Hetz, MD, FACS
COL, MC, US Army (Ret.)

Dr Hetz is a graduate of the US Military Academy at West Point and the Uniformed Services University of the Health Sciences in Bethesda, Maryland. He did his general surgery residency at Dwight David Eisenhower Army Medical Center in Augusta, Georgia. In the first Gulf War (1991), he served as a staff surgeon with the 12th US EVAC Hospital. In 2004, Dr Hetz was Commander of the 31st Combat Support Hospital in Balad, Iraq. He retired from the US Army in 2006. Dr Hetz remains on the general surgery teaching staff and is the Director of Medical Education at William Beaumont Army Medical Center in El Paso, Texas.